Paediatrics

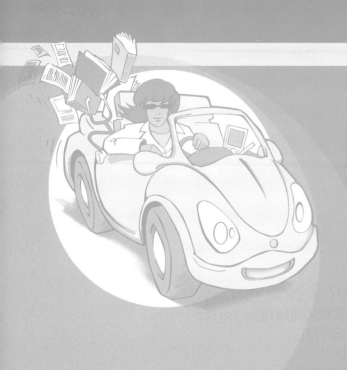

First and second edition authors:

Christine Budd

Mark Gardiner

David Pang

Tim Newson

CRASH COURSE

Third Edition

Paediatrics

Series editor
Daniel Horton-Szar
BSc (Hons), MBBS (Hons), MRCGP
Northgate Medical Practice
Canterbury
Kent, UK

Faculty advisor
Tim Newson
B Med Sci, BMBS, MRCP (UK), MRCPCH
Consultant Paediatrician
Kent & Canterbury Hospital
Kent, UK

Shyam Bhakthavalsala
MBBS, MRCPCH
Specialist Registrar, William Harvey Hospital, Ashford, Kent, UK

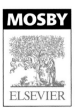

MOSBY
ELSEVIER

Edinburgh • London • New York • Oxford • Philadelphia • St Louis • Sydney • Toronto 2008

MOSBY
ELSEVIER

Commissioning Editor	Alison Taylor
Development Editor	Kim Benson
Project Manager	Nancy Arnott
Page design	Sarah Russell
Icon illustrations	Geo Parkin
Cover design	Stewart Larking
Illustration management	Merlyn Harvey

First edition 1999
Second edition 2004
Third edition 2008

ISBN: 978-0-7234-3462-7

British Library Cataloguing in Publication Data
A catalogue record for this book is available from the British Library

Library of Congress Cataloging in Publication Data
A catalog record for this book is available from the Library of Congress

Note
Knowledge and best practice in this field are constantly changing. As new research and experience broaden our knowledge, changes in practice, treatment and drug therapy may become necessary or appropriate. Readers are advised to check the most current information provided (i) on procedures featured or (ii) by the manufacturer of each product to be administered, to verify the recommended dose or formula, the method and duration of administration, and contraindications. It is the responsibility of the practitioner, relying on their own experience and knowledge of the patient, to make diagnoses, to determine dosages and the best treatment for each individual patient, and to take all appropriate safety precautions. To the fullest extent of the law, neither the Publisher nor the Authors assumes any liability for any injury and/or damage to persons or property arising out or related to any use of the material contained in this book.

The Publisher

ELSEVIER your source for books, journals and multimedia in the health sciences
www.elsevierhealth.com

Working together to grow
libraries in developing countries

www.elsevier.com | www.bookaid.org | www.sabre.org

ELSEVIER   BOOK AID International   Sabre Foundation

The publisher's policy is to use **paper manufactured from sustainable forests**

Printed in China

Preface

This new edition of Crash Course in Paediatrics has kept the same successful format of previous editions. We have updated chapters with important developments in paediatrics since the last edition. There is an extended self assessment section. There has been an adaptation of the hints and tips boxes which highlight points that can assume great importance in clinical practice, to hopefully enhance their relevance. This remains a text that emphasizes the practical aspects of paediatrics and will be invaluable to aid students on paediatric attachments to clinical areas.

This book has been written for the undergraduate but its format and practical emphasis means it will be of use for doctors on a paediatric attachment in their foundation years or at the beginning of their careers in paediatrics either in hospital or community.

Tim Newson
Shyam Bhakthavalsala

More than a decade has now passed since work began on the first editions of the Crash Course series, and over four years since the publication of the second editions. Medicine never stands still, and the work of keeping this series relevant for today's students is an ongoing process. These third editions build upon the success of the preceding books and incorporate a great deal of new and revised material, keeping the series up to date with the latest medical research and developments in pharmacology and current best practice.

As always, we listen to feedback from the thousands of students who use Crash Course and have made further improvements to the layout and structure of the books. Each chapter now starts with a set of learning objectives, and the self-assessment sections have been enhanced and brought up to date with modern exam formats. We have also worked to integrate material on communication skills and gems of clinical wisdom from practising doctors. This will not only add to the interest of the text but will reinforce the principles being described.

Despite fully revising the books, we hold fast to the principles on which we first developed the series: Crash Course will always bring you all the information you need to revise in compact, manageable volumes that integrate pathology and therapeutics with best clinical practice. The books still maintain the balance between clarity and conciseness, and provide sufficient depth for those aiming at distinction. The authors are junior doctors who have recent experience of the exams you are now facing, and the accuracy of the material is checked by senior clinicians and faculty members from across the UK.

I wish you all the best for your future careers!

Dr Dan Horton-Szar
Series Editor

Contents

Contents

Glossary

Acute epiglottitis life threatening emergency, caused by infection with *H. influenzae* leading to inflammation of the epiglottis and upper airway obstruction.

Acute glomerulonephritis acute inflammation of the glomeruli leading to fluid retention, hypertension, haematuria and proteinuria.

Acute otitis media an acute inflammation of the middle ear due to a viral or bacterial infection.

Apnoea of prematurity episodes of apnoea seen in preterm infants due to immaturity of the respiratory centre.

Attention deficit hyperactivity disorder a condition characterized by lack of attention beyond normal for the child's age, hyperactivity and impulsiveness.

Autistic spectrum disorder a range of conditions usually with onset earlier than 3 years, characterized by impaired social interaction, impaired communication and a restricted pattern of behaviour.

Breath holding attacks episodes characterized by a screaming infant or toddler holding his/her breath in expiration, goes blue and limp for a few seconds followed by rapid recovery.

Bronchiolitis acute inflammation leading to narrowing of the bronchioles and lower airways, most commonly caused by respiratory syncytial virus.

Caput succedaneum diffuse swelling of the scalp in a neonate that crosses the suture lines, caused by oedema.

Cephalhaematoma subperiosteal haemorrhage into the scalp bones in a neonate, usually associated with birth trauma.

Cerebral palsy a disorder of motor function due to a non-progressive lesion of the developing brain; the manifestations may evolve as the child grows, although the lesion itself remains the same.

Chronic lung disease of prematurity Preterm infant needing oxygen beyond 36 weeks corrected gestation or beyond 28 days of age.

Congenital adrenal hyperplasia a group of disorders caused by a defect in the pathway that synthesizes cortisol from cholesterol, often presenting with female virilization, salt wasting and cortisol deficiency.

Craniosynostosis premature fusion of the cranial sutures.

Croup acute inflammation of the upper airways (larynx, trachea and bronchi) most commonly caused by parainfluenza virus.

Cushing syndrome syndrome caused by glucocorticoid excess either due to exogenous replacement or endogenous overproduction, characterized by short stature, truncal obesity, skin striae and hypertension.

Developmental dysplasia of the hip progressive malformation of the hip joint leading to varying degrees of actebular dysplasia and dislocation of the femoral head; previously known as congenital dislocation of the hip.

Exomphalos abdominal contents herniate through the umbilical ring, covered in a sac formed by the peritoneum and amniotic membrane.

Febrile fit seizure episode associated with fever in a child between 6 months and 6 years of age in the absence of intracranial infection or any other neurological disorder.

Gastroschisis a developmental defect of the abdomen where whole or part of the bowel and viscera, without a covering sac, protrude through a defect in the abdomen adjacent to the umbilicus.

Gillick principle a child under 16 years of age can give consent for a treatment if he or she is of sufficient understanding to make an informed decision and does not wish the parent to be asked.

Global developmental delay a significant delay in two or more developmental domains.

Guillain–Barré syndrome acute demyelinating polyneuropathy, often following a viral or bacterial infection, typically characterized by hyporeflexia and an ascending paralysis.

Haemolytic uraemic syndrome clinical syndrome caused by verocytotoxin producing *E. coli* O157:H7, resulting in microangiopathic haemolytic anaemia, thrombocytopenia and renal failure.

Haemophilia A X-linked recessive coagulation disorder due to reduced or absent factor VIII.

Haemophilia B X-linked recessive disorder of coagulation caused by deficiency of factor IX.

Henoch–Schönlein purpura a multisystem vasculitis of small blood vessels, affecting skin, kidneys, joints and the gastrointestinal tract.

Idiopathic thrombocytopenic purpura immune mediated destruction of platelets leading to thrombocytopenia, for which no other cause is evident.

Inborn errors of metabolism any inherited disorder that results from a defect in the normal biochemical pathways.

Infantile colic recurrent episodes of inconsolable crying of unknown aetiology, often accompanied by drawing up of the legs, seen in the first few months of life.

Infantile spasms (West syndrome) a rare kind of epilepsy which has its onset in late infancy and is characterized by myoclonic spasms and a typical EEG (hypsarrhythmia).

Irritable hip transient inflammation of the lining of the hip joint (transient synovitis), usually following a viral infection.

Juvenile idiopathic arthritis arthritis involving one or more joints in a child, persisting for more than 6 weeks after excluding other causes; previously known as juvenile chronic arthritis/juvenile rheumatoid arthritis.

Kawasaki disease a systemic vasculitis causing fever, redness of eyes, lymphadenopathy, mucosal involvement and rash with a potential for late coronary aneurysms.

Legg–Calve–Perthes disease idiopathic avascular osteonecrosis of the femoral head seen in children between 3 and 12 years of age.

Low birth weight weight less than 2500 g.

Muscular dystrophies group of disorders characterized by progressive degeneration of muscle in the absence of any storage material.

Necrotizing enterocolitis inflammation and necrosis of the intestine, commonly seen in preterm infants and often predisposed by early and rapid introduction of formula feeds.

Neonatal encephalopathy a combination of abnormal consciousness, tone and reflexes, respirations, feeding and seizures in the early neonatal period due to various reasons, not necessarily from intrapartum asphyxia.

Neonatal screening this is done by the neonatal spot blood test, screening for phenylketonuria, hypothyroidism, cystic fibrosis, MCADD deficiency and certain haemolytic anaemias.

Nephrotic syndrome clinical condition characterized by proteinuria, hypoalbuminaemia and oedema.

Neural tube defect range of conditions caused by a failure of fusion of the neural plate, resulting in defects of the vertebra and/or the spinal cord.

Neurodegenerative disease disorders of the central nervous system characterized by delayed development and a loss of acquired skills (developmental regression).

Nocturnal enuresis involuntary voiding of urine during sleep beyond 5 years of age.

Otitis media with effusion (OME) persistent fluid in the middle ear due to recurrent middle ear infections or poor Eustachian tube ventilation.

Patent ductus arteriosus a vessel connecting the aorta to the left pulmonary vein, that usually closes a few hours after birth.

Persistent fetal circulation high pulmonary vascular resistance leading to right to left shunt across the duct and at the atrial level, in the absence of any other congenital heart defect.

Physiological jaundice of the newborn jaundice occurring between 2 and 14 days of life, in a term infant characterized by predominantly unconjugated hyperbilirubinaemia and a total bilirubin less that 350 µmol/L, in the absence of other causes.

Preterm less than 37 completed weeks' gestation.

Pyelonephritis infection of the upper urinary tract involving the renal pelvis.

Pyrexia of unknown origin documented protracted fever for more than 7 days without a diagnosis despite initial investigations.

Reflex anoxic seizures episodes, usually provoked by pain, where an infant or toddler turns pale and loses consciousness, sometimes associated with a few jerky movements followed by rapid recovery.

Respiratory distress syndrome respiratory distress, usually in a preterm infant, due to surfactant deficiency.

Retinopathy of prematurity abnormal vascular proliferation of the retina occurring in preterm infants in response to various injuries, especially hyperoxia.

School refusal an unwillingness to attend school, usually due to separation anxiety, stressors like bullying or adverse life events; these children usually tend to be good academically, but oppositional at home.

Short stature a height below 0.4th centile for age.

Slipped upper femoral epiphysis uncommon condition characterized by progressive slippage of the femoral head from the neck at the epiphysis, most commonly seen in obese teenagers.

Small for gestational age Birth weight less than 10th centile for gestational age.

Still's disease a systemic variant of juvenile rheumatoid arthritis characterized by high fever, typical rash, lymphadenopathy, hepatosplenomegaly and serositis.

Stridor predominantly inspiratory noise due to narrowing of the extrathoracic airways.

Tetralogy of Fallot cyanotic congenital heart disease characterized by a large VSD, pulmonary stenosis, overriding of the aorta and right ventricular hypertrophy.

Thalassaemia a group of haemolytic anaemias characterized by defective globin chain synthesis.

Transient tachypnoea of the newborn a transient condition characterized by tachypnoea and respiratory distress due to delayed reabsorption of lung fluid.

Transposition of great arteries cyanotic congenital heart disease where the aorta arises from the right ventricle and the pulmonary artery arises from the left ventricle, usually associated with an ASD, VSD or a PDA.

Wheeze predominantly expiratory noise due to obstruction of the intrathoracic airways.

THE PATIENT PRESENTS WITH

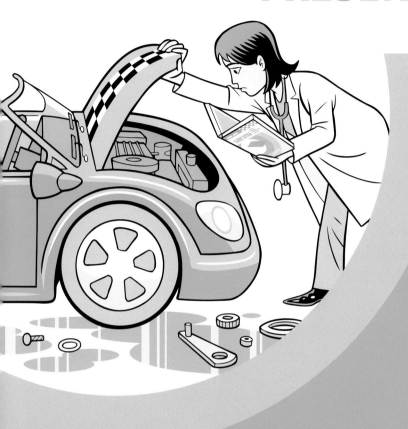

Fever or rash

Objectives

At the end of this chapter, you should be able to

- Assess a child with fever.
- Understand the common types of rash in children.
- Identify the warning signs in a child with fever and rash.
- Learn a systematic approach to a child with petechial rash.

THE FEBRILE CHILD

Fever is a common presenting symptom in children and can be a major challenge to paediatricians. Most of the causes are due to benign, self-limiting, viral infections but skill is needed to distinguish these from serious infection (Fig. 1.1). The latter has the potential to deteriorate rapidly so it is essential that it is identified as early as possible.

Fever is defined as a central temperature of greater than 38°C. Electronic tympanic membrane thermometers correlate moderately well with rectal temperature and are adequate for most practical purposes.

History

How long has the child been febrile?

A duration of more than a week or two suggests diseases such as tuberculosis (TB), malaria, typhoid and autoimmune non-infectious disorders.

Are there any localizing symptoms?

An infection in certain systems will advertise itself:

- Cough or coryza: suggest respiratory tract infection.
- Vomiting and diarrhoea: suggest gastrointestinal tract infection, although vomiting alone is non-specific.
- A painful limb: suggests infection of the bones or joints.
- Lower abdominal pain: suggests urine infection but lobar pneumonia can also present this way.

- Headache, photophobia and neck pain: suggest meningism.

Younger children (<2 years of age) might not localize symptoms and fever might be the only symptom.

Has there been recent foreign travel?

Malaria or typhoid can be overlooked if recent travel abroad is not disclosed in the history.

Examination

Is the child systemically unwell?

The active, playing and communicative child is unlikely to have sepsis. However, any ill child must have an assessment of the airway, breathing and circulation, and of the vital signs. Clues to serious sepsis include (see Fig. 1.7):

- Poor peripheral perfusion.
- Persistent tachycardia.
- Lethargy or irritability.

Assume sepsis in all febrile infants aged <3 months until proved otherwise.

Are there local signs of infection?

Tonsillitis, otitis media, pneumonia, meningitis and septic arthritis can all be revealed on examination

Common causes of a fever	
Minor illnesses	**Major illnesses**
Upper respiratory infection	Meningitis
Non-specific viral infections and rashes	Pneumonia
Gastroenteritis without dehydration	Urinary tract infection Septicaemia

Fig. 1.1 Common causes of a fever.

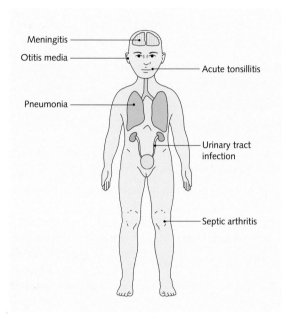

Fig. 1.2 Fever: important sites of local bacterial infection.

(Fig. 1.2); a rash might be diagnostic. Look for a bulging fontanelle in meningitis.

Investigations

In a well child in whom a confident clinical diagnosis has been possible, no investigation is required. However, certain investigations are appropriate in any ill febrile child. These include:

- Markers of inflammation: white cell count (raised or low in overwhelming sepsis), differential (neutrophil predominance in bacterial infection) and C-reactive protein. These are useful if there is uncertainty in diagnosis or for serial measurement of a septic

child, however, they cannot rule out serious infection.

A seriously ill child might initially have normal blood inflammatory markers.

- Samples for microbiological examination: blood cultures, urine for microscopy and culture, throat swab and cerebrospinal fluid. Polymerase chain reaction (PCR) is becoming increasingly useful as it provides high sensitivity and specificity.
- Imaging: a chest X-ray (CXR) should be considered if there is any suspicion of lower respiratory tract infection.
- A 'septic screen'; infants suspected of severe infection without localizing signs on examination are investigated with a standard battery of investigations before starting antibiotic therapy. These include: blood culture, full blood count (FBC), CRP, lumbar puncture, urine sampling and CXR.

Aide-mémoire to identify serious sepsis

ILLNESS—Irritability, Lethargy, Low capillary refill, Neutropenia or neutrophilia, Elevated or low temperature suggests Serious Sepsis.

Management

If a benign viral infection is suspected then only symptomatic therapy is needed. In the very young, or those who look ill, antibiotics are started before the results of diagnostic testing because quickly ruling out serious infection is often impossible; treatment can be tailored when the results are back. Treating the fever with antipyretics might reduce febrile convulsions.

Pyrexia of unknown origin (PUO)

The designation PUO should be reserved for a child with a documented protracted fever (more than 7 days) and no diagnosis despite initial investigation (Fig. 1.3). It is frequently misapplied to any child presenting with a fever of which the cause is not immediately obvious. Most are infectious and 40–60% will resolve without diagnosis. Particular

Type	Cause
Infective	Pyelonephritis Osteomyelitis Abscesses Endocarditis Tuberculosis Typhoid CMV HIV Hepatitis Malaria
Inflammatory	Kawasaki disease Rheumatoid arthritis Crohn disease
Malignancy	Leukaemia, lymphoma
Factitious fever	Only recorded by patient

Fig. 1.3 Causes of pyrexia of unknown origin (PUO).

patterns of fever and response to treatment can be helpful in making important diagnosis (e.g, Kawasaki disease, juvenile chronic arthritis).

THE CHILD WITH A RASH

Children often present with a rash that might, or might not, be associated with systemic signs. An exact diagnosis is often not possible but a few rashes are associated with serious systemic disease. Careful clinical history and examination are again essential and investigation is reserved only for certain cases.

History

The history of a rash should ascertain the following:

- Duration, site of onset, evolution and spread.
- Does it come and go (e.g. urticaria)?
- Does the rash 'itch' (e.g. eczema, scabies)?
- Has there been any recent drug ingestion or exposure to provocative agents (e.g. sunlight, food, allergens, detergents)?
- Are any other family members or contacts affected (e.g. viral exanthems, infestations; see Chapter 10)?
- Are there any other associated symptoms (e.g. sore throat, upper respiratory tract infection)?
- Is there any family history (e.g. atopy, psoriasis)?

Examination

Check for non-dermatological features such as:

- Fever.
- Mucous membranes.
- Lymphadenopathy.
- Splenomegaly.
- Arthropathy.

Describe the rash in 'dermatological language', observing the morphology, arrangement and distribution of the lesions.

Morphology

Describe the shape, size and colour of the lesions. There might be:

- Macules, papules or nodules.
- Vesicles, pustules or bullae.
- Petechiae, purpura or ecchymoses.

Arrangement

Are the lesions scattered diffusely, well circumscribed or confluent?

Distribution

The distribution is important (Fig. 1.4). It can be local or generalized (flexor surfaces: eczema; extensor surfaces: Henoch–Schönlein purpura (HSP) or psoriasis) or might involve mucous membranes (measles, Kawasaki disease, Stevens–Johnson syndrome).

It is important to note the distribution as well as the morphology of a rash.

Palpation

Feel the rash for scale, thickness, texture and temperature; dry skin suggests eczema.

Investigations

Investigations are rarely required but might include skin scrapings for fungi or scabies.

Causes of a rash

The main causative categories are shown in Fig. 1.5.

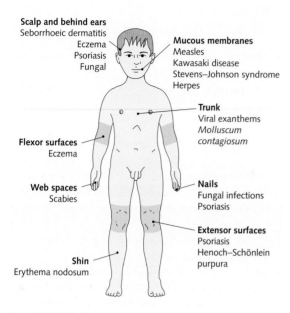

Fig. 1.4 Distribution of rashes.

Causes of a rash	
Type	**Cause**
Infection	Viral Toxin related Streptococcal Meningococcal
Infestations	Scabies
Dermatitis	Eczema Vasculitis
Allergy	Drug-related Urticaria
Haematological	Bleeding disorders

Fig. 1.5 Causes of a rash.

Diagnostic features of the more common generalized rashes

The common generalized rashes are: maculopapular rash, vesicular rash, haemorrhagic rash and urticarial rash.

Maculopapular rash

This is most likely to be caused by a viral exanthem but might be a drug-induced eruption. Common diagnostic features are:

- Measles: prodrome of fever, coryza and cough. Just before the rash appears, Koplik's spots appear in the mouth. The rash tends to coalesce.
- Rubella: discrete, pink macular rash starting on the scalp and face. Occipital and cervical lymphadenopathy might precede the rash.
- Roseola infantum: occurs in infants under 3 years. After 3 days of sustained fever, a pink morbilliform (measles-like) eruption appears as the temperature subsides. It is caused by human herpesvirus (HHV)-6 or HHV-7.
- Enteroviral infection: causes a generalized, pleomorphic rash and produces a mild fever.
- Glandular fever: symptoms include malaise, fever and exudative tonsillitis. Lymphadenopathy and splenomegaly are commonly found.
- Kawasaki disease: causes a protracted fever, generalized rash, red lips, lymphadenopathy and conjunctival inflammation.
- Scarlet fever: causes fever and sore throat. The rash starts on the face and can include a 'strawberry' tongue.

Vesicular rash

Common causes of vesicular rash are:

- Chickenpox: successive crops of papulovesicles on an erythematous base; the vesicles become encrusted. Lesions present at different stages. The mucous membranes are involved.
- Eczema herpeticum: exacerbation of eczema with vesicular spots caused by a herpes infection.

Haemorrhagic rash

Due to extravasated blood these lesions do not blanch on pressure. Lesions are classified by size:

- Petechiae (smallest).
- Purpura.
- Ecchymoses (largest).

Common diagnostic features are:

- Meningococcal septicaemia: petechial or purpuric rash (might be preceded by maculopapular rash).
- Acute leukaemia: look for pallor and hepatosplenomegaly.
- Idiopathic thrombocytopenic purpura: the child looks well but might have petechial rash with, or without, nose bleeds.

- Henoch–Schönlein purpura: distribution is usually on the legs and buttocks. Arthralgia and abdominal pain might be present.
- Bleeding disorders : haemophilia, Von Willebrand disease and Ehlers–Danlos usually present with easy bruising and prolonged bleeding following trivial trauma.

Take care to think of child abuse in traumatic bruising.

Non-blanching or rapidly spreading rash suggests meningococcal sepsis.

Urticarial rash

Urticaria (hives), a transient, itchy rash characterized by raised weals, appears rapidly and fades; it can recur. Causes include:

- Food allergy, e.g. shellfish, eggs, cows' milk.
- Drug allergy, e.g. penicillin: note that <10% of penicillin allergies are unsubstantiated.
- Infections, e.g. viral: this is the most common and is often self-limiting.
- Contact allergy, e.g. plants, grasses, animal hair.

Two other distinctive rashes that occur in childhood and require special consideration are erythema multiforme and erythema nodosum.

Erythema multiforme

A distinctive, symmetrical rash characterized by annular target (iris) lesions and various other lesions including macules, papules and bullae. The severe form with mucous membrane involvement is Stevens–Johnson syndrome. Causes include infections (most commonly herpes simplex, mycoplasma or Epstein–Barr virus) and drugs. Mostly it is idiopathic and self limiting.

Erythema nodosum

Red, tender, nodular lesions usually occur on the shins. Important causes include streptococcal infections and TB.

THE CHILD WITH FEVER AND PETECHIAL RASH

The most important differential diagnosis in this common scenario is serious sepsis especially meningococcal disease which requires immediate treatment.

However there are many other important causes of fever and petechiae including:

- Infections: viral infections (enteroviruses and influenza); meningococcal disease; bacteraemia with *Streptococcus pneumoniae* and *Haemophilus influenzae*.
- Other diseases: Henoch–Schönlein purpura, ITP, acute leukaemia.
- Mechanical causes: trauma; forceful coughing/vomiting with petechiae seen in the distribution of the SVC—face and neck; non-accidental injury.

The majority of children presenting with fever and petechiae do not have serious sepsis. Figure 1.6 shows an algorithm that is useful in identifying serious sepsis.

Indicators of serious sepsis
(see Fig. 1.7)

- Unwell child: tachycardia, tachypnoea, cold extremities, poor capillary refill, irritability, lethargy.
- Purpura >2 mm and spreading.
- Abnormal blood results WCC <5 or >20; neutrophilia or neutropenia; high CRP.

Management of early meningococcal disease/septicaemia

Principles of management are:

- Oxygen, obtaining good venous access, immediate administration of fluid resuscitation, administration of a third generation cephalosporin (cefotaxime 50 mg/kg or ceftriaxone 80 mg/kg), early senior intensive care input.
- Investigations: full blood count, blood culture, coagulation screen, meningococcal PCR, C reactive protein, renal function, liver function and throat swab.

Fig. 1.6 Algorithm for clinical decision making in child presenting with fever and petechiae.

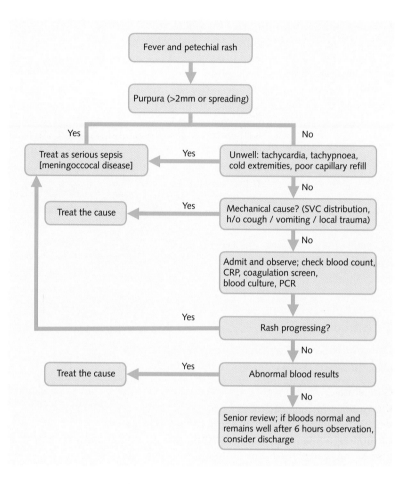

Worrying signs of serious bacterial sepsis
All children less than 3 months old
Bulging fontanelle
White cell count greater than 20 × 10⁹/L or less than 4 × 10⁹/L
Presence of shock
Decreased conscious level or lethargy
Persistent tachycardia
Apnoea
Non-blanching rash

Fig. 1.7 Worrying signs of serious bacterial sepsis.

Further reading

Brogan PR, Raffles A. The management of fever and petechiae: making sense of rash decisions. *Archives of Disease in Childhood* 2000; **83**: 506–507.

Hart CA, Thompson APJ. Meningococcal disease and its management in children. *British Medical Journal* 2006; **333**:685–690.

Heart, lung or ENT problems

Objectives

At the end of this chapter, you should be able to

- Understand common cardiac and respiratory symptoms and signs.
- Evaluate a child with a murmur.
- Identify respiratory distress in a child.
- Differentiate stridor from wheeze.
- Understand common upper airway symptoms.

HEART

Congenital heart malformations account for most of the cardiovascular disease seen in paediatric practice. Rare causes include rheumatic fever, viral myocarditis or pericarditis, and arrhythmias. Kawasaki disease is now the leading cause of acquired heart disease in children in the developed world. Heart disease presents in a limited number of ways:

- An abnormality detected on prenatal ultrasound.
- A murmur noted on routine examination in an asymptomatic infant or child.
- Arrhythmia and/or syncope.
- Sudden collapse.
- Cardiac failure with or without low cardiac output.

History

Cardiac symptoms include:

- Poor feeding, cough and difficulty breathing—cardiac failure in babies.
- Syncope: caused by arrhythmias and on rare occasions by severe aortic stenosis (AS).
- Older children might describe palpitations.
- Recurrent chest infections.
- Failure to thrive.
- Rapid weight gain from oedema.

Rapid weight gain is an early sign of cardiac failure in infants.

Examination

The major physical signs are:

- Cyanosis.
- Murmurs.
- Signs of cardiac failure.

Cyanosis

Several varieties of congenital heart disease might present with central cyanosis (a 'blue' baby) at, or soon after, birth. Central cyanosis is visible if the concentration of deoxygenated haemoglobin (Hb) in the blood exceeds 5 g/dL. Peripheral cyanosis—blueness of the hands and feet (due to a sluggish peripheral circulation)—is a normal finding in babies who are cold, crying or unwell from some non-cardiac cause.

Central cyanosis due to congenital heart disease is distinguished from that due to respiratory disease by the failure of right radial artery pO2 to rise above 15 kPa after breathing 100% O_2 for 10 min. Differential cyanosis in the limbs indicates the

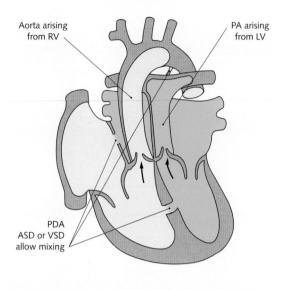

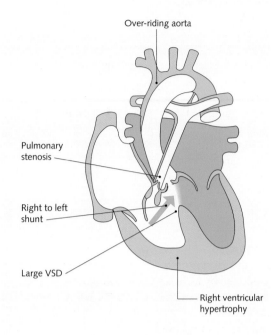

Fig. 2.1 Transposition of the great arteries. There has to be mixing between the two circulations to be compatible with life. As the foramen ovale and the ductus arteriosus begin to close, progressive cyanosis develops.

Fig. 2.2 Tetralogy of Fallot: the stenosis of the pulmonary valve causes resistance to flow and shunting of blood through the large ventricular septal defect.

presence of right to left shunting across the ductus arteriosus.

Causes

In most patients, there is an abnormality that allows a portion of the systemic venous return to bypass the lungs and enter the systemic circulation directly (i.e. a right to left shunt). These can be classified as:

1. Lesions with abnormal mixing: desaturated systemic venous blood is mixed with oxygenated pulmonary venous blood so that the blood discharged into the systemic circulation is not fully saturated. Pulmonary vascularity is increased and pulmonary plethora is apparent on chest X-ray (CXR), e.g. transposition of the great arteries (TGA) (Fig. 2.1).
2. Lesions with inadequate pulmonary blood flow: these infants often have right outflow tract obstruction and depend on blood flowing to the lungs from left to right across a patent ductus arteriosus (PDA). Severe cyanosis develops when the duct closes, pulmonary vascularity is diminished and oligaemic lung

fields are apparent on CXR, e.g. Fallot's tetralogy (Fig. 2.2).

Murmurs

Cardiac murmurs are common in children of all ages. The majority of these are not associated with pathology (innocent murmurs) and clinical examination will allow most to be distinguished from structural cardiac disease.

Evaluation of a murmur

A murmur is merely one component of the information obtained by examination of the cardiovascular system and cannot be interpreted in isolation. Important features of a murmur include the:

- Timing: is it systolic or diastolic? (most murmurs in children are systolic; diastolic murmurs are rare and always pathological).
- Character: is it pansystolic or ejection systolic?
- Loudness: this is graded out of 6; grade 4 and above can be palpated (thrill).
- Radiation: a murmur that radiates from its site of maximal loudness is more likely to be significant.

Innocent murmurs

The hallmarks of an innocent murmur
are:

- An asymptomatic child.
- A normal cardiovascular examination including
  normal heart sounds.
- Systolic or continuous (a diastolic murmur by
  itself is never innocent).
- No radiation.
- Variation with posture.

In most children with a murmur, the heart is normal
and the murmur is innocent. Innocent murmurs are
generated by turbulent flow in a structurally normal
cardiovascular system (CVS). There are two main
varieties of innocent murmur, the ejection murmurs
and the venous hums.

The ejection murmurs are:

- Generated in the outflow tract of either side of
  the heart.
- Soft, blowing, systolic.
- Heard in the second or fourth left intercostal
  space.

The venous hums:

- Are generated in the head and neck veins.
- Are continuous low-pitched rumble.
- Are heard beneath the clavicle.
- Disappear on lying flat.

An innocent murmur is more likely to be noted
during tachycardia, e.g. with fever, anaemia or
exercise.

Significant murmurs

A murmur with any of the following features is
significant:

- Symptoms: syncope, episodic cyanosis.
- CVS signs: abnormal pulses, heart sounds,
  blood pressure (BP) or cardiac impulse.
- Murmur: diastolic, pansystolic, radiating to the
  back or associated with a thrill.

Significant murmurs, which can be difficult to distinguish from an innocent murmur, include those
caused by pulmonary stenosis (PS) and PDA. Refer
for echocardiography if in doubt.

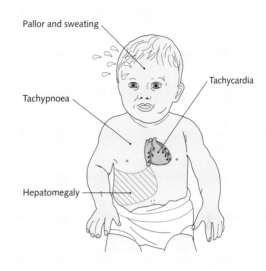

Fig. 2.3 Signs of cardiac failure in an infant.

Cardiac failure

Cardiac failure is rarely seen in paediatric practice
and is usually encountered in babies. The clinical
features are different from those in adults, i.e. babies
do not climb stairs or need extra pillows at night!
Feeding is the only exertion they undertake and, not
being ambulant bipeds at this time of life, their
ankles do not swell up.

Clinical features of cardiac failure

- Symptoms: the parents might notice poor
  feeding and breathlessness, excessive sweating
  and recurrent chest infections. There might be
  failure to thrive.
- Signs: tachycardia, cool periphery, tachypnoea
  and hepatomegaly. CVS signs can include a
  third heart sound, murmur and abnormal
  pulses (Fig. 2.3).

Causes of cardiac failure

This may be due to pressure overload (obstructive
lesions) or volume overload (left to right shunts):

- Obstructive lesions usually present in neonates
  (e.g. severe coarctation of the aorta [COA] or
  hypoplastic left heart syndrome).

- Volume overload usually presents in infants. The left to right shunt increases (e.g. ventricular septal defects [VSD], PDA) as the pulmonary vascular resistance falls.

Cardiac failure can be confused with the more common respiratory causes of tachypnoea, e.g. bronchiolitis or wheezing associated with a viral infection. A CXR will clarify the situation. Less common causes of cardiac failure include supraventricular tachycardia and viral myocarditis.

Investigations for cardiac failure

Useful investigations include:

- CXR will show an enlarged heart with pulmonary congestion.
- Electrocardiogram (ECG) will be suggestive of the underlying heart defect.
- Echocardiography shows the underlying heart defect, as well as poor contractility of the ventricles.

LUNG

Several noises of great diagnostic value emanate from the respiratory tract. A cough is the most obvious. Stridor and wheeze—two other noises associated with breathing and caused by airway narrowing—are also of vital importance.

Paediatric airway anatomy

The paediatric airway differs from the adult and older child; the:

- Tongue is larger.
- Larynx is higher and more anterior.
- Larynx is funnel-shaped.
- Trachea is short.
- Narrowest portion is at cricoid (vocal cords in adults).
- Epiglottis is horseshoe-shaped.

Neonates are obligate nose breathers until 5 months of age, although 40% of term babies will convert to oral breathing if nasal obstruction occurs. See Chapter 28 for physiological respiratory differences.

Respiratory distress

This term is loosely applied to indicate an increased work of breathing. This may be in the form of fast breathing; use of accessory muscles of breathing—intercostal and subcostal recessions, flaring of alae nasi; cyanosis and grunting.

Tachypnoea (fast breathing) is usually a rate (in breaths per minute) of:

- >60 in neonates.
- >50 in infants.
- >40 in under fives.
- >30 in older children.

Cough, stridor and wheeze

Cough

A cough is a reflex, involuntary explosive expiration that is a primary defence mechanism of the respiratory tract. In most instances, cough is due to an acute upper respiratory viral infection, but there are important causes of chronic cough. The cough itself is rarely diagnostic except in two instances:

1. The 'barking' cough of croup (acute laryngotracheobronchitis).
2. The paroxysmal prolonged bouts of coughing, sometimes ending in a sharp intake of breath (the 'whoop'), that occur in pertussis (whooping cough) and certain viral infections.

History of cough

Find out the following information:

- Duration of the cough: this is usually brief, e.g. less than 1 week. A chronic cough, (>3 weeks duration) indicates chronic infection, suppurative lung disease, post-viral cough, receptor sensitivity, asthma, whooping cough, inhaled foreign body or TB. Abrupt onset of symptoms sometimes with a history of choking suggests inhaled foreign body.
- Type of cough—whether dry, moist or productive: the majority is dry (e.g. post-viral infection, asthma); a moist or productive cough raises the possibility of suppurative lung disease, e.g. cystic fibrosis (a productive cough is rare in children as sputum produced is swallowed).
- Association with wheeze: cough without wheeze in children is rarely due to asthma.
- Trigger factors: passive smoking, exposure to daycare, nocturnal cough or cough on exposure to animals and atopy.

Common causes of a cough are shown in Fig. 2.4. Note that many children with neurological

Fig. 2.4 Causes of cough.

Causes of cough		
Type of cough	Cause	Clues to diagnosis
Acute	Viral respiratory infection	Coryzal symptoms
	Bronchiolitis	Wheeze in <1 year
	Pneumonia	Fever and dyspnoea
	Foreign body	Sudden onset
Chronic	Asthma	Associated wheeze
	Tuberculosis	Tuberculosis contact
	Pertussis	Lymphocytosis, apnoea
	Suppurative lung disease, e.g. cystic fibrosis	Productive cough
	Hyper-reactive cough receptors	Usually after upper respiratory tract infection

Fig. 2.5 Causes of stridor.

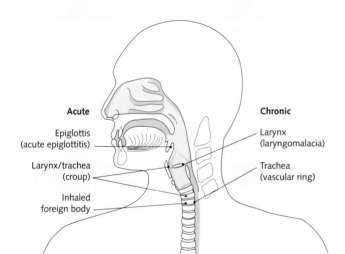

Acute

Epiglottis (acute epiglottitis)

Larynx/trachea (croup)

Inhaled foreign body

Chronic

Larynx (laryngomalacia)

Trachea (vascular ring)

disorders, e.g. severe cerebral palsy, cannot cough well and this is one of the reasons for their susceptibility to respiratory infections.

Apnoea

This is the cessation of breathing for at least 20 seconds or associated with a fall in heart rate. Its presence can signify significant respiratory or neurological disease and acute life-threatening events, especially in infants. It is common in preterm infants due to immaturity of the respiratory centres.

Stridor and wheeze

Differences between stridor and wheeze

Stridor is a noise associated with breathing due to narrowing of the extrathoracic airway, i.e, the upper airway; wheeze is a noise associated with breathing due to narrowing of the intrathoracic airway. Either noise can occur at any phase of the respiratory cycle. The differences are:

- Stridor is usually worse on inspiration when extrathoracic airways naturally collapse.
- Wheeze is usually worse on expiration when intrathoracic airways naturally collapse.

It is very important to make a clear distinction between these signs as the likely cause and management of stridor is very different from that of wheeze. Stridor implies an upper airway obstruction, which could be life threatening.

Stridor

There are two types of stridor: the acute and the persistent (Fig. 2.5).

Causes of acute stridor:

- Acute laryngotracheobronchitis (croup).
- Acute epiglottitis.
- Inhaled foreign body.
- Angioneurotic oedema (rare), anaphylaxis.

Causes of persistent stridor in an infant are:

- Laryngomalacia ('floppy' larynx).
- Anatomical obstructions, e.g. vascular ring (rare).

The different features of epiglottitis and croup reflect the differences in pathology. In epiglottitis, there is rapid onset of supraglottic swelling (the swollen epiglottis is painful and makes swallowing difficult) and bacteraemia. In croup, involvement of the larynx generates the characteristic hoarse voice and barking cough.

Features of epiglottitis:
- Appearance: toxic.
- Cough: slight/absent.
- Voice: muffled.
- Drooling: yes.
- Able to drink: no.

Features of croup:
- Appearance: well.
- Cough: barking.
- Voice: hoarse.
- Drooling: no.
- Able to drink: yes.

Wheeze

The usual causes are viral lower respiratory tract infections and asthma. In children <1 year old, the tiny airways are easily narrowed by oedema and secretions, making wheeze a common feature of infections that involve the bronchi and bronchioles. In children >2 years old, asthma is the most common cause of wheeze. Asthma might have its onset in the first year of life, however, it can be difficult to distinguish from the episodic wheezing induced by recurrent viral infections of the lower respiratory

tract. Distinct patterns of wheezing are recognized in childhood asthma: infrequent episodic (75%), frequent episodic (20%) and persistent (5%).

Less common causes of recurrent or acute wheezing in childhood include:

- Cystic fibrosis associated with failure to thrive and frequent chest infections.
- Laryngeal pathology: abnormal voice or cry.
- Gastro-oesophageal reflux: excessive vomiting.
- Inhaled foreign body: sudden onset is the clue.

Respiratory distress may be due to a cardiac cause. History of an underlying heart problem, failure to thrive, presence of murmurs, abnormal position of the cardiac apex, hepatomegaly and cyanosis not improving despite 100% oxygen should alert to the possibility of a heart defect.

EAR, NOSE AND THROAT (ENT)

Infections of the ears and the throat are very common in childhood and ENT examination is therefore essential in any febrile child.

A small child might not localize pain to the ear. The ears must be examined carefully in any febrile child.

Ear

Pain or discharge

Earache is usually caused by infection of the middle ear (acute otitis media). Less common causes include otitis externa, a foreign body or referred pain from teeth. A discharge might be of wax or purulent material (from otitis externa, otitis media with perforation, or a foreign body).

Hearing impairment

Hearing impairment is classified into two main types: conductive and sensorineural hearing loss (SNHL). The causes of both are illustrated in Fig. 2.6.

- Conductive hearing loss is very common and usually due to otitis media with effusion (OME, also known as 'glue ear'). Over half of all preschool children have at least one episode of OME. A much smaller percentage has persistent OME with hearing impairment, which can delay language acquisition. Impedance tests are used to assess middle ear function (Fig. 2.7); they are not a direct measure of hearing.

Any child with delayed speech must have a hearing test:
- Speech uses frequencies of 400–4000 Hz.
- Hearing thresholds (in decibels = db):
  >70 db = profound hearing loss.
  20–70 db = mild/severe hearing loss.
  <20 db = normal hearing.

Causes of impaired hearing	
Type	**Cause**
Conductive	Otitis media with effusion Foreign body Wax

Sensorineural	Congenital infection
	Prematurity (<32/40)
	Risk factors: hypoxia
	               jaundice
	               ototoxic drugs
	Meningitis
	Genetic (rare)

Fig. 2.6 Causes of impaired hearing.

- Sensorineural hearing loss is less common. Routine screening is now introduced in the UK (Fig. 2.8). Not all cases will be detected in the neonatal period as, for example, congenital infections and some genetic causes of SNHL are progressive and cannot be detectable at this age.
- Acquired hearing loss occurs after CNS infections, e.g. meningitis, and all affected children should have their hearing tested after the acute illness has resolved (Fig. 2.9). Treatment with cochlear implantation might be required.

Impedance tympanometry

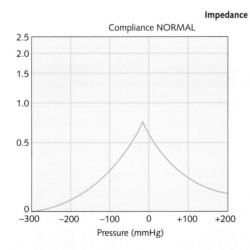

Compliance NORMAL

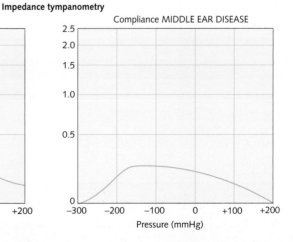

Compliance MIDDLE EAR DISEASE

Fig. 2.7 Impedance tympanometry. This tests for middle ear disease. Sound is transmitted across the tympanic membrane if it is compliant (i.e. equal pressure either side). The test measures reflected sound at different pressures. In serous otitis media, compliance is reduced at all pressures because of the fluid present resulting in a flattened curve.

- Parental suspicions about possible hearing loss should be taken seriously, with early referral for audiological testing.
- Children with significantly impaired language development, behavioural problems or those with a history of repeated middle ear disease should also be referred.

Nose

Noses can discharge or bleed. The common cold accounts for most acute watery discharges. A chronic discharge might be due to allergic rhinitis or a unilateral foreign body.

Causes of epistaxis (nose bleeds) include:

- Trauma.
- Nose picking.
- Bleeding disorders (especially low platelets).

Fig. 2.8 Tests of auditory function.

	Test of auditory function	
Age	**Test**	**Indication**
Newborn	Otoacoustic emission Brainstem-evoked potential audiometry response cradle	Presence of high-risk factors, e.g. prematurity Newborn screening
7–9 months	Parental questionnaire distraction test	Used prior to newborn screening
18–24 months	Speech discrimination tests Threshold audiometry (<3 years) Impedance audiometry	Children with suspected hearing loss Children with repeated middle ear disease
School entry	'Sweep test' (modified pure tone audiogram – Fig. 2.9)	Screen all children

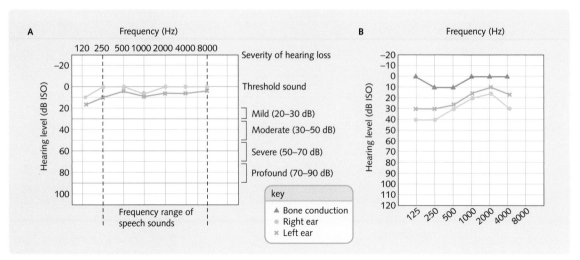

Fig. 2.9 Audiogram demonstrating: (A) normal hearing and (B) bilateral conductive hearing loss. In (B), there is a 20–40 dB hearing loss in both the right and left ears.

Throat

Sore throat (pharyngitis)

- Constitutional upset, tonsillar exudate and lymphadenopathy suggest a bacterial infection: group A β-haemolytic streptococci is a common pathogen ('strep. throat').
- Rarely, a peritonsillar abscess (quinsy) might develop and require incision and drainage.
- Epstein–Barr virus (infectious mononucleosis) is an important cause of exudative tonsillitis.

Snoring and obstructive sleep apnoea (OSA)

Snoring is a common symptom in children but in some is associated with significant OSA. History of apnoea with arousals during sleep and unusual sleep positions can indicate OSA. Daytime symptoms include chronic mouth breathing, behavioural problems and occasionally daytime sleepiness. Severe OSA can result in failure to thrive, right heart failure and cor pulmonale. Those children at high risk of OSA include children with craniofacial problems and Down syndrome.

Gut or liver problems

Objectives

At the end of this chapter, you should be able to

- Understand common symptoms of gastrointestinal disease.
- Assess a child with a gastrointestinal complaint.
- Differentiate among common gastrointestinal problems.

GUT

Disorders of the gut present with a limited number of symptoms, including abdominal pain, vomiting, diarrhoea or constipation, failure to thrive and bleeding.

Abdominal pain

Acute abdominal pain

The most important issue is to identify conditions needing urgent surgical intervention (Figs 3.1 and 3.2).

History

In babies, abdominal pain is inferred from episodic screaming and drawing up of the legs. In older children, important features in the history are:

- Duration: pain lasting more than 4 hours is likely to be significant.
- Location: pain further away from the umbilicus is more likely to be significant (early appendicitis is an exception to this).
- Nature: constant or intermittent/colicky.
- Associated symptomatology: vomiting (is there obstruction or gastroenteritis?), stools (pain and bloody stools suggest intussusception in an infant, inflammatory bowel disease in older children), dysuria (urinary tract infection), cough (pneumonia), anorexia (a normal appetite is a sign of well-being).

Physical examination

Careful systemic examination is important if the many traps for the unwary are to be avoided. Look for:

- Fever: present in appendicitis, mesenteric adenitis and urinary tract infections (UTIs).
- Jaundice: infectious hepatitis causes abdominal pain.
- Rash: the abdominal pain of Henoch–Schönlein purpura (HSP) might precede the characteristic purpuric rash.
- Respiratory tract: is there a lower lobe pneumonia?
- Hernial orifices: is there a strangulated hernia?
- Genitalia: is there a torsion of the testis?

Investigations

- Full blood count (FBC): a neutrophil leucocytosis might be present in acute appendicitis or bacterial infection of the urine, lung or throat. A sickling test should be considered in children of African or Afro-Caribbean origin.
- Urinalysis: dipstick for glucose and ketones, urine microscopy and culture.
- Imaging: a plain abdominal film although rarely needed, might reveal constipation, renal calculi or signs of intestinal obstruction. Abdominal ultrasound might reveal obstructive uropathy, an appendix mass intussusception or ovarian cysts.
- Urea and electrolytes: in a vomiting child, electrolyte disturbances must be identified.
- Blood glucose.
- CRP.

Surgical causes of acute abdominal pain	
	Clinical clues
Acute appendicitis	Pattern of migration and right iliac fossa tenderness
Intussusception	Episodic pattern
Torsion of testes	Clinical examination
Strangulated inguinal hernia	Groin mass

Fig. 3.1 Surgical causes of acute abdominal pain.

Medical causes of acute abdominal pain	
Abdominal causes	Systemic causes
Colic	Diabetic ketoacidosis
Constipation	Sickle-cell disease
Mesenteric adenitis	Henoch–Schönlein purpura
Gastroenteritis	Lower lobe pneumonia
Hepatitis	
Pancreatitis	
Acute pyelonephritis/UTI	

Fig. 3.2 Medical causes of acute abdominal pain.

Recurrent abdominal pain

In most children, recurrent abdominal pain does not have an organic cause and a positive diagnosis of 'functional' abdominal pain can be made without investigations (Fig. 3.3) in most.

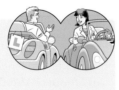

Extensive investigation often reinforces anxieties in the parents and child and should be discouraged.

If a diagnosis of functional abdominal pain is made, it is important to emphasize that the pain is often real and not faked, but without an identifiable physical cause.

There is a long list of rare causes of recurrent abdominal pain (Fig. 3.4). Careful history and examination will usually provide a clue. Further investigations to exclude a possible organic cause may include:

Features of 'functional' recurrent abdominal pain
• Pain is periumbilical, worse on waking, and short-lived
• No associated appetite loss or bowel disturbance
• Family history of migraine, irritable bowel syndrome, or recurrent abdominal pain
• Healthy, thriving child with normal physical examination

Fig. 3.3 Features of 'functional' recurrent abdominal pain.

Rare 'organic' causes of recurrent abdominal pain
UTI
Urinary calculus
Obstructive uropathy
Inflammatory bowel disease
Duodenal ulcer
Malrotation
Recurrent pancreatitis

Fig. 3.4 Rare 'organic' causes of recurrent abdominal pain.

- Urine microscopy and culture.
- Plain abdominal film.
- Abdominal ultrasound.
- FBC, erythrocyte sedimentation rate (ESR).
- *Helicobacter pylori* serology or hydrogen breath test.

- Acute appendicitis is uncommon under 2 years.
- Consider intussusception in vomiting infants aged 6–12 months.
- Not all abdominal pain originates in the abdomen.
- Diabetic ketoacidosis is often associated with abdominal pain.
- Consider gynaecological causes in a teenage girl.

Vomiting

Vomiting is a non-specific symptom associated with a wide variety of conditions but can also be a normal finding in well babies. A complete clinical assessment often distinguishes the normal possets from serious pathology. Vomiting may also indicate disease outside the gastrointestinal tract.

History

Important points to establish include:

- Does the vomit contain blood or bile? Biliary vomiting needs a surgical opinion and further investigations.
- Is it projectile? It is quite common for babies to posset and bring up small quantities of ingested milk. Projectile vomiting, on the other hand, may indicate pyloric stenosis.
- Duration: is vomiting an acute or a persistent problem?
- Associated symptoms: is vomiting accompanied by fever, abdominal pain, constipation or diarrhoea?

Examination

Examine for the following:

- Signs of dehydration.
- Fever.
- Abdominal distension (visible peristalsis), tenderness or masses.
- Hernial orifices and genitalia.

Common and important causes are discussed below.

The neonate

Vomiting can be a sign of systemic infection (e.g. meningitis, UTI) or certain inborn errors of metabolism (e.g. congenital adrenal hyperplasia).

Surgical causes include bowel obstruction, which can be either small or large bowel obstruction. This is often associated with abdominal distension and no bowel motions. Visible peristalsis might be seen.

Causes of small bowel obstruction include:

- Duodenal atresia (associated with Down syndrome).
- Malrotation with volvulus.
- Strangulated inguinal hernia.
- Meconium ileus due to cystic fibrosis.

Causes of large bowel obstruction include Hirschsprung's disease (absence of the myenteric plexus in the rectum and colon). Passage of meconium is often delayed beyond 48 hours.

Infants: 1 month to 1 year

The commonest cause of persistent vomiting in babies up to 1 year is gastro-oesophageal reflux due to functional immaturity of the lower oesophageal sphincter that resolves spontaneously. Thickening the feeds and positioning head up after feeds are useful manoeuvres. Severe reflux is uncommon (it occurs in cerebral palsy and babies with chronic lung disease) and might be complicated by failure to thrive, oesophagitis and recurrent aspiration pneumonia.

Acute medical causes of vomiting include:

- Gastroenteritis.
- Respiratory tract infections such as tonsillitis, otitis media and whooping cough.
- UTI.
- Meningitis.

Important surgical causes include pyloric stenosis and intussusception:

- Pyloric stenosis causes non-bile-stained projectile vomiting, most commonly in baby boys between the age of a few weeks and 3 months.
- The peak age of intussusception is around 6–9 months. It presents with episodic severe abdominal pain and irritability and is associated with pallor and eventually shock and passage of bloodstained 'redcurrant jelly' stools.

Older children

Acute vomiting can occur in infections as described or might be one of the symptoms of acute appendicitis or abdominal migraine. Rare but important causes include raised intracranial pressure, malrotation of the intestine, inborn errors of metabolism and eating disorders such as bulimia nervosa.

Haematemesis

The differential diagnosis for vomiting blood varies with the age of the child. In the first few days of life it is usually caused by swallowed maternal blood. Later on, the main causes are oesophagitis and gastritis. Oesophageal varices are a cause in liver disease but peptic ulcers in children are uncommon. Haematemesis can also occur due to a tear in the oesophageal mucosa due to forceful vomiting (Mallory–Weiss syndrome).

Diarrhoea

Acute diarrhoea

The most common cause is infective viral gastroenteritis. It commonly occurs in combination with vomiting.

Infective causes of acute diarrhoea
Viral
Rotavirus
Small round structured virus (SRSV)
Adenovirus
Bacterial
E. coli
Campylobacter spp.
Salmonella spp.
Shigella spp.
Vibrio cholerae
Protozoa
Giardia lamblia
Entamoeba histolytica
Cryptosporidium parvum

Fig. 3.5 Causes of acute diarrhoea.

Assessment of dehydration			
Signs and symptoms	Mild <5%	Moderate 5–10%	Severe >10%
Decreased urine output	+	+	+
Dry mouth	+/−	+	+
Sunken eyes or depressed fontanelle	+/−	+	+
Decreased skin turgor	−	+/−	+
Tachypnoea	−	+/−	+
Tachycardia	−	+/−	+
Prolonged capillary refill time	−	+/−	+
Appearance	Alert	Alert/lethargic	Lethargic

Fig. 3.6 Assessment of dehydration.

Some infections cause pathology in the lower gastrointestinal (GI) tract. In this case, there might be no vomiting and diarrhoea—often with blood and mucus—dominates the clinical presentation (Fig. 3.5). Bloody diarrhoea should raise suspicion of specific pathogens and of non-infective conditions such as intussusception and inflammatory bowel disease.

Bloody diarrhoea—consider:
- Infective causes: *Campylobacter*, *Shigella*, amoeba.
- Intussusception: especially 6–9 months.
- Haemolytic–uraemic syndrome: check renal function and blood pressure.
- Ulcerative colitis (rare).

Causes of chronic diarrhoea	
Infective causes	Giardiasis Amoebiasis
Food intolerance	Disaccharides—lactose intolerance Proteins—cow's milk protein intolerance
Malabsorption	Coeliac disease (gluten enteropathy) Cystic fibrosis
Inflammatory bowel disease	Crohn's disease Ulcerative colitis

Fig. 3.7 Causes of chronic diarrhoea.

On examination, high fever suggests a bacterial gastroenteritis, especially *Shigella* infection. Assessment of dehydration is most important (Fig. 3.6).

Chronic diarrhoea

The most common cause of persistent loose stools in a well, thriving, preschool child is so-called 'toddler diarrhoea'. A maturational delay in intestinal motility causes intermittent explosive loose stools with undigested vegetables often present ('peas and carrots' syndrome). An acute diarrhoeal episode might become protracted (duration >2 weeks) because of 'postgastroenteritis' syndrome due to secondary lactose intolerance. Watery diarrhoea returns when a normal diet, including milk, is reintroduced. Stools give a positive Clinitest result for reducing substances. Some infective agents, such as *Giardia*, also cause protracted diarrhoea.

Chronic diarrhoea in a child who is failing to thrive raises the possibility of several important diagnoses (Fig. 3.7). A description of the stools might suggest steatorrhoea (pale, bulky and offensive) and the presence of blood or mucus suggests infective causes or inflammatory bowel disease.

Physical examination

This includes assessment of dehydration (including weight) and then identifying the cause of diarrhoea. Look for any evidence of malabsorption—anaemia, poor weight gain, abdominal distension and buttock wasting. A thriving child with no associated symptomatology is unlikely to have significant disease. Faecal soiling due to constipation and overflow can be mistaken for diarrhoea (confirm by rectal examination).

Investigations

These are directed towards the suspected cause:

- Stool microscopy and culture.
- Tests for reducing substances.
- Tests for nutrient malabsorption—Hb estimation, serum iron and red cell folate.
- Jejunal biopsy (coeliac disease).
- Sweat test (cystic fibrosis).

Constipation

The term 'constipation' refers to infrequent passage of stools, passage of abnormally hard stools or pain or discomfort on defecation. It might be accompanied by soiling caused by involuntary passage of faeces (overflow incontinence) or voluntary defecation in an unacceptable place (encopresis).

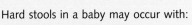

Hard stools in a baby may occur with:
- Inadequate milk intake.
- Overstrength formula feeds.
- Changing to cow's milk.

In infants and children, constipation is often acute and transient though there is a wide normal variation in stool pattern. Constipation might follow an acute febrile illness and can be prolonged if the hard stools cause a small, superficial anal tear.

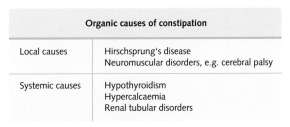

Organic causes of constipation	
Local causes	Hirschsprung's disease Neuromuscular disorders, e.g. cerebral palsy
Systemic causes	Hypothyroidism Hypercalcaemia Renal tubular disorders

Fig. 3.8 Organic causes of constipation.

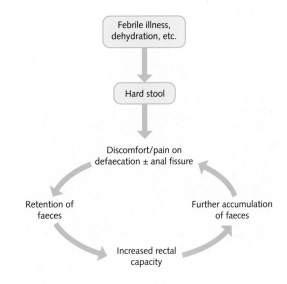

Fig. 3.9 The cycle of simple constipation.

Organic causes of constipation are rare (Fig. 3.8). An organic cause is more likely in infants, with onset at birth or when constipation occurs in the context of additional problems such as failure to thrive.

In childhood, the most common cause of chronic constipation is so-called 'simple' constipation (Fig. 3.9) associated with acquired megacolon. Short-segment Hirschsprung's disease might present late and should be considered in severe or intractable constipation (Fig. 3.10).

History

Enquire about:

- Frequency and consistency of stools.
- Presence of pain or blood on defecation.

Fig. 3.10 Differences between simple constipation and Hirschsprung's disease.

Differences between simple constipation and Hirschsprung's disease		
	Simple constipation	Hirschsprung's disease
Frequency	Common	Rare—1 : 4500 live births
Onset	Late	85% in first month of life
Passage of meconium	Normal (<24 h)	Delayed
Soiling	Usual	Uncommon
Abdomen	Faecal mass	Distended
Rectum	Loaded and distended	Narrow and empty

- Presence or absence of soiling (in children).
- Any history of delay in passage of meconium.

Physical examination

Check for the following:

- Systemic signs of failure to thrive or dehydration.
- Abdominal distension, palpable descending colon.
- Presence of anal fissure.
- Rectal examination: anal tone, rectum empty or loaded?

Failure to thrive

The phrase 'failure to thrive' is used to describe an inadequate weight gain during the first year of life. Although this might be associated with poor linear growth and short stature, it is better to consider this as a separate problem.

The rate of weight gain obtained by plotting serial weights on a centile chart over a period of time is more important, since a single observation is difficult to interpret. It is also important to remember that birth weight is determined by the intrauterine environment, and the weight of a large infant may drop from its birth centile to a lower, genetically determined centile (catch down) in the first year.

Poor weight gain is a common cause of parental anxiety. If the child's growth steadily follows the centile curve, it is likely to be normal even if it is below the 2nd centile, if he /she is otherwise well. Normal small infants have small appetites, a feature that can cause inappropriate parental anxiety.

Recognition of the constitutionally small child:

- Small parents.
- Low birth weight for gestational age.
- Proportionally small: low centile for height, weight and head circumference.
- Normal height and weight velocities.
- Asymptomatic.
- Normal physical examination.

Globally, the most common cause of failure to thrive is inadequate intake of food (i.e. starvation). In the UK, most cases have a non-organic cause and are associated with psycho-social and environmental deprivation. Organic causes include inadequate food intake, defective absorption of food from the

Fig. 3.11 Causes of failure to thrive.

Causes of failure to thrive	
Organic	Non-organic
Inadequate food intake: • Breast feeding—insufficient milk, poor technique • Bottle feeding—milk too dilute • Insufficient diet offered • Anorexia: due to chronic illness • Unable to feed: cleft palate, cerebral palsy • Vomiting: gastro-oesophageal reflux Malabsorption: • Coeliac disease • Cystic fibrosis • Short gut (post-operative) Protein-losing enteropathy: • Cow's milk protein intolerance Increased energy requirements: • Chronic illness—cystic fibrosis, congenital heart disease, chronic renal failure	• Psycho-social/enviromental deprivation • Inadequate or inappropriate feeding is usually a component

GI tract (malabsorption), protein loss from the gut and increased energy expenditure (Fig. 3.11).

Extensive investigation is not usually required. The constitutionally small normal child should be recognized (see Hints & Tips) and non-organic failure to thrive can be positively diagnosed. A brief hospital admission to document weight gain on a measured dietary intake might be helpful.

LIVER

Liver disease is uncommon in childhood and usually manifests as jaundice or hepatomegaly.

Jaundice

Jaundice is a yellowish discoloration caused by an increase in circulating bilirubin. The bilirubin can be unconjugated or conjugated, depending on the aetiology (Fig. 3.12). Mild jaundice is best detected in the sclerae rather than the skin.

Infectious hepatitis is the most common cause of acute jaundice in the older child. However, jaundice is encountered most commonly in the newborn period, at which time its causes range from trivial physiological changes to severe liver disease requiring early recognition and intervention.

Neonatal jaundice

See Chapter 9.

Jaundice after infancy

Jaundice in childhood usually has an infective cause. Viral hepatitis accounts for most, but other pathogens can involve the liver. Infective hepatitis can be caused by:

• Hepatitis viruses: hepatitis A is the most common cause of jaundice after the neonatal period.
• Epstein–Barr virus (EBV).
• Malaria or bilharzia.
• Leptospirosis (Weil's disease).

Liver injury can be caused by a variety of drugs (e.g. sodium valproate, halothane) and, in overdose, paracetamol and iron are toxic to the liver. Jaundice with pallor suggests a haemolytic episode (e.g. glucose-6-phosphate dehydrogenase deficiency, spherocytosis or haemolytic uraemic syndrome). Malaria is an important cause in tropical regions.

Fig. 3.12 Bilirubin metabolism.

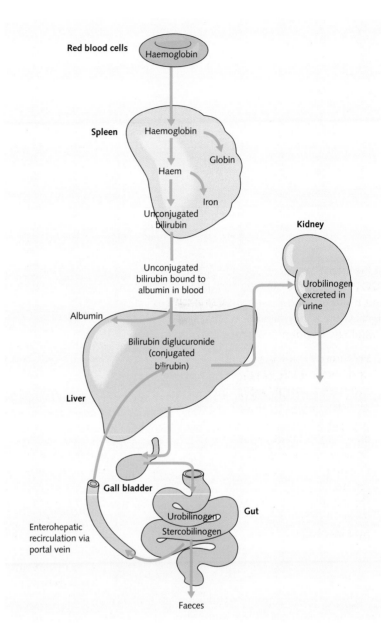

Hepatomegaly after infancy

Isolated hepatomegaly is uncommon. In association with jaundice, the causes include biliary atresia and infective hepatitis. In babies, hepatomegaly is an important feature of cardiac failure.

Hepatosplenomegaly can occur in advanced liver disease and in a number of important haematological diseases (e.g. leukaemia, thalassaemia) and rare storage disorders (e.g. mucopolysaccharidosis).

Haematuria or proteinuria

In the infant or younger child, urinary tract infection (UTI) is the most common disorder encountered and it often presents without specific symptoms or signs. Urine abnormalities might also indicate renal pathology. Important symptoms are:

- Polyuria (frequency) or enuresis: suggesting UTI or diabetes mellitus. Polyuria suggests an increased urine output (diabetes mellitus, diabetes insipidus) or excessive water intake, whereas frequency does not necessarily mean an increased urine output.
- Dysuria: suggesting UTI.
- Oliguria: suggesting dehydration or acute renal failure.
- Discoloured urine (Fig. 4.1).
- Fever with or without rigors: rule out UTI or pyelonephritis.

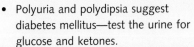

- Polyuria and polydipsia suggest diabetes mellitus—test the urine for glucose and ketones.
- Excessive drinking is a more common cause of polyuria and polydipsia in a toddler than diabetes insipidus.
- Polyuria might present as secondary enuresis.

Important signs are:

- Hypertension: suggesting glomerulonephritis.
- Oedema: suggesting nephrotic syndrome.
- Palpable bladder or kidneys: suggest anatomical abnormalities.

HAEMATURIA

Test strips are very sensitive. Haematuria should be confirmed by urine microscopy and is defined as >10 red blood cells (RBCs) per high power field. The causes are listed in Fig. 4.2.

History

Find out the following:

- Duration and recurrence.
- Dysuria and frequency: suggest UTI.
- Associated loin pain: suggests pyelonephritis if associated with fever or renal stones, especially if the pain is colicky.
- Recent foreign travel: suggests schistosomiasis.
- Recent sore throat or skin infection: suggests post-streptococcal glomerulonephritis.
- Family history of haematuria or deafness: suggests Alport syndrome.

Examination

Examine for:

- Fever: suggests UTI.
- Oedema: suggests nephrotic syndrome. In nephritis oedema is usually mild though haematuria is more common.
- Hypertension: suggests acute nephritis/chronic renal scarring or chronic renal insufficiency.
- Typical rash and joint swelling: suggests Henoch–Schönlein purpura.
- Bruises and purpura: suggests idiopathic thrombocytopenic purpura.
- Abdominal mass: suggests Wilms' tumour.

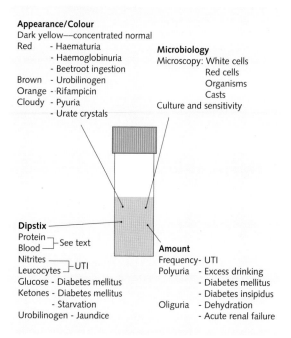

Appearance/Colour
Dark yellow—concentrated normal
Red - Haematuria
 - Haemoglobinuria
 - Beetroot ingestion
Brown - Urobilinogen
Orange - Rifampicin
Cloudy - Pyuria
 - Urate crystals

Microbiology
Microscopy: White cells
 Red cells
 Organisms
 Casts
Culture and sensitivity

Dipstix
Protein ⎤
Blood ⎦ See text
Nitrites ⎤
Leucocytes ⎦ UTI
Glucose - Diabetes mellitus
Ketones - Diabetes mellitus
 - Starvation
Urobilinogen - Jaundice

Amount
Frequency - UTI
Polyuria - Excess drinking
 - Diabetes mellitus
 - Diabetes insipidus
Oliguria - Dehydration
 - Acute renal failure

Fig. 4.1 Information available from urine.

Causes of haematuria	
Glomerular	**Non-glomerular**
Presence of red cell or white cell casts and proteinuria suggests a glomerular source of the blood—glomerulonephritis: • Acute, poststreptococcal • Henoch–Schönlein nephritis • IgA nephropathy (Berger's disease) • Alport syndrome (familial deafness and nephritis)	Infection: • Bacterial UTI • TB • Schistosomiasis Trauma Stones Wilms tumour Bleeding disorders, esp: thrombocytopenia

Fig. 4.2 Causes of haematuria.

Causes of proteinuria	
Transient	**Persistent**
Fever Exercise Orthostatic—proteinuria During the day (stops When recumbent at night)	Nephrotic syndrome ($>1\ g/m^2/24\ h$) UTI Glomerulonephritis

Fig. 4.3 Causes of proteinuria.

UTI can present with fever and no clues to its origin, especially in infants and young children. Urine microscopy and culture should be undertaken in any infant with unexplained fever.

• Persistent proteinuria or haematuria for >6 months.
• Unexplained abnormal renal function.
• Chronic glomerulonephritis.
• Nephrotic syndrome if the child is <1 year or >12 years old at onset.
• Steroid-resistant nephrotic syndrome.

Investigations

The choice of investigations depends on the renal pathology suspected:

• Microscopy and culture of urine.
• Imaging: nuclear medicine and ultrasound scans.
• Haematology: full blood count (FBC), coagulation screen and sickle-cell screen.
• Biochemistry: urea and electrolytes (U&E), creatinine (Cr), Ca^{2+}, PO_4^{3-} and urate.
• Throat swab.
• Anti-streptolysin O titre (ASOT), C3 and hepatitis B antigen.

Transient, benign haematuria can occur but is a diagnosis of exclusion. A renal biopsy might be indicated when there is a need for a diagnosis:

PROTEINURIA

Transient, mild proteinuria is mostly benign. The nephrotic syndrome causes persistent heavy proteinuria. The causes of proteinuria are listed in Fig. 4.3. Normal children produce $<60\ mg/m^2/24\ h$ of protein in the urine.

Definition

• Early morning urine protein/creatinine ratio >20 mg/mmol.
• Greater than 5 mg/kg in a 24-h urine sample.

Examination

Physical examination should include evaluation for signs of renal disease (especially the nephrotic syndrome), which include:

- Oedema: especially periorbital, scrotal, leg and ankle.
- Ascites.
- Pleural effusions (unusual).
- Blood pressure: low or high.

Investigations

The investigations include:
- Urine dipstix (Fig. 4.4).
- Early morning protein creatinine ratio.

Albustix values	
Stix reading	Albumin concentration g/L
+	0.3
+ +	1.0
+ + +	3.0
+ + + +	>20

Fig. 4.4 Albustix values.

- Renal function: U&E, Cr.
- Plasma albumin and lipids.
- Midstream urine for microscopy, culture and sensitivity.
- Throat swab, ASOT, anti-DNaseB.
- Complement C3, C4.

Objectives

At the end of this chapter, you should be able to

- Understand the common types of paroxysmal events in children.
- Take history and examine a child with suspected epilepsy.
- Understand the common causes of headache.
- Evaluate an unconscious child.

Important symptoms are:

- Paroxysmal episodes (fits, faints, and funny turns).
- Headache.
- Vomiting and ataxia.

Important signs are:

- Focal neurology.
- Altered consciousness or coma.

Global or specific developmental delay can be a manifestation of neurological disease, as can abnormalities of head size or shape; these are discussed in Chapters 8 and 17.

FITS, FAINTS AND FUNNY TURNS

Transient episodes of altered consciousness, abnormal movements or abnormal behaviour are a common presenting problem. The first task is to distinguish true epileptic seizures (fits) from faints and funny turns. An accurate account from a witness is essential.

History

Provoking events

Find out exactly when and where the episode occurred.

Description of the episodes

Get an exact description of:

- Any altered consciousness or awareness?
- Abnormal movements (involving limbs or face?).
- Altered tone (rigidity or sudden fall?).
- Altered colour (pallor or cyanosis?).
- Eye movements (did they 'roll up'?).
- Duration of the episode?
- Any trigger factor, e.g. flashing lights?

Other important features to establish in the history include:

- Previous history: was the birth normal, was there any developmental delay, has there been any recent head injury?
- Family history: both epilepsy and febrile convulsions run in families.

The paroxysmal episodes (faints and funny turns) that must be distinguished from epileptic seizures are listed in Fig. 5.1 and described below.

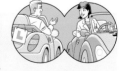

While taking history, it is very useful to take them through the event from the beginning. Parents can often demonstrate the fit. When the nature of the fit is not clear, it is extremely useful if parents can record the event on video (a mobile phone with video recording facility can be handy).

Differential diagnosis of seizures by age	
Age	**Differential diagnosis**
Infants	Jitteriness Benign myoclonus Apnoeas Gastro-oesophageal reflux
Toddlers	Breath-holding attacks Reflex anoxic seizures Rigors
Children	Vaso-vagal syncope (faints) Tics Day-dreaming Migraine Panic attacks, tantrums Night terrors

Fig. 5.1 Differential diagnosis of seizures by age.

Seizures (fits)

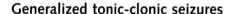

- A 'seizure' is a transient episode of abnormal and excessive neuronal activity in the brain.
- The term 'epilepsy' refers to the tendency to recurrent seizures.

Generalized tonic-clonic seizures

These are characterized by:

- Tonic phase of rigidity with loss of posture followed by clonic movements of all four limbs.
- Loss of consciousness.
- Duration: 2–20 minutes.
- Postictal drowsiness.

Febrile seizures are usually of this sort.

Meningitis or encephalitis must be considered in all children with fever and seizure. Febrile convulsions are a diagnosis of exclusion.

Absence seizures

These are characterized by:

- Brief unawareness lasting a few seconds.
- No loss of posture.
- Immediate recovery.
- Might be very frequent.
- Associated with automatisms (e.g. blinking and lip-smacking).

Partial seizures

These are characterized by:

- Involvement of only a part of the body.
- May be associated with an aura.
- May spread to involve the entire body—secondary generalized epilepsy.
- Consciousness may be retained (simple partial seizure) or lost (complex partial seizures).

Faints (vasovagal syncope)

Features include the following:

- Usually occurs in teenagers.
- Provoked by emotion, hot environment.
- Preceded by nausea and dizziness.
- Sudden loss of consciousness and posture.
- Rapid recovery.

Funny turns

Breath-holding attacks

These have the following characteristics:

- They are provoked by temper or frustration usually in children between 6 months and 6 years of age.
- The screaming toddler holds his or her breath in expiration, goes blue, then limp and then makes a rapid spontaneous recovery.

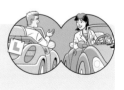

It is important to advise parents not to reinforce these behaviours by paying too much attention to the child.

Reflex anoxic seizures

These have the following characteristics:

- They are provoked by pain (usually a mild head injury) or fear.

- The infant or toddler becomes pale and loses consciousness (reflecting syncope, secondary to vagal-induced bradycardia).
- The subsequent hypoxia might induce a tonic-clonic seizure.

Rigors

Rigors are transient exaggerated shivering in association with high fever.

Examination

The well child

Physical examination is often normal in a well child with idiopathic epilepsy (the majority). However, particular attention should be paid to:

- Skin: neurocutaneous syndromes are associated with epilepsy, especially tuberous sclerosis and neurofibromatosis.
- Optic fundi: fundal changes might be apparent in congenital infections and neurodegenerative diseases.

The convulsing child

Physical examination of an infant or child presenting acutely with generalized tonic-clonic seizures (convulsions) has a different emphasis, reflecting the likely causes (Fig. 5.2). Important features on examination include:

- Fever: febrile convulsions or intracranial infection.
- Anterior fontanelle: tense or bulging if the intracranial pressure (ICP) is raised.
- Meningism.
- Optic fundi: papilloedema in raised ICP (changes might occur in congenital infections and neurodegenerative diseases).
- Focal neurological signs.
- Altered level of consciousness.

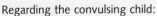

Regarding the convulsing child:
- Remember ABC: airway, breathing, circulation.
- Always measure blood glucose urgently in a convulsing child to identify and treat hypoglycaemia.

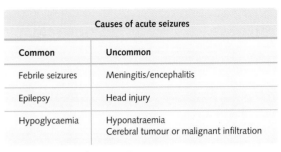

Causes of acute seizures	
Common	Uncommon
Febrile seizures	Meningitis/encephalitis
Epilepsy	Head injury
Hypoglycaemia	Hyponatraemia Cerebral tumour or malignant infiltration

Fig. 5.2 Causes of acute seizures.

HEADACHE

An acute headache commonly occurs as a non-specific feature of any febrile illness but can be a feature of meningitis. Recurrent headaches are very common in children and their causes range from the trivial to the sinister (Fig. 5.3); serious causes are rare.

History

Important features include:

- Site: frontal, temporal, bilateral or unilateral?
- Intensity: severe, throbbing?
- Duration and frequency?
- Provoking factors: stress, food?
- Associated symptoms: weakness, paraesthesia, nausea or vomiting?

Simple tension headaches

These are characterized by the following:

- Symmetrical and band-like in nature.
- Gradual onset, duration less than 24 hours.
- No associated nausea or vomiting.
- Often recur frequently.
- Affect 10% of school children.

Migraine

- Can be unilateral and throbbing in nature.
- With or without visual aura, area of visual loss or fortification spectra.
- Associated nausea, vomiting, abdominal pain.
- Duration several hours.
- Trigger factors—stress or relaxation, foods (cheese, chocolate).
- Family history.

Fig. 5.3 Causes of recurrent headache.

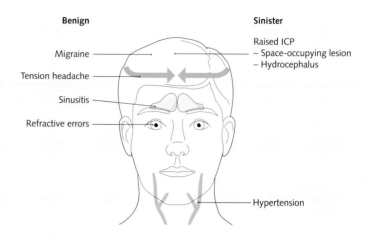

Migraine can be classified as:
- Common: no aura.
- Classical: aura preceding headache.
- Complex: associated neurological deficit, e.g. hemiplegia, ophthalmoplegia.

Headache is rarely caused by a brain tumour but 70% of children with a brain tumour present with headache. The headache might wake the child at night, is worst in the morning and associated with vomiting. Most are in the posterior fossa and cause raised ICP.

Headache from raised intracranial pressure

- Worse in recumbent position, i.e. during the night or early morning.
- Associated with nausea and vomiting.
- Pain is usually mild and diffuse.
- Personality changes may develop.

Examination

Attention should be paid to the following signs in a child with recurrent headache:

- Blood pressure: hypertension (e.g. aortic coarctation is a rare cause of headache).
- Pulse: radial–femoral delay (coarctation).
- Visual acuity: refractive errors cause headache.
- Papilloedema: a late sign of raised ICP.
- Focal neurological deficit: especially cerebellar signs (posterior fossa tumour).

THE UNCONSCIOUS CHILD

The acute development of a diminished level of consciousness is a medical emergency. In the majority of cases a systemic problem rather than a primary brain disorder is responsible (Fig. 5.4). The cause might be evident from the history but, if not, clinical evaluation is the key after emergency management. For investigation and management see Chapter 26. It is important not to perform lumbar puncture in an acutely comatose child as raised intracranial pressure is likely. It can always be performed later if a diagnosis is required.

Examination

Systemic examination

This is the priority:

- ABC: airway, breathing, and circulation.
- Temperature.

Causes of coma	
Cause	Differential diagnosis
Infection	Meningitis Encephalitis
Trauma	Head injury
Metabolic	Hypoglycaemia
Primary CNS disorder	Seizures
Drugs	Opiates Lead

Fig. 5.4 Causes of coma.

Glasgow coma scale			
Score	Eye opening	Best motor response	Best verbal response
1	No response	No response	No response
2	Open to pain	Extension	Non-verbal sounds
3	Open to verbal command	Inappropriate flexion	Inappropriate words
4	Open spontaneously	Flexion with pain	Disorientated and conversing
5		Localizes pain	Orientated and conversing
6		Obeys command	

Fig. 5.5 The Glasgow coma scale: top score = 15.

- Blood glucose.
- Hypertension, bradycardia, irregular respiration (signs of coning).
- Signs of physical abuse or injury.

Neurological examination

For a neurological examination, check the AVPU score; there are four categories:

- A = alert.
- V = responds to voice.
- P = responds to pain (the Glasgow Coma Scale (GCS) is usually less than 8 at this point).
- U = unresponsive.

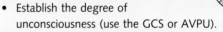

When a child is comatose:
- Establish the degree of unconsciousness (use the GCS or AVPU).
- Assess and treat the ABCs and hypoglycaemia.
- Look for signs of raised intracranial pressure.
- Establish the possible causes and decide which need immediate treatment.

Check also:

- The Glasgow coma scale (Fig. 5.5).
- The pupils: these might be small (suggests opiate or barbiturate poisoning), large (suggests a postictal state) or unequal (suggests severe head injury or intracranial haemorrhage).
- For meningism.
- The fontanelle.

Further reading

Kirkham FJ. Non-traumatic coma in children. *Archives of Diseases of Childhood* 2001; **85**:303–312.

Musculoskeletal problems

Objectives

At the end of this chapter, you should be able to

- Assess a limping child.
- Understand the common causes of limb and joint pains.
- Understand the normal postural variations in children.

Disorders of the musculoskeletal system can present in a variety of ways. The common presenting symptoms include:

- Limb or joint pain.
- Fever.

Important signs are:

- Limp.
- Altered posture.
- Point tenderness.
- Reduced range of movement.

LIMP

A limp is an abnormality of gait (the term applied to the rhythmic movement of the whole body in walking). It can be painful or painless, and the cause varies with age (Fig. 6.1).

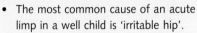
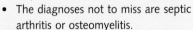

- The most common cause of an acute limp in a well child is 'irritable hip'.
- The diagnoses not to miss are septic arthritis or osteomyelitis.

History

The history should establish:

- Duration: chronic pain is unlikely to be caused by infection.
- Any prodromal illness (e.g. sore throat) or trauma.
- Presence and location of any pain.

Examination

Physical examination can begin by observing the child walking, if this can be done without distress. Important physical signs include:

- Fever: suggests bone or joint infection.
- Skin rashes.
- Range of movement.
- Point tenderness or signs of inflammation.
- Unequal leg length.
- Spinal abnormality, e.g. hairy patch.
- Neurological signs: check tone, power and tendon reflexes.

Investigations

Useful investigations may include:

- Imaging: X-rays, ultrasound of the joint.
- Nuclear medicine: isotope bone scans.
- Full blood count, acute phase reactants.
- Blood cultures (if febrile).

THE PAINFUL LIMB

Pain in a limb can arise from the bone, joint or soft tissues. In the lower limbs, pain might be associated with a limp (see above). Pain in a joint (arthralgia) is considered separately.

Recurrent limb pain

So-called 'growing pains' are common in the lower limbs. Their features are listed in Fig. 6.2.

An important rare cause of limb pain, especially at night, is malignant deposits in the bone (e.g. leukaemia).

Causes of a limp	
Age group	**Cause**
All ages	Trauma Septic arthritis/osteomyelitis
1–2 years	Congenital dislocation of the hip (developmental dysplasia of the hip) Cerebral palsy
3–10 years	Transient synovitis (irritable hip) Perthes disease Rarities: • JIA • Leukaemia
11–15 years	Slipped upper femoral epiphysis Osgood–Schlatter's disease Rarities: • Bone tumours • JIA • Hysteria

Fig. 6.1 Causes of a limp.

Features of growing pains
Common between 7 and 11 years of age Occurs in evening and night Predominantly lower limbs Normal examination **Never:** Functional disability Limp Morning symptoms

Fig. 6.2 Features of growing pains.

Limb pain of acute onset

In a young infant this might present as pseudo-paralysis. Important causes include:

- Trauma.
- Osteomyelitis or septic arthritis.
- Sickle-cell disease ('painful crisis').

Trauma is usually accidental (e.g. sports injury) but non-accidental injury should also be a consideration. Osteomyelitis usually presents with a painful, immobile limb in a febrile child. The long bones around the knee are the most common site of infection.

THE PAINFUL JOINT

Arthralgia usually reflects inflammation, i.e. arthritis. Diagnostic possibilities depend on whether the

Causes of acute monoarthralgia	
Cause	**Clinical clues**
Septic arthritis	Fever and inability to move
Irritable hip	Recent cold
Haemophilia	Easy bruising
Juvenile idiopathic arthritis	Chronic pain and swelling
Trauma	Immediate symptoms-- no chronicity

Fig. 6.3 Causes of acute monoarthralgia.

Causes of polyarthritis	
Type	**Cause**
Inflammatory	Juvenile idiopathic arthritis Systemic lupus erythematosus Henoch-Schönlein purpura
Infectious/reactive	Viral Mycoplasma Rheumatic fever

Fig. 6.4 Causes of polyarthritis.

presentation is acute or insidious, and whether one or several joints are involved. Causes of an acutely painful joint are shown in Fig. 6.3.

Septic arthritis is a medical emergency—joint destruction can occur within 24 h if untreated. X-rays are not helpful in early diagnosis and aspiration of the joint space is indicated if septic arthritis is suspected.

Polyarthritis might have an acute onset but is more likely to run a chronic and relapsing course. Causes to consider are shown in Fig. 6.4.

Inequalities of limb length

This is caused by shortening or overgrowth in one or more bones in the leg. Causes include trauma, neuromuscular disorders and congenital malformations. Treatment is surgical.

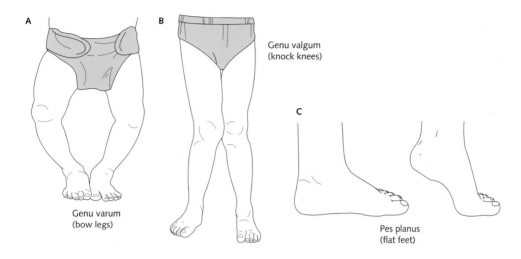

Fig. 6.5 Normal postural variants: (A) genu varum (bow legs), (B) genu valgum (knock knees), (C) pes planus (flat feet). Note the medial longitudinal arch appears when standing on tiptoe.

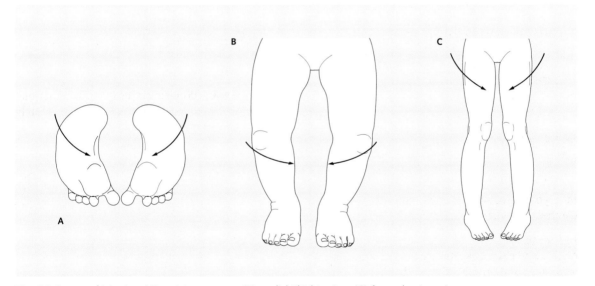

Fig. 6.6 Causes of intoeing: (A) metatarsus varus, (B) medial tibial torsion, (C) femoral anteversion.

NORMAL POSTURAL VARIANTS

These are common and most resolve without treatment (Fig. 6.5). They include:

- Bow legs (genu varum): common in infants and toddlers up to 2 years.
- Knock knees (genu valgum): the physiological knock-knee pattern is seen during the third and fourth years.

- Flat feet (pes planus): often present in toddlers.
- Intoeing: metatarsus varus in infants, medial tibial torsion in toddlers, femoral anteversion in children (Fig. 6.6).

Pathology should be suspected if there is:

- Rapid or severe progression.
- A positive family history.
- Asymmetry.

Pallor, bleeding, splenomegaly or lymphadenopathy

In childhood, disorders of the blood or bone marrow often present with striking physical signs rather than complex symptomatology. The pallor of anaemia is the most common sign but abnormal bruising or bleeding, enlargement of the spleen or liver, or a propensity to infection can all reflect an underlying haematological problem.

PALLOR

It is easy to miss mild degrees of anaemia, especially in those patients with pigmented skin. Pallor is best diagnosed by observing the conjunctiva and palmar creases. Note that peripheral vasoconstriction also causes pallor, e.g. shock.

Anaemia

The history and physical examination will often provide a good idea of the likely cause (Fig. 7.1). Few symptoms will occur unless the haemoglobin decreases below 7–8 g/dL, except in acute blood loss. Infants born preterm have a physiological anaemia at the age of 2 months that can reach as low as 7 g/dL.

Mean haemoglobin (g/dL) values in infancy and childhood are:

- 2 weeks   16.8 (13.0–20.0).
- 3 months   12.0 (9.5–14.5).
- 6 months to 6 years   12.0 (10.5–14.0).
- 7–12 years   13.0 (11.0–16.0).

History

This should include enquiry about:

- The presence of chronic diseases, especially renal or prematurity.
- Gastrointestinal symptoms.
- Dietary history: adequate iron intake? Most anaemia in childhood is due to iron deficiency.
- Family history: relatives with inherited disorders such as sickle-cell disease, thalassaemia or hereditary spherocytosis

It is sometimes difficult to elicit a family history of inherited anaemias. A family history of frequent blood transfusions is a useful pointer towards an inherited anaemia.

Examination

Age and ethnic group

Causes of anaemia are very age dependent and inherited anaemias show a racial preponderance:

- Afro-Caribbean ancestry: sickle-cell disease.
- Mediterranean and Asian ancestry: thalassaemia.

Associated signs

- Jaundice: suggests acute haemolysis.
- Petechiae or bruising: suggest marrow failure.

Fig. 7.1 Causes of anaemia in infants and children.

Causes of anaemia in infants and children	
Cause	**Type**
Decreased red cell production Iron deficiency anaemia	Nutritional Occult blood loss (Meckel's diverticulum) Malabsorption (coeliac disease)
Haemoglobinopathy	β-thalassaemia
Marrow replacement	Malignant disease—acute leukaemia Marrow aplasia
Chronic disease	Renal failure, inflammatory disorders
Reduced red cell life span (haemolytic anaemia) Intrinsic red cell defects	Abnormal membrane–spherocytosis Abnormal haemoglobin—sickle cell disease, thalassaemia Enzyme deficiencies–G6PD (X-linked), pyruvate kinase Immune-mediated:
Extrinsic disorders	• ABO, rhesus incompatibility • Auto-immune diseases • Bacterial infections • Malaria Microangiopathy—haemolytic uraemic syndrome Hypersplenism
Excessive blood loss Gastrointestinal	Hookworm infestation Meckel's diverticulum
Iatrogenic	Excessive venesection in babies
Epistaxis	Recurrent, severe
Menstruation	

- Splenomegaly: suggests haemolysis, haemoglobinopathy or marrow failure.

Investigation

The most important initial investigation is examination of the peripheral blood (full blood count; FBC) to confirm reduced haemoglobin concentration and document red cell indices (Fig. 7.2). Additional valuable information from the FBC includes:

- Reticulocytes: an increase suggests haemolytic anaemia; a decrease suggests marrow aplasia.
- Pancytopenia: a reduction in all cell types suggests marrow failure or hypersplenism.
- A peripheral blood film can also reveal abnormal cells (blasts) commonly seen in leukemias.

Depending on the initial results, further investigations to clarify the cause might include:

Red cell indices and film
MCV (mean corpuscular volume): • Microcytic anaemia suggests iron deficiency, thalassaemia • Macrocytic anaemia (normal in neonates) suggests folate, vitamin B_{12} deficiency (rare)
MCHC (mean corpuscular haemoglobin concentration): • Hypochromic anaemia suggests iron deficiency, thalassaemia
The film may reveal: • Sickle cells—sickle-cell disease • Microcytic, hypochromic cells—iron deficiency • Spherocytes—hereditary spherocytosis

Fig. 7.2 Red cell indices and film.

- Serum iron, ferritin and total iron-binding capacity.
- Coombs' test: this is positive in haemolysis caused by immune mechanisms.
- Red cell folate, vitamin B_{12}.

- Haemoglobin electrophoresis.
- Red cell enzyme estimation: glucose-6-phosphate dehydrogenase (G6PD), pyruvate kinase.
- Bone marrow aspiration.

BLEEDING DISORDERS

Normal haemostasis requires integrity of the coagulation factors, functional platelets and their interaction with the vessels. Disorders of the coagulation system may be hereditary or acquired. In the past, the coagulation cascade was thought to contain intrinsic and extrinsic pathways; however, it is now thought to comprise a common pathway involving tissue factor activation, with a central role for thrombin and membrane-associated complexes (Fig. 7.3).

Clinical evaluation

The history and examination should answer the following questions:

- Is there a generalized haemostatic problem?
- Is it inherited or acquired?
- What is the likely mechanism: vascular, platelets, coagulation or a combination?

Investigations will be required to establish the precise nature of the underlying abnormality.

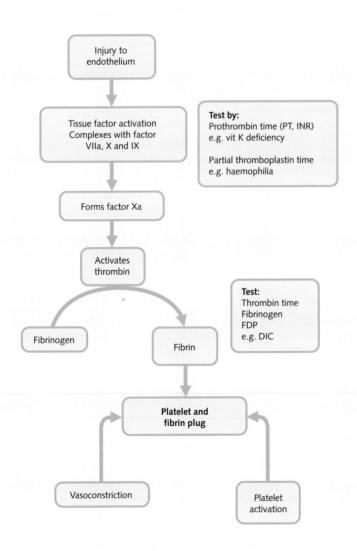

Fig. 7.3 Coagulation cascade: tests and defects.

History

- Age of onset: inherited disorders usually present in infancy but, if mild, may not be detected until adulthood.
- If the child has had a haemostatic challenge such as tonsillectomy without excessive bleeding then a bleeding disorder is unlikely.
- Family history: note that up to one-third of cases of haemophilia are from spontaneous mutation.

Bruising—normal and abnormal:
- Mobile toddlers commonly have multiple bruises on shins but bruises in non-mobile infants need further evaluation.
- Mongolian blue spots in infants can be mistaken for bruising.
- Newborns often have petechiae around the face and forehead.

Examination

The commonest clinical manifestation is excessive bleeding into the skin but spontaneous bleeding into other sites like nasal mucosa (epistaxis), gums, joints (haemarthrosis) and the genitourinary tract (haematuria) can also occur. Spontaneous bleeding from multiple sites suggests a generalized haemostatic disorder.

A petechial or purpuric rash in a febrile child must raise the possibility of meningococcal sepsis.

- Bleeding into skin and mucous membranes: platelet or vascular disorder.
- Bleeding into muscles or joints: coagulation disorder.

Manifestation of skin bleeding

The terms used vary with the size of lesion. Test small lesions using a transparent glass to see if they blanch. Failure to blanch indicates extravasated blood.

- Petechiae: small red spots the size of a pinhead.
- Purpura: confluent petechiae.
- Ecchymosis: a large area of extravasated blood (a synonym for a bruise).
- Haematoma: extravasated blood that has infiltrated subcutaneous tissue or muscle to produce a deformity.

An important differential diagnosis of excessive bruising is non-accidental injury. There are some very important causes of a petechial/purpuric rash (see Chapter 1).

Investigations

Laboratory investigation of a suspected bleeding disorder initially includes:

- Blood film.
- Renal and liver function.
- Platelet count: normal is $150–450 \times 10^9/L$ (spontaneous bleeding can occur at counts below $30 \times 10^9/L$).
- Coagulation screen: prothrombin time, activated thromboplastin time and thrombin time. Further investigation for tissue factors should be done by a tertiary haematological centre.

Causes of bleeding disorders

The causes are set out in Fig. 7.4 and arranged according to the underlying basic mechanism. Most causes are acquired:

- The most common vascular problem encountered is Henoch–Schönlein purpura (see Chapter 1).
- Bruising with thrombocytopenia in a well child is most commonly due to idiopathic thrombocytopenic purpura.
- Inherited coagulation disorders are uncommon but haemophilia must be considered in a male infant or child with a bleeding tendency.

Bleeding disorders in chidhood		
Defect	Inherited	Acquired
Vascular defects	Hereditary haemorrhagic telangiectasia (rare) Ehlers–Danlos syndrome (rare)	Henoch–Schönlein purpura Scurvy (vitamin C deficiency) Cushing's disease Meningococcal septicaemia
Platelet defects • Thrombocytopenia	Rare	Immune-mediated: • Idiopathic thrombocytopenic purpura (most common) Peripheral consumption: • Disseminated intravascular coagulation (DIC) • Haemolytic–uraemic syndrome Marrow failure: • Aplastic anaemia • Acute leukaemia
• Abnormal function	Rare	Drug-induced, e.g. aspirin, dipyridamole
Coagulation defects	Haemophilia A (factor VIII) Haemophilia B (factor IX, Christmas disease) Von Willebrand disease	Vitamin K deficiency: • Haemorrhagic disease of newborn • Malabsorption • Liver disease Drugs—anti-coagulant therapy with warfarin, heparin

Fig. 7.4 Bleeding disorders in childhood.

- It is important to rule out bleeding disorders when considering bruising in the context of non-accidental injury.

SPLENOMEGALY

In neonates and very thin children, the tip of the spleen is often palpable. The spleen can enlarge during acute infections and in various haematological diseases. Enlargement of both liver and spleen together suggests a different aetiology from that associated with isolated splenomegaly (Figs 7.5 and 7.6).

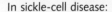

Differential diagnosis of a left-sided abdominal mass:
- Splenomegaly.
- Renal masses: Wilms' tumour, hydronephrosis.
- Neoplasia: neuroblastoma (non-renal), lymphoma.

In sickle-cell disease:
- Splenomegaly is present in early life but splenic infarction subsequently reduces the spleen in size.
- The immunological function of the spleen is always impaired, regardless of size.

History

- Systems review: this might elicit symptoms related to the many infective causes.
- Family history: inherited anaemias, storage disorders, e.g. Gaucher's disease.

Examination

Note coexistent lymphadenopathy, hepatomegaly, pallor (anaemia), fever or rash. In infectious mononucleosis, care must be taken in palpating the spleen because it can rupture.

Fig. 7.5 Causes of splenomegaly.

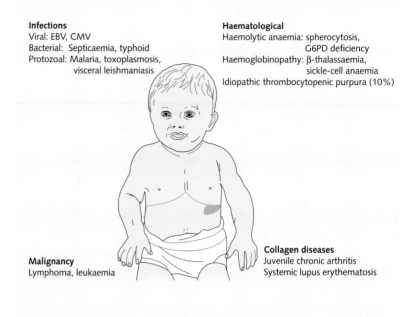

Infections
Viral: EBV, CMV
Bacterial: Septicaemia, typhoid
Protozoal: Malaria, toxoplasmosis,
          visceral leishmaniasis

Haematological
Haemolytic anaemia: spherocytosis,
                    G6PD deficiency
Haemoglobinopathy: β-thalassaemia,
                   sickle-cell anaemia
Idiopathic thrombocytopenic purpura (10%)

Malignancy
Lymphoma, leukaemia

Collagen diseases
Juvenile chronic arthritis
Systemic lupus erythematosis

Fig. 7.6 Causes of hepatosplenomegaly.

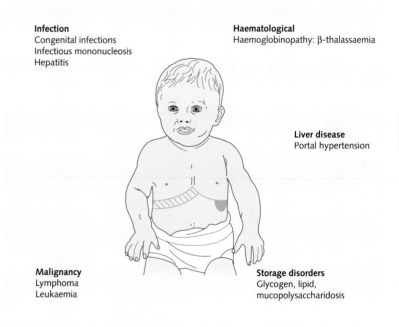

Infection
Congenital infections
Infectious mononucleosis
Hepatitis

Haematological
Haemoglobinopathy: β-thalassaemia

Liver disease
Portal hypertension

Malignancy
Lymphoma
Leukaemia

Storage disorders
Glycogen, lipid,
mucopolysaccharidosis

Investigations

- Abdominal ultrasound scan (USS).
- Infections: monospot, blood cultures, film for malaria parasites.
- Haematological: FBC, blood film, reticulocyte count.
- Malignancy: bone marrow aspiration.
- Liver disease: liver function tests (LFTs), hepatitis serology.

Causes of generalized lymphadenopathy

Cause	Example
Infection	Infectious mononucleosis Rubella Toxoplasmosis Cytomegalovirus HIV infection
Malignancy	Acute leukaemia Lymphoma
Immunological	JCA Sarcoidosis (rare) Kawasaki disease Atopic eczema

Fig. 7.7 Causes of generalized lymphadenopathy.

Causes of cervical lymphadenopathy

Type	Features
Acute, short duration	Reactive and secondary to local infection in throat or scalp: Cervical adenitis—bacterial infection in gland
Persistent, non-inflamed	Reactive and secondary to local infection: • Tuberculous adenitis—TB, atypical mycobacteria • Neoplasia—lymphoma, neuroblastoma

Fig. 7.8 Causes of cervical lymphadenopathy.

LYMPHADENOPATHY

Lymph node enlargement, particularly in the cervical region, is a common clinical problem in children. Cervical lymph nodes are normally palpable in many children and has to be distinguished from pathological enlargement.

Local infection is the commonest cause of transient regional lymphadenopathy but uncommon sinister causes of persistent or progressive lymphadenopathy do exist (Figs 7.7–7.9).

History

The history should establish:

- Duration: less than 4 weeks in most infections; more than 1 year less likely to be neoplastic.
- Constitutional symptoms: e.g. weight loss, fever, night sweats.

Features of worrying lymph nodes

Rapid growth
Skin ulceration
Fixation to skin or fascia
>3 cm with hard consistency
Greater than 3 cm for more than 6 weeks despite treatment

Fig. 7.9 Features of worrying lymph nodes.

- Rash: associated rash suggests viral exanthemata.
- Pets: toxoplasmosis or cat scratch fever.
- Travel contacts and family history of TB.
- Drugs: phenytoin, carbamazepine.

Examination

Palpate all nodal sites: look for regional or generalized lymphadenopathy. Examine the nodes:

- Size: greater than 1 cm diameter is more likely to be significant. Small, mobile nodes are less likely to be significant than large, firm, fixed nodes.
- Erythema and tenderness: suggest bacterial adenitis.
- Drainage region: ENT and scalp for cervical nodes.
- Skin: infective lesions, atopic eczema and exanthemata.
- Abdomen: hepatosplenomegaly.

Also note systemic signs such as weight loss and pallor.

Investigations

The diagnosis is apparent in most children and further investigations are unnecessary in the following common clinical situations:

- Transient node enlargement with local infection.
- Lymphadenopathy in the context of diagnosed systemic illnesses such as rubella, Epstein–Barr virus, atopic eczema and Kawasaki disease.

By contrast, lymphadenopathy presenting in the following clinical contexts requires investigation to establish an underlying diagnosis.

Persistent significant cervical lymphadenopathy

Initial tests are:

- FBC: to determine infection.
- Chest X-ray: to check for TB, lymphoma.
- Tuberculin skin test: if positive this suggests mycobacteria tuberculosis but weak false positives can be caused by non-tuberculous mycobacteria.

If malignancy is suspected, a lymph node biopsy might be indicated.

Cervical nodes are quick to enlarge but are slow to resolve with local infection. Consider TB or malignancy in persistent and progressive cervical lymphadenopathy.

Generalized lymphadenopathy

Constitutional symptoms and hepatosplenomegaly might or might not be present.

Initial tests
- FBC plus differential.
- Monospot and Epstein–Barr IgM antibodies.
- Chest X-ray.
- Abdominal USS.
- Bone marrow aspiration might be necessary.
- Lymph node biopsy might be necessary.

Lymphadenitis

Acutely infected nodes are tender with associated redness and increased warmth. If untreated, they can form an abscess—indicated by the presence of fluctuance. An ultrasound of the node will help to identify an abscess which may need surgical drainage. Uncomplicated lymphadenitis is treated with antibiotics.

Short stature or developmental delay

Objectives

At the end of this chapter, you should be able to

- Understand the normal pattern of growth in children.
- Take appropriate history and examine children with short stature.
- Identify children with global and specific developmental delay.

GROWTH

Four phases of growth are recognized:

1. Infantile phase (birth to 1 year): dependent on nutrition.
2. Childhood phase (1 year to 5 years): dependent on growth hormone.
3. Mid-childhood phase (5 years to puberty): increased levels of adrenal androgens influence growth.
4. Pubertal phase: growth spurt caused by increased levels of sex steroids.

Growth is assessed by measuring three specific parameters:

- Height (or length in children <18 months).
- Weight.
- Head circumference.

Centile charts showing the normal range of values for these measurements from before birth to adulthood are available (see Part II). Problems with inadequate weight gain ('failure to thrive') and abnormal head growth (microcephaly and macrocephaly) are considered elsewhere. An approach to the evaluation of 'short stature' is presented here. In preterm infants the corrected age (chronological age minus number of weeks preterm) should be used until 2 years of age.

Short stature

A pragmatic definition of short stature requiring further evaluation is:

- A height below the 0.4th centile for age.
- A predicted height less than the mid-parental target height.

- An abnormal growth velocity as indicated by the height changing by more than the width of one centile band over 1–2 years.

It is important to observe the velocity of growth over 1–2 years in an otherwise well child with short stature. If the growth velocity is normal, further investigations are unnecessary and parents can be reassured. The best way to do this is to plot the child's growth on the centile chart to give a visual image of his/her growth.

The causes of short stature are shown in Fig. 8.1.

History

This should elicit information about:

- Early childhood illness and systemic disorders.
- Parental height: the genetic height potential is estimated by calculating the target centile range (TCR) from the mid-parental height (MPH).
- Family history: inherited skeletal dysplasias.

To estimate the adult height potential, calculate the mid-parental height (MPH):

- Father's height plus mother's height divided by 2.

Then adjust for the sex of the child:

- Boys: add 7 cm.
- Girls: subtract 7 cm.

Identify the mid-parental centile, i.e. the centile nearest to the MPH. The target centile range (TCR) is encompassed by MPH:

- ±10 cm in boys.
- ±8.5 cm in girls.

Causes of short stature
Familial short stature
Constitutional delay of pubertal growth spurt
Endocrine disorders: • Growth hormone deficiency • Hypopituitarism • Hypothyroidism • Cushing syndrome/steroid excess
Chromosomal disorders/syndromes: • Turner syndrome • Silver–Russell syndrome
Skeletal dysplasias: • Achondroplasia
Emotional/psychosocial deprivation
Chronic illness: • Congenital heart disease • Cystic fibrosis • Cerebral palsy • Chronic renal failure

Fig. 8.1 Causes of short stature.

Fig. 8.2 Short stature algorithm.

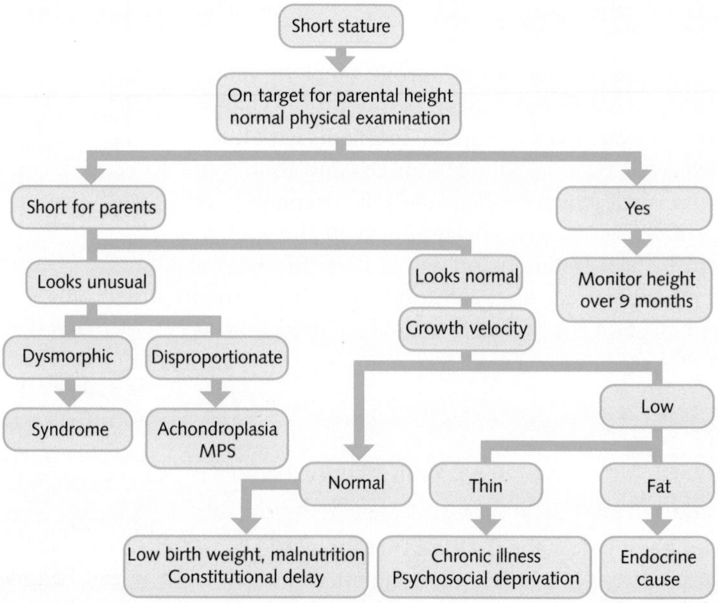

Examination

Examine the following:

- Height: measure accurately with a wall-mounted, calibrated stadiometer.
- Growth velocity: a minimum of two measurements, 6 months apart is required. Adjust to cm/year and plot at midpoint in time.
- Dysmorphic features: these might identify a syndrome (see Hints & Tips).
- Weight (see Hints & Tips).
- Visual fields and fundi: might indicate a pituitary tumour.
- Stage of puberty.

An approach to the evaluation of short stature is shown in Fig. 8.2.

Investigations

Investigations that might be of value include the following:

- Bone age: estimated from X-rays of the left wrist (delayed skeletal maturity in constitutional pubertal delay).
- Karyotype: chromosomal analysis to identify Turner syndrome (45, X0) in short girls.

- Skeletal survey: in disproportion (skeletal dysplasias).

- Endocrine investigations: thyroid function tests (T4, TSH) and growth hormone (secretion is pulsatile so a provocation test, e.g. exercise or insulin-induced hypoglycaemia, is necessary to identify deficiency).

- Skull X-ray: for suspected craniopharyngioma.

- MRI—looking at pituitary

Syndromes associated with short stature:
- Turner syndrome: neck-webbing, wide-spaced nipples, low hairline in a girl.
- Prader–Willi syndrome: obesity, hypotonia and, in boys, small genitals.
- Skeletal dysplasias: disproportionate limbs and trunk—short limbs (achondroplasia) or short trunk (mucopolysaccharidosis; MPS).

Height should be monitored over 6–12 months in response to parental concern regardless of current centile.

Warning signs of developmental delay by age	
Year	Sign
First 8 weeks	Not smiling in response Poor eye contact Head lag Silent baby—no coos, gurgles
8 months	Poor interaction Not sitting with support Not babbling
Second 18 months	Not recognizing own name Not walking three steps alone Not using first words
24 months	Not giving/receiving affection Unable to build a three-brick tower Not linking two words
Third	Unable to play Unsteady gait Not using more than 50 words

Fig. 8.3 Warning signs of developmental delay by age.

DEVELOPMENTAL DELAY

Normal development depends on genetic potential and on the environment: nature and nurture. There is a wide variation in normal rates of development in all spheres. Delay can be global or specific; normal development is described in Part II.

Delay can present through:

- Parental concern.
- Routine surveillance.
- Concern of teacher, health visitor, etc.

A list of warning signs shown in developmental delay by age is given in Fig. 8.3.

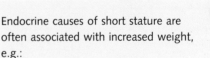

Endocrine causes of short stature are often associated with increased weight, e.g.:
- Hypothyroidism.
- Growth hormone deficiency.
- Steroid excess.

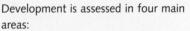

Development is assessed in four main areas:
- Gross motor.
- Vision and fine motor.
- Hearing and speech.
- Social behaviour.

Global delay

An intellectually impaired child is delayed in all aspects of development, but not all children with general delay are intellectually impaired; 40% will have a chromosomal abnormality, 5–10% will have developmental malformations and 4% will have a metabolic cause.

History

This should encompass:

- Birth history: details of pregnancy and birth including prematurity and hypoxia.

- Family history: of learning disability.
- Developmental milestones.
- Social history: risk factors, e.g. psychosocial deprivation.

Examination

You should examine the following:

- Developmental assessment.
- Appearance: dysmorphic features in syndromes associated with delay, e.g. Down syndrome, Williams syndrome, fragile X syndrome.
- Head circumference: microcephaly.

Investigations

These are directed towards identifying a specific aetiology (Fig. 8.4) and will include:

- Karyotype: Down syndrome, fragile X syndrome.
- Thyroid function tests.
- Congenital infection screen.
- Plasma and urine amino and organic acids.
- Brain imaging: MR spectroscopy.

It is important to distinguish developmental delay from actual regression. Loss of previously acquired skills suggests a serious inherited neurodegenerative disorder.

Causes of global developmental delay	
Type	**Causes**
Perinatal	Hypoxic-ischaemic Intracranial haemorrhage Teratogens
Metabolic	Hypothyroidism Inborn errors of metabolism
Infection	Meningitis Encephalitis
Genetic Neurodegenerative disease	Chromosome disorders Tay–Sachs syndrome Adrenoleucodystrophy

Fig. 8.4 Causes of global developmental delay.

Specific developmental delay

Two common and important examples of delayed development in specific areas are walking and speech.

Delayed walking

The percentage of children who are walking unsupported is:

- 50% by 12 months.
- 90% by 15 months.

Further assessment is indicated if a child is not walking unsupported by age 18 months. Many will be normal late walkers, especially if a 'bottom shuffler', but a small percentage will have an underlying problem (Fig. 8.5).

Examination

- Hips: signs of dislocation (waddling gait, leg length discrepancy, limited abduction).
- Tone, power, and tendon reflexes in all limbs.
- Locomotion: 'commando crawler' or 'bottom shuffler'?

Investigations

If indicated:

- Imaging of hips or spine.
- Creatine kinase for Duchenne muscular dystrophy.

Speech and language delay

The development of normal speech and language requires:

- Adequate hearing.
- Cognitive development.
- Coordinated sound production.

Causes of late walking	
Normal variants	**Organic causes**
Familial 'Bottom shuffler' 'Commando crawler'	Cerebral palsy Congenital dislocation of the hip Duchenne muscular dystrophy (boys)

Fig. 8.5 Causes of late walking.

Speech refers to the meaningful sounds that are made, whereas language encompasses the complex rules governing the use of these sounds for communication. Language can be further divided into language comprehension and language expression, and independent delays can occur in either aspect. As might be expected, the development of language is highly dependent on general intellectual development.

Normal speech and language development:
- 6 months: babbles.
- 12 months: says 'mama' or 'dada', understands simple commands and responds to name.
- 18 months: single words with meaning.
- 2 years: speaks in phrases.
- 4 years: conversation.

The causes of delay in speech and language development include:

- Hearing impairment.
- Environmental factors: lack of stimulus.
- Global delay: the most common cause.
- Psychiatric disorders: autism.
- Familial.

It is worth distinguishing between delay and actual disorders of speech and language such as stammering, dysarthria due to mechanical problems (e.g. cleft palate) or neuromuscular problems (e.g. cerebral palsy).

Check the hearing in any child with delayed speech.

Objectives

At the end of this chapter, you should be able to:

- Understand the common feeding problems in newborns.
- Define respiratory distress in newborns.
- Identify the common causes of neonatal respiratory distress.
- Identify fits in newborns.
- Understand the common congenital malformations in newborns.

Important presenting problems in the term newborn infant include:

- Feeding difficulties.
- Vomiting.
- Jaundice.
- Breathing difficulties.
- Seizures.
- Congenital malformations.
- Ambiguous genitalia.

FEEDING DIFFICULTIES

Difficulties in establishing feeding can occur with both breast- and bottle-fed newborn infants.

Weight gain in infants

All babies, except those babies with intrauterine growth retardation, lose weight in the first week. Full term infants should regain their birth weight by day 7–10 and preterm babies by day 14.

Reluctance to feed in an infant who has previously fed normally might indicate severe disease. It is also important to note the quantity and frequency of feeds and plot the baby's weight on a centile chart

Breastfeeding

Breastfeeding should be encouraged by antenatal education and then supported until it is established. Potential problems include:

- Latching on: chin forward and head tilted back (the baby's, not the mother's!). The areola should be in the baby's mouth as this encourages successful feeding and avoids damage to the nipple.
- Cracked nipples: occurs commonly and is more likely if the baby does not latch on well.
- Breast engorgement: prevented by demand feeding and alleviated by expression after feeding.
- Intestinal hurry: frequent loose stools are common on day 4 or 5 when the supply of milk is plentiful. This is normal.

Bottle-feeding

Problems that might occur include:

- Incorrect reconstitution: bowel problems and electrolyte abnormalities.
- Inadequate sterilization: gastroenteritis.

Milks differ in composition and age-specific milks should be used.

VOMITING

Babies often regurgitate (posset) small amounts of milk during and between feeds. This is of no pathological significance and should not be confused with vomiting (the forceful expulsion of gastric contents through the mouth).

Vomiting in the newborn might reflect systemic disease or intestinal obstruction. It is important to establish whether the vomit is:

- Milk.
- Bile-stained.
- Blood-stained.
- Frothy, mucoid.

Important causes are listed in Fig. 9.1. Bile-stained vomit suggests intestinal obstruction. Blood in the vomit might be of maternal or infant origin. This can be differentiated by alkali denaturation test (Apt Test). Plain abdominal X-ray is the most useful investigation (supine and lateral decubitus views; Fig. 9.2).

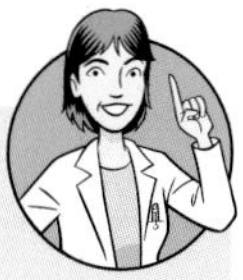

Blood-stained vomit in the newborn might be due to:
- Swallowed maternal blood—predelivery or from a cracked nipple.
- Trauma from a feeding tube.
- Haemorrhagic disease of the newborn—vitamin K deficiency.

JAUNDICE

Neonatal jaundice

Physiological jaundice occurs in most newborns, especially preterms. A combination of increased red cell breakdown and immaturity of the hepatic enzymes causes unconjugated hyperbilirubinaemia. It is exacerbated by dehydration, which can occur if establishment of feeding is delayed.

Fig. 9.1 Vomiting in the newborn.

Vomiting in the newborn	
Cause	Features/examples
Intestinal obstruction	Small bowel: • Duodenal atresia/stenosis (30% have Down syndrome) • Malrotation with volvulus • Meconium ileus (cystic fibrosis) Large bowel: • Hirschsprung's disease • Rectal atresia
Tracheo-oesophageal fistula	Frothy mucoid vomiting occurs if a feed is given
Infections: • Gastroenteritis • Urinary tract infection • Septicaemia • Meningitis	Often non-specific
Necrotizing enterocolitis	Preterm infants
Raised intracranial pressure	Bulging fontanelle
Congenital adrenal hyperplasia	Ambiguous genitalia in a female infant

Onset of jaundice in the first 24 hours of life is always pathological; the causes are listed in Fig. 9.3. Recognition and treatment of severe neonatal unconjugated hyperbilirubinaemia is important to avoid kernicterus (brain damage due to deposition of bilirubin in the basal ganglia). Evaluation of persistent conjugated hyperbilirubinaemia is important to allow early (<6 weeks) diagnosis and treatment of biliary atresia.

- Onset of jaundice in the first 24 hours of life is always pathological.
- Consider biliary atresia in an infant with persistent neonatal jaundice due to conjugated hyperbilirubinaemia and pale stools (rare but treatable).

Definition of physiological jaundice:
- Onset after 24 hours of birth.
- Resolves within 2 weeks.
- More than 85% unconjugated.
- Total bilirubin <350 µmol/L.

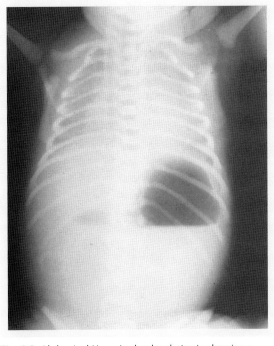

Fig. 9.2 Abdominal X-ray in duodenal atresia showing a 'double bubble' from distension of the stomach and duodenum. Air is absent distally.

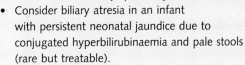

Fig. 9.3 Causes of neonatal jaundice.

Causes of neonatal jaundice	
Onset	**Cause**
Less than 24 hours old	Excess haemolysis: • Immune-mediated—rhesus or ABO incompatibility • Intrinsic RBC defects—G6PD, pyruvate kinase deficiency, or hereditary spherocytosis Congenital infections
Between 24 hours and 2 weeks old	Physiological jaundice Breast milk jaundice Infection, e.g. UTI Excess haemolysis, bruising, or polycythaemia
Persistent jaundice after 2 weeks old	Unconjugated: • Breast milk jaundice • Infections, e.g. UTI • Excess haemolysis, e.g. ABO incompatibility, G6PD deficiency • Hypothyroidism (screened for in newborn) • Galactosaemia Conjugated (>15% of total bilirubin): • Biliary atresia • Neonatal hepatitis

BREATHING DIFFICULTIES

In the newborn, breathing difficulties are referred to as respiratory distress. The signs of respiratory distress are:

- Tachypnoea: respiratory rate over 60/min.
- Recession: subcostal or intercostal.
- Nasal flaring.
- Expiratory grunting.
- Cyanosis.

Common breathing difficulties

The most common cause of breathing difficulties in the newborn is the respiratory distress syndrome due to surfactant deficiency, a condition largely confined to preterm infants. The major causes of respiratory distress in term infants are shown in Fig. 9.4.

Respiratory distress syndrome (RDS)

Only 1% of cases of RDS occurs in the term neonate. Such infants are often difficult to ventilate but do respond to surfactant therapy, in a similar manner to the preterm with RDS.

Transient tachypnoea of the newborn (TTN)

TTN is believed to be caused by a delay in the normal reabsorption of the lung fluid at birth and is more common after caesarean section. The chest X-ray (CXR) might show a streaky appearance with fluid in the horizontal fissure; it usually resolves within 48 hours.

Meconium aspiration

Approximately 10% of term neonates pass meconium before birth; it is rare in preterm babies. It

Causes of respiratory distress in term infants	
Pulmonary	Non-pulmonary
Transient tachypnoea of newborn	Septicaemia
Pneumonia	Severe anaemia
Meconium aspiration	Congenital cardiac disease
Respiratory diaphragmatic hernia	
Choanal atresia	
Pneumothorax	

Fig. 9.4 Causes of respiratory distress in term infants.

is often associated with birth asphyxia. Meconium should be cleared from the oropharynx and airway if the baby is floppy with poor respiratory efforts, but not if the baby is active and vigorous. Inhalation of meconium results in bronchial obstruction and collapse, chemical pneumonitis and secondary infection—all leading to respiratory distress. There is also a high incidence of air-leak (pneumothorax, pneumomediastinum) and pulmonary hypertension.

Pneumonia

Risk factors include premature labour and prolonged rupture of the membranes (over 24 hours). Group B streptococcal infection is an important cause of early onset pneumonia.

Pneumothorax

Pneumothorax occurs spontaneously in about 1% of term infants and resolves spontaneously. The cause is mostly iatrogenic in ventilated babies. Diagnosis is by CXR and transillumination in neonates.

Persistent fetal circulation

High pulmonary vascular resistance causes right to left shunting at both atrial and ductal levels with severe cyanosis. It can occur as a primary disorder but is more commonly a complication of birth asphyxia, meconium aspiration or respiratory distress syndrome. A CXR might show pulmonary oligaemia. Diagnosis is suggested by differences in PaO_2 on pre- and postductal arterial blood gases (ABGs) and confirmed by echocardiography.

Diaphragmatic hernia

In this uncommon malformation ($1:4000$ births), a hole in the diaphragm (usually on the left) allows the abdominal contents to herniate into the chest. Most are diagnosed on antenatal ultrasound scan. Initial resuscitation involves early intubation and nasogastric aspiration (to avoid inflation of the bowel). Surgical repair is then undertaken once the neonate is stable. If not diagnosed on antenatal ultrasound, it usually presents with failure to respond to resuscitation at birth. The apex beat and heart sounds are displaced to the right with poor air entry on the left. The relatively high mortality is accounted for by the inevitable pulmonary hypoplasia due to compression of the fetal lung.

Congenital malformations of the lung

Respiratory distress may arise from various congenital malformations, like pulmonary hypoplasia, sequestration, cystic adenoid malformation of the lung, congenital lobar emphysema, etc.

Chylothorax

This is another rare cause of respiratory distress and occurs due to accumulation of lymphatic fluid in the pleural cavity, either spontaneously due to a developmental anomaly of lymphatic drainage or iatrogenic from birth trauma or thoracotomy.

NEONATAL SEIZURES

Seizures are more common in the neonatal period than any other time of life because the neonatal brain is mostly excitatory. The manifestations of neonatal seizures are rather different from those in older children and it can be difficult to distinguish true seizures from normal baby movements.

Neonatal episodes that are *not* seizures include:

- Jitteriness: the movement is a tremor—rhythmic movements of equal rate and amplitude (in seizures, clonic movements have a fast and slow component). There are no ocular phenomena. It is sensitive to external stimuli and is stopped by holding.
- Benign myoclonus: shock-like jerks when asleep.
- Stretching, sucking movements.

The main types of seizure are:

- Subtle seizures: eye deviation, apnoeas, autonomic phenomenas and oral movements.
- Clonic seizures: seen as focal rhythmic and slow jerking; generalized clonic seizures are not seen in neonates.
- Myoclonic seizures: rapid isolated jerks.
- Tonic seizures: manifest as flexor or extensor posturing.

The perinatal and birth history together with clinical examination will often indicate the cause.

Initial investigations

- Blood glucose, electrolytes, Ca^{2+}, Mg^{2+}.
- Cerebrospinal fluid (CSF) analysis for infection.
- Cranial ultrasonography for haemorrhages.

As indicated:

- Inborn error of metabolism: blood ammonia, lactate and amino acids, urine amino acids, organic acids, IV pyridoxine test.
- Congenital infection screen.
- Cranial imaging: ultrasonography is widely used in neonatal units; computed tomography (CT) or magnetic resonance imaging (MRI) (more sensitive) are used if a cause could not be identified.

A detectable cause is present in the majority and varies with the time of onset (Fig. 9.5). The most common causes are neonatal encephalopathy, intracranial haemorrhage, CNS infection and congenital abnormality.

CONGENITAL MALFORMATIONS

Up to 70% of major congenital malformations can now be detected antenatally using ultrasound and can affect any of the major organ systems. Some of the most important are described below.

Causes of neonatal seizures	
Hypoxia	
Electrolyte and metabolic abnormalities	Hypoglycaemia Inborn errors of metabolism
CNS	Haemorrhage Infection Structural abnormality
Drug withdrawal	Opiates Benzodiazepines
Genetic disease	Neurocutaneous diseases
Hyperbilirubinaemia	Bilirubin encephalopathy

Fig. 9.5 Causes of neonatal seizures.

Congenital refers to any condition present at birth. The cause might be genetic, environmental, infectious or idiopathic. Parents are often worried if a condition is the result of something they did during pregnancy and also the chances of its recurrence in subsequent children. It is important to provide genetic counselling in the presence of such malformations.

Craniofacial disorders

Cleft lip and palate

This affects about 1:1000 babies. It manifests as:

- Cleft lip alone: 35%.
- Cleft lip and palate: 25%.
- Cleft palate alone: 40%.

Inheritance is polygenic but some are associated with maternal anticonvulsant therapy. A cleft lip is usually diagnosed at the 18- to 20-week scan but isolated cleft palates are difficult to diagnose antenatally. Some affected infants can be breastfed and special long teats or other feeding devices might help bottlefed infants. Surgical repair is carried out at 6–12 months of age on the palate, and either early (first week) or late (3 months) on the lip.

Pierre Robin anomaly

This is an association of micrognathia, posterior displacement of the tongue and midline cleft of the soft palate. Prone positioning maintains airway patency until growth of the mandible is established. The cleft is surgically repaired.

Gastrointestinal disorders

Oesophageal atresia

The incidence is 1:3500 live births. A tracheo-oesophageal fistula (TOF) is usually present (Fig. 9.6). As the fetus is unable to swallow during intra-uterine life, there is associated polyhydramnios. Diagnosis should be established before the first feed by attempting to pass a feeding tube into the stomach and checking its location by X-ray. Forty per cent of cases have other associated abnormalities, e.g. as part of the VACTERL association:

- Vertebral.
- Anorectal.
- Cardiac.
- Tracheo-oesophageal.
- Renal.
- Limb (radial).

Abdominal wall defects

Gastroschisis (1:5000)

The bowel protrudes without any covering sac through a defect in the anterior abdominal wall

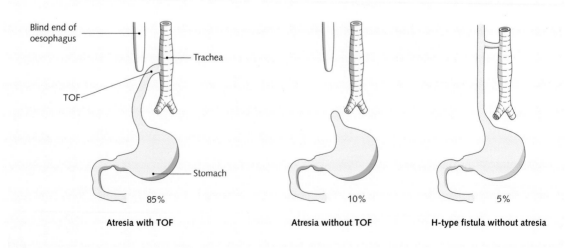

Blind end of oesophagus		
Trachea		
TOF		
Stomach		
85%	10%	5%
Atresia with TOF	Atresia without TOF	H-type fistula without atresia

Fig. 9.6 Oesophageal atresia and tracheo-oesophageal fistula (TOF).

adjacent to the umbilicus. This is usually an isolated anomaly.

Exomphalos (1:2500)

The abdominal contents herniate through the umbilical ring and are covered with a sac formed by the peritoneum and amniotic membrane. It is often associated with other major congenital abnormalities.

Neural tube defects

These arise from failure of fusion of the neural plate in the first 28 days after conception. The incidence in the UK has fallen dramatically in the last 25 years because of improved maternal nutrition, folic acid supplementation and better antenatal screening.

Folic acid supplements should ideally be taken preconception and all pregnant women are advised to take them during the first trimester.

There are three main types:

- Spina bifida occulta.
- Meningocele.
- Myelomeningocele.

They are usually in the lumbosacral region (Fig. 9.7).

Spina bifida occulta

The vertebral arch fails to fuse. There might be an overlying skin lesion such as a tuft of hair or small dermal sinus. Tethering of the cord (diastomyelia) can cause neurological deficits with growth.

Meningocele

This is uncommon (5% of cases). The smooth, intact, skin covered cystic swelling is filled with CSF. There is no neurological deficit and excision and closure of the defect is undertaken after 3 months.

Myelomeningocele

This accounts for more than 90% of overt spina bifida. These are usually open, with the unfused neural plate, exposed meninges and leaking CSF. Neurological deficits are always present and can include:

- Motor and sensory loss in the lower limbs.
- Neuropathic bladder and bowel.

In addition, there is often scoliosis and associated hydrocephalus due to the Arnold–Chiari malformation (herniation of the cerebellar tonsils through the foramen magnum). Surgery is for preventing infection and not to restore neurological function.

Congenital talipes equinovarus (club foot)

The entire foot is fixed in an inverted and supinated position (Fig. 9.8). This should be distinguished from 'positional talipes', in which the deformity is mild and can be corrected with passive manipulation.

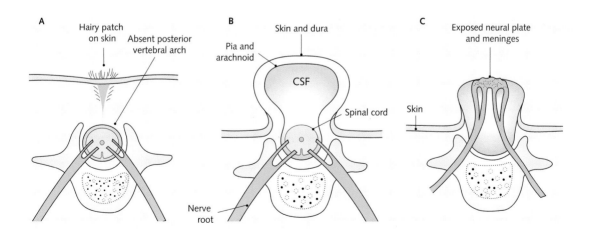

Fig. 9.7 Neural tube defects. Spina bifida occulta (A); meningocele (B); myelomeningocele (C).

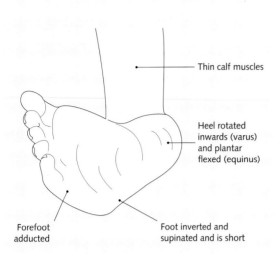

Fig. 9.8 Talipes equinovarus (club foot).

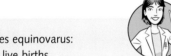

Features of talipes equinovarus:
- 1.5 per 1000 live births.
- Male to female ratio: 2:1.
- 50% bilateral.
- Multifactorial inheritance.
- Associated with oligohydramnios, congenital hip dislocation and neuromuscular disorders, e.g. spina bifida.

AMBIGUOUS GENITALIA

On occasion, it is not possible to give an immediate answer to the question 'Is it a boy or a girl?' The most common cause of ambiguous external genitalia is congenital adrenal hyperplasia (CAH) leading to a virilized female (see Chapter 21).

- Congenital adrenal hyperplasia (CAH) leading to virilization of a female infant is the most common cause of ambiguous genitalia.
- In two-thirds of children with CAH, a life-threatening, salt-losing adrenal crisis occurs at 1–3 weeks of age requiring urgent IV treatment with saline and glucose. This might be the first indication in boys.

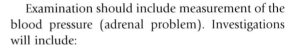

Establishing the definitive cause of ambiguous genitalia takes time and it is important not to attempt to guess the future sex of rearing. Parents also need to be reassured that the baby will be either male or female and not intersex, though it may take some time to determine that. Expert counselling is required.

Examination should include measurement of the blood pressure (adrenal problem). Investigations will include:

- Urgent chromosomal analysis-karyotype.
- Ultrasound imaging of pelvic organs and adrenal glands.
- Electrolyte and endocrine investigations (17-hydroxyprogesterone is increased in CAH).

The chromosomal sex does not necessarily determine the sex of rearing. In many intersex conditions, it is preferable to raise the child as a female because it is easier to fashion female external genitalia than to create a functioning penis.

Further reading

Levene M, Evans D. Neonatal seizures. *Archives of Disease in Childhood. Fetal Neonatal Edition* 1998; **78**:F70–F75.

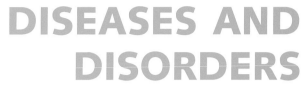

DISEASES AND DISORDERS

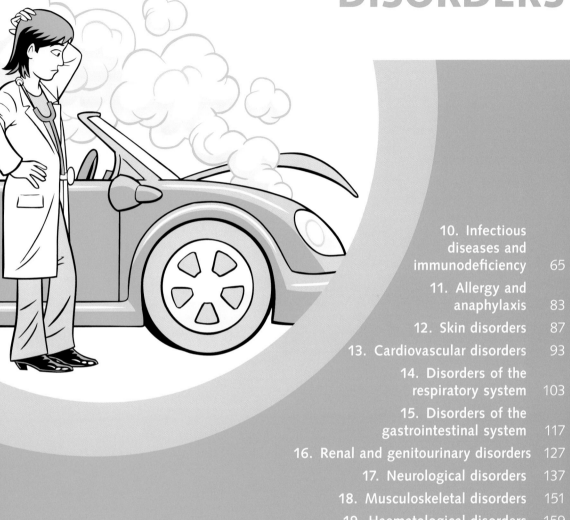

Infectious diseases and immunodeficiency

Objectives

At the end of this chapter, you should be able to

- Differentiate among the common viral exanthems.
- Understand the common infectious diseases affecting children.
- Identify the symptoms and signs of Kawasaki disease.
- Know the common causes of immunodeficiency in children.

Despite the spectacular successes achieved by public health measures and immunization programmes in preventing infectious diseases, these remain a major cause of mortality and morbidity in childhood:

- In the developing world, 12 million children under 5 years of age die each year from the combined effects of malnutrition and infections such as gastroenteritis, pneumonia, measles and malaria.
- In the developed world, major diseases such as diphtheria and polio have been effectively eliminated, and the infection rates of others such as invasive disease caused by *Haemophilus influenzae* type B, measles, mumps, rubella and pertussis are greatly reduced.

In the UK there has been a resurgence of many of these diseases due to a reduction in immunization coverage following adverse media reports on their safety. The worldwide resurgence of tuberculosis (TB), together with the growing impact of human immunodeficiency virus (HIV) infection in childhood, leaves no room for complacency.

VIRAL INFECTIONS

Viral exanthems

The term 'exanthem' is applied to diseases in which a rash is a prominent manifestation. Classically, six exanthems with similar rashes were described. They are numbered in the order in which they were described and are listed in Fig. 10.1. The second disease is, of course, bacterial in origin and the fourth disease is no longer recognized as an entity.

Measles 'first disease'

Incidence and aetiology

Measles is caused by infection with a single-stranded RNA virus of the *Morbillivirus* genus. The incidence in England and Wales declined dramatically after vaccination was introduced (1968), from a pattern of epidemics every 2 years, with up to 800 000 cases a year in the 1960s, to 50 000–100 000 cases a year in the 1980s. Following the introduction of the MMR (measles, mumps, rubella) vaccination in 1988, notifications fell further to just 10 000 cases in 1993. However, outbreaks are now being seen because the immunization rate fell after public concerns about the safety of MMR vaccination.

Clinical features

Fever, cough, coryza and conjunctivitis are followed (in some cases) by the pathognomonic Koplik's spots on the buccal mucosa and, after 3 or 4 days, by an erythematous maculopapular rash. The rash spreads downward from the hairline to the whole body, becomes blotchy and confluent and might desquamate in the second week.

Measles is highly infectious. Transmission is by droplet spread and the incubation period is about 10 days. Children should stay off school for 1 week after appearance of the rash.

Measles is very dangerous in immunocompromised children, such as those in remission from acute leukaemia or with HIV. These children are susceptible to giant cell pneumonia and encephalitis. In developing countries, malnutrition and particularly vitamin A deficiency impairs immunity and renders measles a more severe disease. It is estimated that up to 2 million children in developing countries die annually from measles.

Viral exanthems

		Pathogen
First	Measles	Paramyxovirus
Second	Scarlet fever	Group A β-haemolytic streptococcus
Third	Rubella	Togavirus
Fourth	'Duke's disease'	—
Fifth	Erythema infectiosum	Parvovirus B19
Sixth	Roseola infantum	Human herpesvirus 6

Fig. 10.1 Viral exanthems.

Complications

Acute complications include febrile convulsions, otitis media, tracheobronchitis and pneumonia due either to the primary virus infection or bacterial superinfection (Fig. 10.2). Rarely, severe encephalitis occurs (1 : 5000 cases) about 8 days after onset of the illness. The mortality is 15% and severe neurological sequelae occur in 40% of survivors. (Subacute sclerosing panencephalitis, SSPE, is a very rare immune-mediated neurodegenerative disease that can occur 7–10 years after measles.)

Diagnosis

Diagnosis can be confirmed by detection of specific IgM in serum samples ideally taken from 3 days after the appearance of the rash. The disease is notifiable.

Management

Treatment is symptomatic.

There is a lot of parental anxiety regarding MMR vaccination and its association with autism. However there is no good evidence to suggest such a relation. The apparent relation between MMR vaccination and the onset of autism reflects the natural history of autism since that is the age group when its clinical features are first noticed. Parents must be reassured about the safety of MMR and its benefits outweigh any potential adverse effects.

Complications of measles

Giant cell pneumonia
Conjunctivitis and keratitis
Middle ear infection
Secondary gastrointestinal infections
Encephalitis
Subacute sclerosing panencephalitis

Fig. 10.2 Complications of measles.

Rubella (German measles)

This mild childhood disease is caused by infection with the rubivirus. Its importance lies in the devastating effect maternal infection in early gestation has on the fetus.

Clinical features

Infection is subclinical in up to half of infected individuals. After an incubation period of 14–21 days, a low-grade fever is followed by a pink-red maculopapular rash, which starts on the face and spreads rapidly over the entire body. The rash is fleeting and might have gone entirely by the third day. Generalized lymphadenopathy, particularly affecting the suboccipital and postauricular nodes, is a prominent feature.

Complications

Complications are unusual in childhood but include arthritis (typically affecting the small joints of the hand), encephalitis and thrombocytopenia.

Diagnosis

Diagnosis is clinical and differentiation from other viral exanthems is often difficult. In circumstances in which it is important, detection of rubella-specific IgM in the saliva or serum is necessary to confirm the diagnosis.

Prevention (immunization)

A live, attenuated vaccine has been available for many years. Since 1988, this has been given as part of the MMR vaccine to all children at 13 months of age and a booster between 3 and 5 years of age. Vaccine failure is rare and, in most people, it provides lifelong protection. The presence of IgG, specific for rubella, indicates immunity as a result of prior infection or immunization.

Congenital rubella

Incidence and diagnosis

The risk and extent of fetal damage is mainly determined by its gestational age at the onset of maternal infection. In the first 8–10 weeks the risk is high; beyond 18 weeks' gestation the risk is minimal.

Maternal infection at up to 10 weeks' gestation confers a 90% risk of some degree of damage that is often severe and includes deafness, congenital heart disease and cataracts. Between 13 and 16 weeks' gestation, there is a 30% risk of hearing impairment. Although congenital rubella is now rare in the UK (14 cases notified in the period 1991–1994), the diagnosis is worth consideration in any growth-retarded newborn or child with unexplained sensorineural deafness.

Clinical features

Clinical features of congenital rubella are shown in Fig. 10.3.

Management

All pregnant women and women contemplating pregnancy should be screened for antirubella IgG. Immigrants to the UK from countries where rubella vaccination is not routine are at particular risk of not being immune. Women found to be seronegative on antenatal screening receive immunization after delivery.

Pregnant women exposed to rubella should be tested for antirubella IgG and IgM regardless of previous history or serological testing. A high likelihood of congenital rubella infection early in pregnancy is an indication for offering termination of the pregnancy.

Clinical features of congenital rubella

Growth retardation
Hepatosplenomegaly
Congenital heart disease
- Patent ductus arteriosus
- Pulmonary stenosis
Eye
- Glaucoma
- Cataract
- Retinopathy
Ear
- Sensorineural deafness

Fig. 10.3 Clinical features of congenital rubella.

Erythema infectiosum or slapped cheek disease 'fifth disease'

This is caused by infection with parvovirus B19, a small DNA virus that is the only parvovirus pathogenic to humans. Transmission can occur via respiratory secretions, from mother to fetus, and by transmission of contaminated blood products.

Clinical features

Asymptomatic infection is common. Erythema infectiosum describes the most common disease pattern of fever followed a week later by a characteristic rash. This starts as a red appearance on the face (hence the name 'slapped-cheek disease') and progresses to a symmetrical lacy rash on the extremities and trunk.

The virus suppresses erythropoiesis for up to 7 days. In children with haemolytic anaemia, such as sickle-cell disease or hereditary spherocytosis, parvovirus infection can cause an aplastic crisis. Maternal infection during pregnancy can be transmitted to the fetus and causes hydrops fetalis (due to fetal anaemia and myocarditis), fetal death or spontaneous abortion.

Diagnosis and management

Diagnosis is clinical, but if confirmation is important (e.g. in pregnancy), specific IgM can be detected 2 weeks after exposure. Management is symptomatic.

'Sixth disease': roseola infantum

Roseola infantum is caused by infection with human herpesvirus (HHV)-6 or HHV-7.

Clinical features and diagnosis

Most children acquire the infection between the age of 3 months and 4 years; 65% are seropositive by 1 year of age. There is sudden onset of a high fever (>39°C) with irritability lasting for 3–6 days. The fever then falls abruptly and a widespread maculopapular rash appears on the face, neck and trunk. Other common features include cervical lymphadenopathy, cough and coryza. Up to one-third of febrile convulsions in children <2 years of age are caused by HHV-6.

Diagnosis is clinical and treatment supportive

Rare complications include aseptic meningitis, encephalitis, hepatitis and massive lymphadenopathy.

Fig. 10.4 Human herpesviruses (HHV) and their diseases.

	Human herpesviruses (HHV) and their diseases	
	Virus	Disease
HHV-1	Herpes simplex virus 1	Oral infection and encephalitis
HHV-2	Herpes simplex virus 2	Neonatal and genital infection
HHV-3	Varicella zoster	Chickenpox and shingles
HHV-4	Epstein-Barr virus	Glandular fever
HHV-5	Cytomegalovirus	Congenital infection and in immunosuppression
HHV-6/7		Roseola

Herpes infections

There are eight human herpesviruses. They cause a number of common and important diseases in children. The hallmark of these viruses is their capacity to become latent with subsequent recurrence, causing, for example, shingles (varicella zoster) and cold sores (HSV1).

The human herpesviruses and their corresponding diseases are shown in Fig. 10.4.

Herpes simplex virus 1 (HSV1, HHV-1)

Clinical features

Most primary infections with HSV1 are asymptomatic. The most common clinical manifestation in childhood is gingivostomatitis. The child (usually a toddler) presents with high fever, misery and vesicular lesions on the lips, gums, tongue and hard palate, which might progress to painful, extensive ulceration. The illness can last as long as 2 weeks.

Less commonly, infection can involve the:

- Eye: causing dendritic ulcers on the cornea.
- Skin: causing eczema herpeticum in children with eczema.
- Fingers: causing a herpetic whitlow.
- Brain: causing herpes simplex encephalitis (HSE).

Treatment

Occasionally, IV fluid will be required for gingivostomatitis but in this condition oral aciclovir has only a marginal effect. High-dose IV aciclovir is used in HSE.

The virus becomes latent in the dorsal root ganglion supplying the trigeminal nerve where subsequent reactivation (by UV light, stress or menstruation) can cause labial herpes (cold sores) in later life.

Herpes simplex virus 2 (HSV2, HHV-2)

Transmission of HSV2 from the genital tract of a mother who is often asymptomatic can result in neonatal herpes infection. Neonatal herpes has high mortality and morbidity. It causes a generalized infection with pneumonia, hepatitis and encephalitis, with onset usually in the first week of life. Treatment is high dose IV aciclovir and supportive care.

Elective Caesarean section is indicated when a mother with active genital herpes goes into labour.

Varicella zoster (HHV-3, VZV)

Chickenpox is a common childhood disease caused by primary infection with the varicella zoster virus (VZV). It is highly infectious with transmission occurring by droplet infection (the respiratory route), direct contact or contact with soiled materials. The average incubation period is 14 days.

Clinical features

A brief coryzal period is followed by the eruption of an itchy, vesicular rash. This starts on the scalp or trunk and spreads centrifugally. Crops appear over 3–5 days and the mucous membranes might be involved.

Complications

Complications are unusual in immunocompetent children but can include secondary bacterial infection of the skin with staphylococci or streptococci and an encephalitis (often affecting the cerebellum), which appears 3–6 days after onset of the rash. Chickenpox can, however, be a very severe disease (mortality 20%) in the immunosuppressed child (children on systemic steroids) and in the newborn infant if the mother develops chickenpox just before delivery.

Diagnosis

Diagnosis is clinical but virus isolated from vesicular fluid can be identified by electron microscopy or culture. The period of infectivity is from 2 days before eruption of the rash until all the lesions are encrusted.

Treatment

Treatment is symptomatic. However, the exposed immunosuppressed child should be given varicella zoster immune globulin (VZIG) if known to be sero-negative. VZIG should also be given to newborn babies if the mother develops varicella or herpes zoster in the 7 days before or after birth and to any exposed preterm infant. Acyclovir should be given in severe chickenpox or for clinical infection in an immunocompromised child or newborn infant. Antibiotics are also given concurrently to cover secondary skin infection.

A live, attenuated vaccine does exist but is not currently licensed in the UK, and no country has adopted widespread varicella vaccination.

Herpes zoster (shingles)

This is due to reactivation of latent varicella zoster and is uncommon in childhood. A vesicular eruption occurs in the distribution of a sensory dermatome, mainly in the cervical and sacral regions. In adults they tend to be thoracic and lumbar. Also, unlike adults, postherpetic neuralgia and malignant association are rare. Treatment with antivirals is not routinely indicated.

Epstein–Barr virus (HHV-4, EBV)

The EBV has a particular tropism for the epithelial cells of the oropharynx and nasopharynx, and for B lymphocytes. It is the major cause of infectious mononucleosis syndrome and is also involved in the pathogenesis of Burkitt's lymphoma and nasopharyngeal carcinoma.

Clinical features

Transmission occurs by droplet transmission or directly via saliva ('the kissing disease'). Most people are infected asymptomatically in childhood. Symptomatic infection (infectious mononucleosis or glandular fever) is most common in adolescents. The incubation period is 30–50 days.

Glandular fever is characterized by fever, malaise, pharyngitis (which may be exudative) and cervical lymphadenopathy. Petechiae might be seen on the palate and a sparse maculopapular rash might occur. Splenomegaly is present in 50% of cases and hepatomegaly with hepatitis (usually anicteric) in 10%. A florid rash might develop if amoxicillin is given. The infection can persist for up to 3 months.

Diagnosis

Diagnosis is usually clinical. The blood shows atypical lymphocytes (T cells) and a heterophile antibody, which is the basis of slide agglutination tests like monospot and Paul–Bunnell tests. The latter appears only in the second week and might not be produced in young children. Specific EBV serology—IgM to viral capsid antigen (VCA)—is available and more reliable. The differential diagnosis is from other causes of infectious mononucleosis (cytomegalovirus, toxoplasmosis) and other causes of pharyngitis.

Management

Management is symptomatic. Rarely, massive pharyngeal swelling can compromise the airway. This is helped by corticosteroid treatment.

Cytomegalovirus (HHV-5, CMV)

Cytomegalovirus (CMV) is a common human pathogen. It is transmitted from mother to fetus via the placenta in utero, via the oral or genital routes, and by blood transfusion or organ transplantation.

- CMV is a common congenital infection but rarely causes severe disease.
- CMV is an important cause of sensorineural hearing loss.
- CMV-negative blood must be used for transfusion in immunodeficient patients.

Incidence

In the UK, about half of all pregnant women are susceptible to CMV and about 1% of these will have a primary CMV infection during pregnancy. In almost half of these mothers, the infant will be infected, making CMV the most common congenital infection with an incidence of 3 : 1000 live births. However, most infants with congenital CMV are asymptomatic and develop normally.

Clinical features

Infection is mild or asymptomatic in adults or children with normal immunity. It can cause a mononucleosis syndrome with pharyngitis and lymphadenopathy. Severe congenital infection causes:

- Intrauterine growth retardation.
- Hepatosplenomegaly, jaundice and purpura.
- Microcephaly, intracranial calcification and chorioretinitis.
- Long-term sequelae include cerebral palsy, epilepsy, learning disability and sensorineural hearing loss. Hearing loss might develop later in life without signs of infection in the newborn period.

In the immunocompromised host, CMV can cause severe disease including pneumonitis or encephalitis. It is a particularly important pathogen following organ transplantation.

Diagnosis and treatment

Diagnosis is made by viral isolation, especially from urine or by a strongly positive titre of IgM anti-CMV antibody. To confirm congenital infection, specimens for viral isolation must be taken within 3 weeks of birth.

Treatment with ganciclovir might be effective in immunocompromised patients.

Mumps

Mumps is caused by infection with an RNA virus of the Paramyxovirus family. Routine vaccination at 12–15 months, as a component of the MMR vaccine, has markedly reduced the incidence. Transmission is by droplet spread and the incubation period is 14–21 days.

Clinical features

The clinical manifestations include fever, malaise and parotitis. Pain and swelling of the parotid gland might initially be unilateral. Parotid gland enlargement is more easily seen than felt, between the angle of the mandible and sternomastoid—extending beneath the ear lobe, which is pushed upwards and outwards.

The swelling usually subsides within 7–10 days. Patients are infectious from a few days before the onset to up to 3 days after the enlargement subsides.

The central nervous system is commonly involved. Before vaccination was introduced, mumps was the commonest cause of aseptic meningitis. Up to 50% of patients have CSF lymphocytosis and 10% have signs of a meningoencephalitis.

Complications

Complications include pancreatitis (abdominal pain and raised serum amylase levels) and epididymo-orchitis. The latter is uncommon in prepubertal males and is usually unilateral. Even when it is bilateral, infertility is very rare. A postinfectious encephalomyelitis occurs in 1 out of 5000 cases.

Diagnosis and treatment

Diagnosis is usually clinical; treatment is symptomatic.

Enteroviruses

The human enteroviruses include:

- Coxsackie virus A and B.
- Echoviruses.
- Poliovirus.

Coxsackie viruses can cause aseptic meningitis, myocarditis, pericarditis, Bornholm disease (pleurodynia) and hand, foot and mouth disease.

Polio

Poliovirus is an enterovirus with antigenic types 1, 2 and 3. Immunization has rendered poliovirus infection uncommon in developed countries but it remains endemic in parts of the developing world such as Africa and the Indian subcontinent. Transmission is by the faecal–oral route with an incubation period of 7–21 days.

Clinical features

The clinical features vary:

- Over 90% of cases are asymptomatic.
- 5% have a 'minor illness'—fever, headache, malaise.
- 2% progress to CNS involvement—aseptic meningitis.
- In under 2%, 'paralytic polio' occurs due to the virus attacking the anterior horn cells of the spinal cord.

Diagnosis

Although imported infections and vaccine-associated infections are seen in the UK, they are rare. The differential diagnosis includes other causes of aseptic meningitis and acute paralytic disease such as Guillain–Barré syndrome. Polio is a notifiable disease.

Viral hepatitis

This can be caused by:

- Hepatitis virus A, B, C, D, E or G.
- Arbovirus-yellow fever.
- Cytomegalovirus, Epstein–Barr virus.

Hepatitis A virus (HAV)

This is an RNA virus spread by faecal–oral transmission. The incubation period is 2–6 weeks.

Clinical features

In infants and young children, many infections are asymptomatic or present as a non-specific febrile illness without jaundice. Older symptomatic children develop fever, malaise, anorexia, abdominal pain (from a tender enlarged liver) and jaundice. Dark urine (due to urobilinogen) may precede the jaundice.

Diagnosis

Diagnosis is often made on the combination of clinical features and history of exposure, but might be confirmed by measurement of IgM anti-HAV antibody. Serum transaminases and bilirubin levels are elevated.

Treatment

There is no specific treatment. The majority of children have a mild, self-limiting illness and recover within 2–4 weeks. The most serious but rare complication is fulminant hepatic failure.

Active immunization is available and is mostly used for frequent travellers. Close contacts should be given prophylaxis with intramuscular human normal immunoglobulin (HNIG).

Hepatitis B virus (HBV)

This is a DNA virus of the Hepadnavirus genus. It is a double-shelled particle with an inner core (HBc) and an outer lipoprotein coat comprising the hepatitis B surface antigen (HBsAg).

Transmission is parenteral via blood and other body fluids. In infants, the most important source of infection is vertical perinatal transmission from infected mothers. Most transmission occurs during or just after birth from exposure to maternal blood. The average incubation period is 20 days.

Incidence

HBV is an important cause of liver disease worldwide. The prevalence of infection in the population varies globally. In parts of Africa and Asia, up to 80% of children are infected by adolescence. In the UK, prevalence is under 2% in the indigenous population.

Clinical features

In most children, infection is asymptomatic, although features of acute hepatitis might occur; fulminant hepatic failure occurs in 1% of cases. The most important consequence of infection is the risk of becoming a carrier with subsequent development of cirrhosis or hepatocellular carcinoma. The risk of developing carrier status rises with infection at a young age (reaching 90% in those infected perinatally). Between 30 and 50% of carrier children will develop chronic HBV liver disease.

Diagnosis

Diagnosis is dependent on serological testing for antibodies and antigens related to HBV. Acute HBV infection is associated with the presence of HBsAg and IgM antibodies to HBc antigen. Carrier status is defined as HBsAg persisting for more than 6 months. The presence of HBeAg correlates with high infectivity, whereas the presence of antibodies to HBeAg indicates low infectivity (Fig. 10.5).

Management

There is no specific treatment for acute hepatitis B infection at any age. Interferon α treatment is

Serological markers of HBV infection				
	HBsAg	Anti-HBs	Anti-HBc IgM	Anti-HBc IgG
Acute HBV infection	+	−	+	+
HBV carrier	+	−	+ or −	+
Immune: Previous infection	−	+ or −	−	+
Immune: Immunization	−	+	−	−

Fig. 10.5 Serological markers of hepatitis B (HBV) infection.

under trial in chronic hepatitis caused by HBV infection.

Prevention

Effective immunization is available and is recommended:

- After perinatal exposure.
- For individuals at risk, e.g. doctors, dentists or intravenous drug abusers.
- Postexposure, e.g. needlestick injury.

Perinatal exposure

All pregnant women should have antenatal screening for the HBsAg. All babies born to women known to be HBsAg positive should commence a course of hepatitis B vaccine within 24 hours of birth. Unless the mother is known to be anti-HBe positive, the baby should also receive hepatitis B specific immunoglobulin (HBIG).

BACTERIAL INFECTIONS

Staphylococcal infections

The coagulase-positive bacterium *Staphylococcus aureus* is the main pathogen but coagulase-negative bacteria, e.g. *Staphylococcus epidermidis,* are a major problem in Intensive Care Units. Methicillin-resistant *Staphylococcus aureus* (MRSA) causes problems of nosocomial (i.e. hospital acquired) infection.

Staphylococcus epidermidis is part of the normal skin flora and *Staphylococcus aureus* is found in the nares and skin in up to 50% of children. Infections occur when defences are compromised. Many infections are therefore caused by the body's own bacteria, but transmission between individuals occurs with close contact.

Staphylococcus aureus most commonly causes superficial infection such as boils and impetigo, and occasionally deeper infections, e.g. of the bones, joints, or lungs (Fig. 10.6). Toxin-producing *Staphylococcus aureus* causes scalded skin syndrome and toxic shock syndrome.

Impetigo

This highly contagious skin infection commonly occurs on the face in infants and young children—especially if there is pre-existing skin disease, e.g. eczema.

Infections caused by *Staphylococcus aureus*	
Direct infection	Toxin-mediated
Impetigo	Toxic shock syndrome
Folliculitis/boils	Scalded skin syndrome
Wound infections	Food poisoning
Abscess	
Pneumonia	
Osteomyelitis	
Septic arthritis	

Fig. 10.6 Infections caused by *Staphylococcus aureus.*

Clinical features

Erythematous macules develop into characteristic honey-coloured crusted lesions. Some cases are due to streptococcal infection.

Treatment

Topical antibiotics can be used for mild cases (e.g. mupirocin) but more severe infections require systemic antibiotics (e.g. flucloxacillin). Nasal carriage is an important source of reinfection and can be eradicated by nasal cream containing chlorhexidine and neomycin.

Boils and abscesses

A boil (or furuncle) is an infection of a hair follicle or sweat gland and is usually caused by *Staphylococcus aureus.*

Clinical features

A painful, red, raised, hot lesion develops and usually discharges a purulent exudate heralding spontaneous resolution.

Treatment

Treatment is with systemic antibiotics. Deeper infection can lead to abscess formation in which case incision and drainage are usually required.

Osteomyelitis/septic arthritis

See Chapter 18.

Staphylococcal scalded skin syndrome (SSSS)

This is a potentially life-threatening, toxin-mediated manifestation of localized skin infection.

Clinical features

SSSS results from the effect of epidermolytic toxins produced by certain phage types. They cause blistering by disrupting the epidermal granular cell layer. The lesions look like scalds.

Treatment

Management requires attention to fluid balance and treatment with intravenous flucloxacillin.

Streptococcal infections

Streptococci are Gram-positive cocci. Important pathogenic types include:

- Group A β-haemolytic streptococci (*Streptococcus pyogenes*).
- Group B streptococci.
- *Streptococcus pneumoniae* (pneumococcus).

These bacteria are responsible for a number of common and important paediatric diseases that can be caused by:

- Direct infection.
- Toxins.
- Postinfectious immune-mediated mechanisms (acute glomerulonephritis, rheumatic fever).

Infections caused by streptococci are shown in Fig. 10.7. Most of these are described elsewhere: tonsillitis (see Chapter 14), pneumonia (Chapter 14), meningitis (Chapter 17), glomerulonephritis (Chapter 16) and rheumatic fever (Chapter 13).

Scarlet fever

This occurs in children who have streptococcal pharyngitis. The organism produces a toxin, which causes a characteristic rash.

Infections caused by *Streptococci*	
Organism	Disease caused
Group A Streptococcus	Pharyngitis/tonsillitis Cellulitis Osteomyelitis Septicaemia Toxin-mediated: • Scarlet fever • Erysipelas • 'Toxic shock-like syndrome'
Streptococcus pneumoniae	Otitis media Pneumonia Meningitis Septicaemia
Group B Streptococcus	Neonatal infection, e.g. pneumonia, meningitis, or septicaemia

Fig. 10.7 Infections caused by streptococci.

Clinical features

The clinical features include:

- Tonsillitis.
- Strawberry tongue.
- Palatal petechiae.
- Rash: a widespread, erythematous rash starting on the trunk that becomes punctate and desquamates on resolution after 7–10 days (flushing of the face is often associated with circumoral pallor).
- Fever.

Diagnosis

Diagnosis is clinical, but can be confirmed by isolation of the streptococcus from a throat swab, and by elevated antistreptolysin 0 titres.

Treatment

Treatment is with penicillin (or erythromycin if the patient has penicillin allergy).

Erysipelas

This intradermal infection is caused by toxin-producing *Streptococcus pyogenes*.

Clinical features

The face or leg is the usual area affected. The skin is dusky and vesicles or bullae might develop.

Diagnosis and treatment

Skin swabs and blood cultures might be negative; treatment is with parenteral antibiotics.

Preseptal cellulitis

This presents as unilateral periorbital oedema in a young child, usually after an upper respiratory tract infecton; fever might be present. The common pathogens are *Streptococcus* species and *Haemophilus influenzae* (more common in children under 3 years old).

It is important to distinguish this from the less common, but more serious, orbital cellulitis, in which there is proptosis, limitation of ocular movement and impaired vision.

Treatment is with IV broad-spectrum antibiotics.

Tuberculosis

Incidence and aetiology

Tuberculosis (TB) remains a major global health problem, causing 3–5 million deaths annually. The increasing incidence in patients with HIV, combined with the emergence of multidrug-resistant strains of the causative organism, has generated new concern over this age-old public health problem.

Tuberculosis is more common among the underprivileged, especially in urban areas and the immunocompromised. Its incidence has been rising in the UK. It occurs in all racial groups but high rates are seen in children whose families have come from endemic areas such as:

- The Indian subcontinent (India, Pakistan and Bangladesh).
- Sub-Saharan Africa.

Tuberculosis is caused by infection with the acid-fast, slow-growing bacillus *Mycobacterium tuberculosis*. Children are usually infected by inhalation of infected droplet nuclei from an adult who is a regular or household contact. Children with the disease (even with active pulmonary disease) are almost always non-infectious. Therefore once a child is identified as having TB, notification to public health is essential to identify the index case and contact trace.

Clinical features

The clinical features of TB (Fig. 10.8) reflect the wide variation in outcomes that follow inhalation of the

Fig. 10.8 Course of infection in tuberculosis.

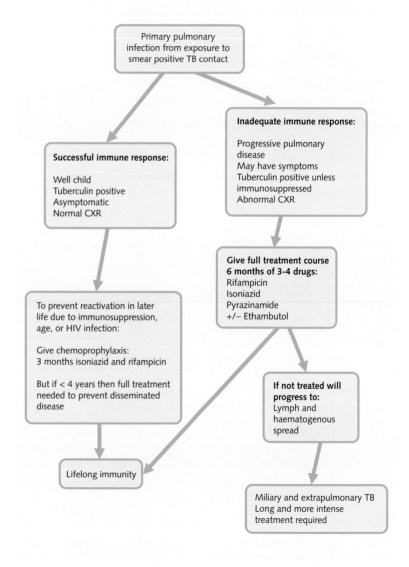

Primary pulmonary infection from exposure to smear positive TB contact

Successful immune response:

Well child
Tuberculin positive
Asymptomatic
Normal CXR

Inadequate immune response:

Progressive pulmonary disease
May have symptoms
Tuberculin positive unless immunosuppressed
Abnormal CXR

Give full treatment course 6 months of 3-4 drugs:
Rifampicin
Isoniazid
Pyrazinamide
+/– Ethambutol

To prevent reactivation in later life due to immunosuppression, age, or HIV infection:

Give chemoprophylaxis:
3 months isoniazid and rifampicin

But if < 4 years then full treatment needed to prevent disseminated disease

If not treated will progress to:
Lymph and haematogenous spread

Lifelong immunity

Miliary and extrapulmonary TB
Long and more intense treatment required

tubercle bacillus or primary infection. Children under 4 years are at particularly high risk of disseminated disease, e.g. TB meningitis.

TB contacts <4 years of age are at high risk of disseminated disease and should be evaluated promptly.

Tuberculous infection: asymptomatic infection

This is most common. A local inflammatory reaction limits disease progression and the disease becomes latent. Reactivation can occur subsequently.

Tuberculous disease: symptomatic infection

Multiplication within macrophages occurs at the peripheral alveolar site (the primary or Ghon focus) and the bacilli spread to the regional lymph nodes causing hilar lymphadenopathy. The peripheral lung lesion and nodes comprise the 'primary or Ghon complex'. Systemic symptoms can then develop, including fever, anorexia, weight loss and cough.

The pulmonary pathology can evolve in several different ways. Bronchial obstruction by enlarged lymph nodes might cause segmental collapse and consolidation. Rarer outcomes include development of a pleural effusion or progressive primary pulmonary TB with cavity formation (in adolescents and adults). Spread into the lymphoid system can result in cervical, supraclavicular or axillary lymphadenopathy.

Haematogenous dissemination

In addition to the above intrathoracic events, haematogenous spread probably occurs in most children, although dormant lesions rather than disease occur in these distant sites. Tubercle bacilli might spread to the bones (especially the vertebral column), joints, kidneys and meninges. Miliary TB is the most severe result of haematogenous spread. It occurs particularly in small infants or immunosuppressed individuals—lesions are found throughout the lungs, liver, spleen and bone marrow.

Diagnosis

This can be difficult and requires a high index of clinical suspicion. A history of close contact to an adult with smear-positive tuberculosis, symptoms (weight loss, night sweats, cough), clinical signs, tuberculin testing, chest X-ray and examination of appropriate specimens by microscopy and culture (gastric washings) can suggest the diagnosis.

Criteria for TB diagnosis include:
- Adult TB contact.
- Signs and symptoms.
- CXR changes.
- Positive Mantoux test.
- Positive cultures (gastric washings or other).

Tuberculin testing

This is done using the Mantoux test in which an intradermal injection of purified protein derivative (PPD) of tuberculin, e.g. 10 units (0.1 mL of 1 : 1000) is made on the volar aspect of the forearm. The site is read after 48–72 hours by measuring the transverse diameter of induration in millimetres. A 5-mm diameter reaction is considered positive, especially if risk factors are present. When previous BCG immunization has been carried out, a reaction of greater than 10 mm is indicative of infection.

Culture and histology

Isolation of *Mycobacterium tuberculosis* by culture is the 'gold standard' but positive cultures are obtained in a minority of children. Early-morning gastric washings on 3 successive days are the best specimens. It takes 6–8 weeks for the bacillus to grow. Microscopy is often negative but histological examination of a lymph node biopsy may reveal caseating granulomata and acid-fast bacilli.

PCR and T-SPOT.TB has been increasingly used in the diagnosis of tuberculosis.

Radiology

TB is suggested by hilar or mediastinal lymphadenopathy, especially if it is unilateral, or in combination with a 'wedge' of collapse or consolidation. Calcification also suggests TB.

Treatment and prevention

A 6-month regimen consisting of four drugs—isoniazid, rifampicin, pyrazinamide and ethambutol for 2 months (or longer, until sensitivities are available) followed by isoniazid and rifampicin for 4 months is used in most instances, except in tuberculous meningitis. In previously untreated white patients who are HIV negative and who have not been in contact with drug-resistant tuberculosis, ethambutol may be omitted in the initial phase. Children with tuberculous infection (asymptomatic with positive Mantoux) but no disease need chemoprophylaxis to prevent future reactivation. In this situation, either a combination of isoniazid and rifampicin for 3 months or isoniazid as a single agent for 6 months is used. The most important preventive measures are prompt treatment of infectious cases and thorough contact tracing.

The BCG (bacilli Calmette–Guerin) vaccine has been used in the UK since the 1950s to protect against TB, especially TB meningitis. Routine BCG immunization of all schoolchildren has been replaced by a more targeted approach since 2005. Currently in the UK, BCG is given to:

- Immigrants from countries with high incidence of TB.
- Mantoux-negative contacts of open TB cases.
- People who intend to live for 1 or more month(s) in a TB endemic country.
- Babies living in areas of UK where the incidence of TB is more than 40 per 100 000 per year.
- Children whose parents or grandparents have lived in a country with a high prevalence of TB.

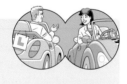

It is important to stress the importance of treatment—these children often become symptom free after the first few weeks and compliance can be poor thereafter, which can lead to clinical infection later on. Parents should be made aware of the risks of inadequate treatment, including emergence of drug resistance.

Typhoid and paratyphoid fever

Typhoid fever is caused by *Salmonella typhi* and paratyphoid by *Salmonella paratyphi*. Both occur worldwide, but mostly in the developing world and the main reservoir is humans; they are invasive,

systemic infections. Salmonellosis occurs after infection with *Salmonella enteritidis* or *Salmonella typhimurium*, which usually cause gastroenteritis (food poisoning) and is more common in the UK than typhoid fever—animals constitute the main reservoir for these strains and nearly half the human infections are transmitted by poultry products. Salmonellae are Gram-negative bacilli.

Transmission of typhoid fever, on the other hand, is by ingestion of food or water contaminated by faeces or urine from an infected person. The incubation period is 1–3 weeks.

Clinical features

The clinical presentation is similar in each case but paratyphoid fever is milder. Typhoid (enteric) fever is characterized by slow onset of fever, malaise, headache and tachypnoea. Signs include splenomegaly, and a characteristic rash of 'rose spots' on the trunk. Unlike adults, children do not usually develop a relative bradycardia. Paratyphoid is a milder illness but diarrhoea is more common.

Diagnosis

Diagnosis is made by culture of organisms from the blood (early in the disease) or from stool and urine (after the first week).

Management

Ceftriaxone for 14 days is effective, as is ciprofloxacin. Family and close contacts should be screened with stool cultures. Three consecutive negative stools signify clearance of infection. Long-term symptomless carriage can occur with a reservoir of infection in the gall bladder and excretion in the faeces.

PARASITIC INFECTIONS

Malaria

Incidence and aetiology

Malaria is a major global health problem with an annual mortality rate between 1.5 and 2.7 million. Although the majority of these are in the sub-Saharan Africa, imported malaria is increasingly reported from the UK.

Malaria is caused by infection with any of the four species of the protozoan parasite *Plasmodium*.

Most of the 300 cases of childhood malaria imported to the UK each year are due to *Plasmodium falciparum*, which accounts for 85% of malaria seen in travellers to Africa. Half of these did not take chemoprophylaxis.

> Fever in a child who has been to a malarious area is malaria until proven otherwise:
> - Most cases are falciparum.
> - *Plasmodium falciparum* requires treatment with quinine.

Transmission is vector-borne via the female anopheles mosquito. The onset is usually 7–10 days after inoculation but might be delayed by months or even years. The feeding female mosquito injects sporozoites, which pass to the liver via the bloodstream. After asexual multiplication in hepatocytes, these emerge as merozoites, which invade, multiply in and destroy the host's red blood cells. Some of the merozoites form gametocytes, which are sucked up by a feeding mosquito; the sexual phase of the life cycle then takes place in the mosquito with the formation of a new generation of sporozoites.

Clinical features

Malaria presents with fever and any child with a fever who has visited a malarious area in the preceding year should be considered to have malaria until proven otherwise. Non-specific symptoms include headache, rigors, abdominal and muscle pains, cough, diarrhoea and vomiting. Common misdiagnoses include viral influenza, gastroenteritis or hepatitis.

Apart from the fever, which is rarely periodic, there are no consistent clinical signs. Splenomegaly, anaemia and jaundice can all occur and a number of signs characterize the severe complication of algid malaria (shock), cerebral malaria (coma, fits) or blackwater fever (haemoglobinuria and renal failure).

Diagnosis

Diagnosis is made by the examination of thick and thin blood films. The former allows rapid scanning of a larger volume of blood per microscopic field. At least three films should be taken as one negative film does not exclude malaria. Both the species and the percentage of parasitaemia should be determined; parasitaemia >2% indicates moderately severe infection.

Management

Children with confirmed or suspected falciparum malaria require hospitalization and treatment with quinine or mefloquine (for those aged over 2 years). This is given orally in uncomplicated disease or intravenously if the parasite count is high or complications are present. In vivax infection, 2–3 weeks of primaquine is needed to clear dormant hypnozoite hepatic infection; falciparum does not have a dormant life cycle.

Travellers to endemic areas should take chloroquine from 1 week before to 4 weeks after travel. It is important to warn them that this does not guarantee protection.

Worms (nematodes)

Four important nematodes infect children:

- *Enterobius vermicularis* (pinworm or threadworm).
- *Ascaris lumbricoides* (roundworm).
- *Ancylostoma duodenale* (hookworm).
- *Toxocara canis*.

Threadworm

This is very common in preschool children. Transmission is via the faecal–oral route. Adult female worms lay their eggs in the perianal area at night. Scratching results in eggs being carried under the fingernails to the mouth and autoinfection.

Clinical features

Children present with perianal pruritus and vulvovaginitis but tissue invasion does not occur and systemic complications are uncommon. The worms appear like white cotton threads and might be visible at the anus.

Diagnosis

Diagnosis can be made by applying transparent adhesive tape to the perianal region in the morning and examining the tape for eggs with a magnifying glass 'the Sellotape test'.

Management

Treatment is with two doses of piperazine 2 weeks apart or a single dose of mebendazole (for children over 2 years). Reinfection is common and can be reduced by keeping fingernails short and wearing close-fitting pants. Family members should be treated even if asymptomatic.

Toxocariasis

Human toxocariasis is mainly caused by infection with *Toxocara canis*, a common gut parasite of dogs. Toxocara eggs are ingested when a child eats soil, play-pit sand or unwashed vegetables contaminated with infective dog or cat faeces.

Clinical features

There are two distinct forms of disease:

- Visceral larva migrans (VLM): characterized by fever, hepatomegaly, wheezing and eosinophilia.
- Occular larva migrans: a granulomatous reaction in the retina causing a squint or reduced visual acuity.

Management

Treatment is with thiabendazole for VLM and steroids for the eye disease. Toxocara infection could be prevented by the regular de-worming of cats and dogs and by not allowing animals to defecate in public places, including sandpits.

KAWASAKI DISEASE

Kawasaki disease (KD), an uncommon systemic vasculitis, is also called mucocutaneous lymph node syndrome. Early diagnosis and treatment might prevent lethal cardiac complications. It has replaced rheumatic fever as the most common cause of acquired heart disease in children.

Early recognition of Kawasaki disease is vital to reduce the risk of cardiac complications:

- The fever is often unresponsive to antipyretics.
- Characteristically, the child is extremely miserable.
- Think of Kawasaki disease in prolonged fever and rash.

Incidence

First described in Japan in 1967, KD affects children mainly between the age of 6 months and 4 years (peak at 1 year). It is much more common in children of Asian origin. In the UK the incidence is 3–4 cases per 100 000.

Clinical features

The aetiology is unknown but the disease process is a vasculitis affecting the small and medium vessels including, most importantly, the coronary arteries leading to aneurysm formation. Subsequent scar formation causes vessel narrowing, myocardial ischaemia or even infarction, and—occasionally—sudden death. A bacterial toxin acting as a 'superantigen' can trigger the vasculitis.

Diagnosis

The diagnosis is based on clinical criteria, which emerge sequentially; five out of six are required to make a diagnosis (Fig. 10.9). Atypical disease is diagnosed if coronary aneurysms are present without all the criteria.

The differential diagnosis includes measles, scarlet fever, rubella, roseola and fifth disease. The following investigations are undertaken if KD is suspected:

- FBC, ESR.
- U&Es, liver function tests.
- Throat swab and ASOT.
- Blood cultures and viral titres.
- Echocardiography.
- ECG.

Thrombocytosis, although common, is a late feature and therefore unhelpful in establishing the diagnosis.

Diagnostic criteria for Kawasaki disease
Fever for 5 days or more
Bilateral (non-purulent) conjunctival injection
Rash—polymorphous
Lips—red, dry, or cracked and strawberry tongue
Extremities:
• Reddening of palms and soles
• Indurative oedema of hands and feet
• Peeling of skin on hands and feet (convalescent phase)
Cervical lymphadenopathy–often unilateral, non-purulent

Fig. 10.9 Diagnostic criteria for Kawasaki disease.

Echocardiography is undertaken to detect coronary artery aneurysm formation. These occur in 30% of untreated cases and typically develop within the first 4–6 weeks of the illness. This investigation is repeated at intervals during the first year.

Treatment

The most effective treatment involves a single dose of IV immunoglobulin (2 g/kg). This reduces both the incidence and severity of coronary artery aneurysm formation if given within the first 10 days.

Aspirin is given concurrently to reduce the risk of thrombosis at a high dose initially (100 mg/kg/day in divided doses) until the pyrexia has resolved. A low dose (3–5 mg/kg/day) is continued for 6–8 weeks. Current evidence on steroid treatment is conflicting and their use is not routinely recommended.

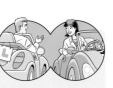

Immunoglobulin is a blood product and parents should be informed of the potential benefits (which is prevention of aneurysm formation) and adverse effects (which can include anaphylaxis).

IMMUNODEFICIENCY

This can be classified into:

- Primary: in which there is an inherited, intrinsic defect in the immune system.

- Secondary: in which a defect in the immune system has been acquired, as occurs in malnutrition, infections (e.g. HIV, measles), immunosuppressive therapy (e.g. steroids, cytotoxic drugs), hyposplenism (e.g. sickle-cell disease, splenectomy).

In acquired immunodeficiency, the cause is usually self-evident. Primary immunodeficiency should be suspected in the following clinical circumstances:

- An excess of infections: this is manifest by severe, unusual or persistent infections, or infections with unusual organisms (Fig. 10.10).
- Unexplained failure to thrive.
- Chronic diarrhoea.

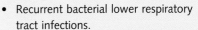

Suspect immunodeficiency in the following circumstances:

- Recurrent bacterial lower respiratory tract infections.
- Neonatal lymphocyte count less than 2.0 × 10^9/L.
- Failure to thrive.

Unusual infection:

- Recurrent or chronic skin infection.
- Recurrent or chronic candidal infections.

Primary immunodeficiencies

These can be inherited as X-linked (affecting boys) or autosomal recessive disorders; 40% are diagnosed in first year of life. Examples are given below.

Fig. 10.10 Immune defects and corresponding susceptibility.

Immune defects and corresponding susceptibility	
Defect	**Susceptibility**
Antibody	Bacteria: *Pneumococcus, Staphylococcus, Streptococcus, Haemophilus influenzae* Viruses: Enteroviruses
Cell-mediated	Viruses: Herpes viruses, measles Fungi: *Candida, Aspergillus, Pneumocystis carinii* Bacteria: *Mycobacteria, Listeria*
Neutrophil function	Bacteria: Gram-positive, Gram-negative Fungi: *Candida, Aspergillus*

X-linked agammaglobulinaemia (Bruton's disease)

There is a failure of B cell development and immunoglobulin production. It presents with severe bacterial infections in the first 2 years of life.

Severe combined immunodeficiency (SCID)

A heterogeneous group of disorders with profoundly defective cellular and humoral immunity (hence the name 'combined'). It presents in the first 6 months of life with failure to thrive, diarrhoea, candidal infections and recurrent, severe and unusual infections. A blood count often shows lymphopenia. Bone marrow transplantation is curative.

Common variable immunodeficiency (CVID)

This term encompasses a heterogeneous group of patients who have low levels of serum IgG and IgA. Usually present in late childhood with recurrent bacterial infection of sinuses or lungs.

Selective IgA deficiency

This is common (1:700 population). Most people with complete absence of IgA are asymptomatic. It is associated with autoimmune diseases in 40%, and also with IgG subclass deficiency. Children deficient in IgG_2, the subclass providing immunity against polysaccharide antigens, might be susceptible to infection with encapsulated organisms (e.g. *Streptococcus pneumoniae*, *Haemophilus influenzae* type B).

Chronic granulomatous disease

An inherited disorder, usually X-linked, in which phagocytic cells fail to produce the superoxide anion. It presents with repeated bacterial and fungal infections involving the skin, lymph nodes, lungs, liver and bones. Granulomas and abscesses form in these sites. Diagnosis is confirmed by failure to reduce nitroblue tetrazolium (NBT test).

The management of primary immunodeficiency is outlined in Fig. 10.11.

Secondary immunodeficiency

Immunosuppressive therapy

Therapeutic drugs, which cause immunosuppression, include:

Management of primary immunodeficiency
The following treatment options are available:
• Antibiotic prophylaxis, e.g. co-trimoxazole, to prevent *Pneumocystis carinii* infection
• Vigorous antibiotic therapy for infections
• Immunoglobulin replacement therapy—regular IV immunoglobulin can be given for severe defects in antibody production
• Bone marrow transplantation
• Gene therapy—this has been successfully performed for SCID caused by adenosine deaminase deficiency

Fig. 10.11 Management of primary immunodeficiency.

- Cytotoxic agents.
- Steroids.

Cytotoxic chemotherapy for malignant disease (e.g. acute leukaemia) causes immunosuppression due to marrow suppression and neutropenia. Febrile children with neutrophil counts less than $0.5 \times 10^9/L$ are at risk for serious and potentially fatal bacterial and fungal infection.

Children on high-dose corticosteroids (e.g. for nephrotic syndrome) are particularly at risk for disseminated chickenpox infection. Children with organ transplants are prone to infection with cytomegalovirus.

Infection

Worldwide, the two most important infections, which cause immunodeficiency, are:

- Measles.
- HIV infection.

Paediatric HIV infection

Human immunodeficiency virus type 1 (HIV-1), the causative agent of acquired immunodeficiency syndrome (AIDS), is transmitted to infants and children by vertical transmission from HIV-infected women or by HIV-contaminated blood or blood products.

Incidence

The WHO estimates that 20 million adults and 1.5 million children have been infected with HIV since the pandemic began; 1500 children in sub-Saharan Africa are infected daily. The incidence of childhood HIV is increasing in the UK but mortality has decreased significantly with new antiviral therapies.

Transmission

The main route of transmission to children is vertically from mother to child: intrauterine, intrapartum or via breastfeeding. Transmission rates vary with geographical area: lower in Europe and higher in Africa. With current management vertical transmission is now <1%.

Diagnosis

All newborns born to HIV-infected women will have circulating maternal HIV antibodies but only a proportion of these are infected with the virus. Passively acquired antibody disappears at 15–18 months of age so this is not a reliable test for infection under 18 months.

Two approaches exist for diagnosis in children younger than 18 months:

- HIV viral culture: the gold standard but not widely available.
- Detection of viral genome by polymerase chain reaction.

Clinical manifestations: progression to AIDS

The incubation period from infection to disease varies but appears to be shorter in perinatally infected children than in adults. Mortality and hospital admissions have decreased since the introduction of combination antiviral therapy.

Changes in immune function are shown in Figs 10.12 and 10.14, and the clinical manifestations in Figs 10.13 and 10.15.

CD4 percentage	
>25%	No evidence of suppression
15–25%	Moderate immunosuppression
<15%	Severe immunosuppression
Viral load	Unlike adults does not correlate well with disease course

Fig. 10.14 Immunological categories.

Noninfectious complication of AIDS	
Neurological	Encephalopathy Motor defects Seizures
Gastrointestinal	Anorexia Nausea Diarrhoea Weight loss
Lymphoid hyperplasia syndrome	Lymphoid interstitial pneumonitis Polyglandular enlargement
Cutaneous	Kaposi's sarcoma

Fig. 10.15 Noninfectious complications of AIDS.

Immunological test results in AIDS
Reduced CD4 count Antigen detection, e.g. p24 Raised IgG antibody HIV DNA/RNA PCR

Fig. 10.12 Immunological test results in AIDS.

Fig. 10.13 Clinical manifestations of HIV infection in children.

Clinical manifestations of HIV infection in children		
Category	Severity	Manifestation
Category N	Asymptomatic	
Category A	Mild	Lymphadenopathy Hepatosplenomegaly Parotitis
Category B	Moderate	Severe bacterial infection Chronic diarrhoea Candidiasis Lymphocytic interstitial pneumonitis (LIP)
Category C	Severe (AIDS)	Wasting (severe failure to thrive) Opportunistic infections, e.g. Pneumocystic carinii pneumonia (PCP) Encephalopathy Severe bacterial infections Malignancy (rare)

Management

Cotrimoxazole prophylaxis against *Pneumocystis carinii* pneumonia is given for children with HIV infection. The primary immunization course should be given. BCG is not recommended but MMR should be deferred only if severely immunosuppressed.

Antiretroviral treatment is recommended when the child becomes symptomatic or there is a low or rapid fall in the CD4 count (<15%). This treatment comprises a combination of reverse transcriptase inhibitors with protease inhibitors.

Coordinated psychological and social support for the whole family is a vital aspect of managing an HIV infected child. Issues include:

- Telling children the diagnosis.
- Retaining confidentiality.
- Two (mother and child) members of the family might be sick or dying at the same time.
- Social or cultural isolation.
- Stigma of diagnosis.
- Major problem with increasing costs of antiviral drugs in developing countries.

Prevention

Zidovudine, given to the mother in pregnancy and during delivery and to the neonate for the first 6 weeks of life reduces the risk of vertical transmission of HIV-1. Caesarean section is recommended but if the maternal viral load is low then vaginal delivery appears to be safe. Antenatal HIV testing therefore confers potential benefits. Education campaigns can reduce but not eliminate the spread of HIV.

Allergy and anaphylaxis

Objectives

At the end of this chapter, you should be able to

- Understand the natural history of allergies.
- Take an appropriate history and perform relevant examination in a child with a suspected allergic reaction.
- Understand the different tests used to diagnose allergies.
- Understand the acute and long-term management of children with anaphylaxis.

Allergy can be defined as a hypersensitive reaction initiated by immune mechanisms. This is mediated primarily by antibodies from the IgE isotype but in some reactions non-IgE mechanisms are responsible. The typical IgE-mediated response is biphasic. This is characterized by an early response (within 20 minutes) and a late response at 3–6 hours. Typical allergic reactions include:

- Asthma.
- Food allergy.
- Allergic rhinoconjunctivitis.
- Atopic eczema.
- Anaphylaxis.

This chapter will cover mainly food allergy and anaphylaxis, as the others are discussed elsewhere.

EPIDEMIOLOGY

The increasing prevalence of allergy in children over the past 20–30 years has led to an increased need for specialized services dealing in childhood allergy. Although part of the increase in cases of allergy stems from greater awareness and reporting, population-based studies have shown a significant rise in allergic diseases. Approximately 6–8% of all children experience food allergy and 6% of all asthmatics have food-induced wheeze. In atopic eczema,

approximately 60% will have a reaction to certain foods.

Many allergies improve as the child grows older.

The natural history of allergy changes with increasing age. In early childhood, food reactions predominate, with manifestations in the skin, respiratory and gastrointestinal tract. With increasing age, inhaled allergens become more important; initially this tends to involve indoor allergens (house-dust mite and pets) and then outdoor allergens (moulds and pollens) later.

Parents often would want to know the long-term outcome of food allergy—85% of children outgrow cow's milk allergy at the age of 3 years but peanut allergy is lifelong.

CROSS-REACTION TO ALLERGENS

It is important to note that children sensitized to one allergen can develop reactions to another even though previous exposure has not occurred. This is because certain allergens share the same binding site (epitope) to IgE and one mimics the other. Examples are:

- Grass and peanut.
- Peanuts, soy beans and lentils.
- Latex and banana.

It is rare to have IgE-mediated reactions to more than three foods and allergy testing results that show cross-reaction should be confirmed by food challenge.

CLINICAL ASPECTS OF ALLERGY

Diagnosis

The aim of the history is to ascertain what allergens the child reacts to and to discover if non-allergy mechanisms might be the cause of symptoms. An example is that 90% of cases of penicillin reaction obtained from the history are not caused by allergic mechanisms. The history should include:

- Age of onset.
- Diurnal and seasonal variations.
- Family history.
- Dietary history.
- Time between exposure and reaction.
- Reproducibility of reaction.
- Housing conditions and school.

Examination of the child must include the skin; ears, nose and throat (ENT); respiratory and gastrointestinal tracts; and some cardiovascular tests (Fig. 11.1). The nutritional status must be noted.

Symptoms that are severe, persistent or recurrent are an indication for allergy testing. This is commonly in the form of skin-prick testing or specific serum IgE levels. Food challenge is the gold standard and is used when doubts remain about the role of particular allergens. There is no lower age limit on testing and it must be noted that the severity of reaction from skin-prick tests or levels of specific IgE have a poor correlation with severity of clinical

Examining a child for allergy	
Respiratory	Asthma/wheeze Stridor and angio-oedema Hoarseness Rhinoconjunctivitis
Gastrointestinal	Nausea, vomitting and diarrhoea Abdominal distension Failure to thrive
Cardiovascular	Hypotension and shock Dizziness
Skin	Pruritus Urticaria Atopic dermatitis Angio-oedema

Fig. 11.1 Examining a child for allergy.

symptoms. Neither of these tests diagnoses non-IgE-mediated reactions and only a food challenge is diagnostic.

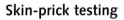

- Skin-prick testing is useful in all ages but not over areas of eczema.
- Food challenge is indicated in cases of doubt.

Skin-prick testing

This is the most common test because it is cheap, quick and has a good safety profile. For most allergens (except soy) a negative test means that it is unlikely that the patient will react to the allergen tested. Unfortunately, a positive test means only a 50–60% chance that the child will react and therefore the test result must be interpreted with a good clinical history. If there is a strong history of food reaction and a positive skin-prick test then a food challenge is not needed to confirm the allergen is responsible for symptoms.

Serum-specific IgE

This is commonly referred to as RAST testing because it describes the type of assay that is performed on the serum. It measures levels of IgE that are food specific. This type of test is useful if skin-prick testing cannot be used (e.g. active eczema, patients on steroids or antihistamines and the drug cannot be stopped). Like skin-prick tests, a negative result is good for ruling out allergens but a positive result is useful only in the context of a positive history.

Food challenge

This is the gold standard and is used when uncertainties about the role of particular allergens or when non-IgE mechanisms are implicated. This is the only investigation that can accurately predict what clinical reactions will occur with food exposure.

Although very helpful in making a diagnosis, allergen challenging can lead to severe reactions including anaphylaxis. Therefore it should be performed in the hospital setting after obtaining informed consent from parents.

MANAGEMENT OF ALLERGY

Children with suspected food allergy should be assessed by a paediatrician experienced in allergy: a specialist nurse and a dietician should be available. Liaison between hospital and community staff, and the education of both family and school play an important part.

A major consideration in management is the anxiety that affects both child and carers. Avoidance of the allergen might be difficult and it is often hard for parents to identify suitable foods; the help of an experienced dietician is essential in these matters. Inhaled allergen avoidance is difficult and various methods are available. Their effectiveness remains controversial, however.

Pharmacological treatment remains standard for asthma and eczema. Antihistamines can be useful and immunotherapy might play a greater role in the future.

ANAPHYLAXIS

Anaphylaxis is a severe allergic reaction that manifests with respiratory difficulty (wheeze or upper airway obstruction) and/or cardiovascular symptoms (shock, hypotension or dizziness).

It is caused by prior exposure to antigen-sensitizing mast cells and basophils, leading to systemic release of inflammatory mediators resulting in capillary leak, mucosal oedema and smooth muscle contraction.

Anaphylaxis can be mediated by IgE, when the term 'allergic anaphylaxis' should be used; when IgE is not implicated or is unclear, the term 'non-allergic anaphylaxis' should be used. The term 'anaphylactoid' is no longer used.

Anaphylaxis has an increasing incidence and, in children, foods are the most common cause, followed by drugs and hymenoptera (bee/wasp) venom. In adults the common causes are drugs, insect venom, foods and latex.

Foods

Foods are the most common cause of anaphylaxis in children. Peanuts are the most common food to cause a reaction.

Insect venom

Anaphylaxis to venom is rare in children but it is associated with the greatest anxiety. The reaction to insect stings decreases with age.

Latex

Anaphylaxis to latex is rare in children and is usually found in those who have had numerous surgical procedures. Note its cross-reaction with banana.

Drugs

Vaccines and penicillins account for the majority of reactions but are rare. Note that MMR immunizations can be given to children with egg allergy, although if there has been previous anaphylaxis to egg, or severe co-existing asthma, the vaccine can be given in hospital. Influenza vaccine should not be given to children with egg allergy.

Recognition

Respiratory difficulty is more common than cardiovascular collapse. Foods tend to cause respiratory and airway symptoms whereas injections and stings cause cardiovascular symptoms. Initial symptoms can be subtle and progression rapid.

Respiratory symptoms and signs

- Cough.
- Stridor, hoarseness and drooling.
- Facial swelling.
- Wheeze.

Cardiovascular symptoms and signs

- Feeling faint/dizziness.
- Syncope.
- Pallor.
- Tachycardia.

Note that the cutaneous signs, such as rash, are not life threatening and might be absent.

Treatment

Treatment is intramuscular adrenaline (epinephrine). This acts on the α-adrenoreceptors to cause peripheral vasoconstriction and on β-receptors to cause bronchodilation and inotropic effects; it also reduces airway swelling. It should be given to all children with respiratory or cardiovascular symptoms. The intramuscular route is preferred because intravenous administration is thought to have contributed in some deaths. IV hydrocortisone and antihistamines should also be administered.

PREVENTION

Allergen avoidance is the only preventive measure and all children with suspected anaphylaxis should be referred for allergy testing. The use of an Epipen, which allows subcutaneous administration of adrenaline, can be life saving but it is essential that carers are trained in its use. Only 32% of parents were able to correctly demonstrate correct use in one study. The Epipen is only one part of managing severe allergic reactions. Management should also include:

- Identifying causes.
- Education on allergen avoidance.
- Treatment plan.
- Training of carers and school.
- Annual re-inforcement.

Epipens in anaphylaxis are useful if carers are trained in their use.

Further reading

Clark AT, Ewen PW. The prevention and management of anaphylaxis in children. *Current Paediatrics* 2002; **12**:370–375.

Host A, Halken S. Practical aspects of allergy testing. *Paediatric Respiratory Reviews* 2003; **4**:312–318.

Ives A, Hourihane J. Evidence-based diagnosis of food allergy. *Current Paediatrics* 2002; **12**:357–364.

Johansson SGO et al. A revised nomenclature for allergy. An EAACI position statement from the EAACI nomenclature task force. *Allergy* 2001; **56**:813–824.

Rosenthal M. How a non-allergist survives an allergy clinic. *Archives of Diseases in Childhood* 2004; **89**:238–243.

ECZEMA (DERMATITIS)

The term 'dermatitis' refers to an inflammation of the skin and is synonymous with eczema (the word eczema literally means 'to boil over'). Three main varieties occur in infants and children:

• Infantile seborrhoeic eczema.
• Atopic eczema.
• Napkin dermatitis.

Infantile seborrhoeic eczema

This mild condition presents in the first 2 months of life with a scaly, non-itchy rash initially on the scalp ('cradle cap'); this might spread to involve the face, flexures and napkin area (Fig. 12.1). Treatment is with emollients and mild topical steroids.

Atopic eczema

Atopic eczema is very common and affects 10–20% of children, usually beginning in the first 6 months of life. There is often a family history of atopic disorders (eczema, asthma and hay fever), reflecting a genetic predisposition that confers an abnormal immune response to environmental allergens. Early diagnosis and treatment of atopic children with antihistamines can reduce the risk of developing asthma in later life.

Clinical features

A dry, red itchy rash occurs that usually starts on, and has a predilection for, the extensor surfaces and face in infants and young children, and the flexures (the antecubital and popliteal fossae) in older children (Fig. 12.2). However, the skin appearance can vary from an acute, weeping papulovesicular eruption to the chronic, dry, scaly, thickened (lichenified) skin that develops in older children. Itching is the most important and troublesome symptom.

Affected children might have an eosinophilia and raised plasma IgE concentration. Histopathological changes include epidermal oedema and vesicle formation, vascular dilatation and cellular infiltration.

Diagnosis

The diagnosis is clinical (see Fig. 12.3 for a comparison of atopic and infantile seborrhoeic eczema). RAST and food challenges are useful in children with associated difficult to manage asthma.

Management

It is important that the skin is kept hydrated and inflammation is reduced. The treatment options are:

• Important general measures.
• Topical preparations.
• Specific treatment for complications such as secondary infection.

Having a child with severe eczema can be quite distressing to parents. In addition to the treatment with steroids and emollients, it is also important to keep the child comfortable by reducing the itch by using cotton fabrics, non-biological detergents and avoiding fabric softeners. Cigarette smoke, dander from furry pets, house dust and grass pollen can also aggravate the condition. Nails should be kept short and excessive heat avoided. Using hand mittens at night will also prevent excessive scratching. Many children eventually grow out of their eczema by their teens.

Mild topical steroids, such as 1% hydrocortisone (ointment rather than cream when the skin is dry), applied to the affected areas twice daily are highly effective. More potent preparations can be used short term for exacerbations but only weak steroids should be applied to the face. Severe eczema can be treated with wet wraps in hospital to maximize hydration.

A new class of drug—topical immunomodulators, e.g. tacrolimus cream—is available and has the advantage of few side effects and low systemic absorption.

Medical management

Topical preparations

The mainstays of management are:

- Emollients.
- Topical steroids.

Emollients moisturize and soften the skin. They are safe and should be used frequently. A daily bath using bath oil and aqueous cream as a soap substitute is advisable, with regular application of an emollient two or three times daily.

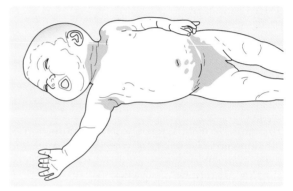

Fig. 12.1 Distribution of infantile seborrhoeic eczema.

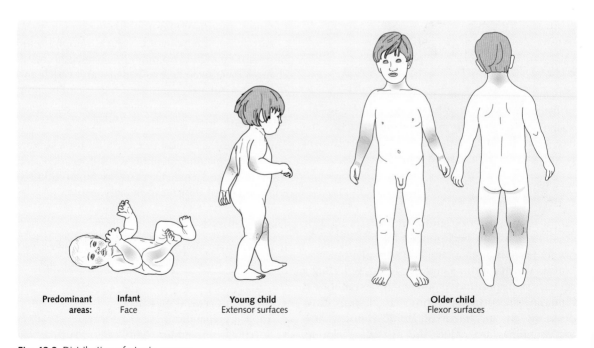

| Predominant areas: | Infant
Face | Young child
Extensor surfaces | Older child
Flexor surfaces |

Fig. 12.2 Distribution of atopic eczema.

Fig. 12.3 Differences between infantile seborrhoeic eczema and atopic eczema.

Differences between infantile seborrhoeic eczema and atopic eczema		
	Infantile seborrhoeic eczema	Atopic eczema
Age	<3 months (usually)	>3 months (usually)
Sleeping	Unaffected	Disturbed
Pruritus	Nil	Significant
Family history of atopy	Usually negative	Often positive
Course	Self-limiting	Chronic, relapsing

In atopic eczema:
- Treat dry skin with emollients.
- Inflamed skin with topical steroids.
- Consider infection if not responding to treatment.

Complications

The most important is secondary infection with either viruses or bacteria. Infection with herpes simplex (eczema herpeticum) is potentially serious and should be treated with aciclovir. Bacterial super-infection is usually caused by staphylococci or streptococci and requires systemic antibiotic treatment.

Atopic dermatitis persists into adulthood in up to 60% of all children and particularly in those with early onset, severe disease and associated asthma and hay fever.

Napkin dermatitis

Rashes in the napkin area are common and can be due to:

- An irritant contact dermatitis (nappy rash).
- Candidiasis.
- Seborrhoeic dermatitis.

Clinical features

Nappy rash

Ordinary nappy rash is due to the prolonged contact of urine and faeces with skin. Particular causes include skin wetness and ammonia from the breakdown of urine by faecal enzymes. The skin is red, moist and might ulcerate. The inguinal folds are spared.

Nappy rash can be prevented by frequent nappy changes (easier with disposable nappies) and barrier creams such as zinc and castor oil cream. Exposure to air can hasten recovery but it is often impractical to implement this at home.

Candidiasis

Candidiasis is also common and is distinguished by bright red skin with satellite lesions and involvement of the skin folds. Candidal infection can be treated with an anticandidal and hydrocortisone preparation, such as miconazole with hydrocortisone.

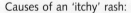

Causes of an 'itchy' rash:
- Atopic eczema.
- Scabies.
- Papular urticaria.
- Urticaria (hives).
- Chickenpox.

INFECTIONS

Bacterial

Bacterial infections of the skin in children include common and important entities such as:

- Impetigo.
- Boils and furuncles.
- Staphylococcal scalded skin syndrome.
- Erysipelas.

These are considered in Chapter 10.

Viral

Viral warts

Hands and feet

The human papilloma virus (HPV) causes viral warts. Two types are seen:

- Skin warts are common on the fingers and soles in school-age children.
- Plantar warts (verrucae) are flat, hyperkeratotic lesions on the soles of the feet.

Most viral warts resolve within a year when immunity develops. Treatment options include:

- Salicylic and lactic acid paint.
- Cryotherapy with liquid nitrogen.

Repeat treatments over many weeks are required.

Other sites

Viral warts also occur in other locations:

- Laryngeal papillomas are found on the vocal cords.
- Genital warts (condylomata acuminata) are papular or frond-like growths in the perineal area.

These can be a sign of sexual abuse in young children.

Molluscum contagiosum

This common eruption in children is caused by the mollusci poxvirus.

Clinical features

Smooth, pearly papules with an obvious central dimple arise in crops (often on the trunk). They are not irritating and are of low infectivity.

Management

The papules resolve spontaneously without scarring usually within 6 months to 2 years and treatment is not required, although cryotherapy can be used if rapid removal is required.

Fungal

These include the dermatophytosis (ringworm) and candidiasis (thrush).

Dermatophytoses (tinea capitis, corporis, pedis and unguium)

Dermatophytes are filamentous fungi that infect the outer layer of the skin and also the hair and nails. They also affect some animal species (e.g. cattle and cats).

Clinical features

Clinical features vary with the site of infection.

Tinea capitis (scalp ringworm)

On the scalp, tinea causes patchy alopecia and occasionally a boggy inflammatory mass called a kerion.

Tinea corporis (body ringworm)

On the trunk, tinea appears as annular lesions with central clearing and a palpable, erythematous border.

Tinea pedis (athlete's foot)

This presents as itchy, scaling and cracking of the skin of the feet, especially between the toes.

Diagnosis

Examination under ultraviolet light (Wood's) shows a green–yellow fluorescence of infected hairs with certain fungal species. Diagnosis can be made by microscopic examination of skin scrapings for fungal hyphae. Culture of the organism is definitive.

Treatment

This varies with the severity of infection:

- Mild infections are treated with topical antifungal preparations such as clotrimazole or miconazole.
- Severe infections require systemic treatment with griseofulvin for several weeks.

Candidiasis (thrush, moniliasis)

Candida albicans, a yeast (budding, unicellular organism), is the most common pathogen. The organism colonizes the skin and mucous membranes. Transmission is via person-to-person contact, contaminated feeding bottles, etc.

Clinical features

In infants, candidal infections frequently involve the oral cavity (thrush) or the napkin area. It is acquired from the mother's vaginal flora. It can also affect the nipples of breastfeeding mothers.

Diagnosis

Diagnosis is clinical:

- Oral thrush presents as white plaques on the tongue and buccal mucosa.
- Monilial dermatitis: localized shiny redness typically affecting moist areas and *not* sparing flexural skin creases (this may occur in the absence of oral thrush).

Management

Topical nystatin is first-line therapy. Oral treatment should be given as well as direct treatment to lesions in perineal disease.

Prevention requires good hygiene and rigorous disinfection of feeding bottles and dummies.

Chronic or recurrent mucocutaneous candidiasis should raise the suspicion of immunodeficiency.

INFESTATIONS

Papular urticaria

This term describes crops of itchy, erythematous papules or small blisters. They are caused by insect bites, most commonly by the fleas or mites from domestic dogs or cats; bedbugs can also be the culprits. Secondary infection might occur.

Scabies

Scabies is caused by the mite, *Sarcoptes scabiei*. It is transmitted by prolonged skin-to-skin contact. In the first infestation, the incubation period can be up to 8 weeks. The fertilized adult female mite burrows deep in the stratum corneum laying two or three eggs a day until she dies after about 5 weeks. The eggs hatch after a few days and larvae move on to the skin surface, maturing into adults in 10–14 days.

Clinical features

The first symptom is pruritus (this is worse at night), which is related to hypersensitivity to the mite or its faeces. The presence of burrows is pathognomonic. Common sites for burrows are the interdigital webs and the anterior aspects of the wrists. In infants, the soles of the feet, head and neck are commonly affected.

The rash consists of vesicles, weals and papules, which may become excoriated and secondarily infected.

Diagnosis

Diagnosis is clinical and might (if necessary) be confirmed by identification of mites or ova in scrapings from burrows or vesicles.

Suspect scabies when:
- There is itching in the family.
- Itchy papules or blisters are present on the soles of the feet.

Treatment

Treatment is permethrin cream 5%. This is for two consecutive days—covering the body from the neck down. In infants, the scalp and face should be included. It can take several weeks for the pruritus to subside after successful treatment as hypersensitivity persists. This can be managed with oral antihistamines and topical steroids.

It is important to treat all contacts. Parents should also be advised to wash all clothes and bedding to prevent reinfection.

Head lice (Pediculosis capitis)

Pediculosis capitis is a blood-sucking arthropod that infests the scalps of up to 10% of school children in some urban areas. Transmission is by head-to-head contact. The head louse prefers clean hair and does not discriminate between social groups.

Clinical features and diagnosis

The louse egg is attached to the base of the scalp hair and is visible as a small, white, grain-like particle. Eggs hatch after a week and the louse lives for 2–3 months. Many infestations are asymptomatic but the most common manifestation is severe itching of the scalp often accompanied by enlarged cervical lymph nodes. Nits are the egg cases and only finding a louse is diagnostic.

Treatment

Treatment is with 0.5% malathion lotion, which should be left on for 12 hours. The hair is then washed with ordinary shampoo and the dead nits removed with a fine-toothed metal comb. All the family should be treated. Clothing and bedding is disinfected by machine washing (cycles over 50°C inactivate lice and nits).

OTHER CHILDHOOD SKIN DISEASES

Pityriasis rosea

This common, acute, benign and self-limiting condition is thought to be of viral origin. It begins with a 'herald patch', an oval or round, scaly, erythematous macule on the trunk, neck or proximal part of limbs. This is followed within 1–3 days by a shower of smaller dull pink macules on the trunk in a so-called 'Christmas tree' pattern following the lines of the ribs. Spontaneous resolution occurs within 6–8 weeks.

No treatment is required.

Acne vulgaris

This is a chronic inflammatory disorder of the sebaceous glands and probably reflects an abnormal response to circulating androgens. It is an almost universal problem of adolescence, peaking in severity at age 16–18 years.

Clinical features

A variety of lesions occur on the face and upper trunk. Characteristically, comedones occur: plugs of keratin and sebum within the dilated orifice of a hair follicle. These can be open (blackheads) or closed (whiteheads). They progress to papules and pustules (bacterial superinfection) and in severe cases to cystic and nodular lesions, which can cause scarring.

Treatment

Treatment options include:

- Topical treatment with keratolytic agents, e.g. benzoyl peroxide.
- Ultraviolet light therapy: exposure to natural sunlight should be encouraged.
- Oral antibiotics: low-dose therapy with minocycline, oxytetracycline (>12 years age) or erythromycin is useful for moderate to severe pustular acne. Antibiotics are given for at least 3 months.
- The vitamin A analogue, 13-*cis*-retinoic acid: for severe acne that has not responded to conventional treatment. This should be prescribed only by a dermatologist.

Urticaria (hives)

Urticaria is a transient, itchy, erythematous rash characterized by the presence of raised weals (hives). It is induced by mast cell degranulation, in which histamine and other vasoactive mediators are released causing vasodilatation and an increase in capillary permeability. Most cases are caused by viral infections but an allergy history is needed to exclude allergic causes.

Clinical features

Urticaria can be accompanied by oedema of the lips and eyes (angioedema). Involvement of the lips and tongue is an emergency because there is a risk of respiratory obstruction. Chronic urticaria can occur and usually clears spontaneously in about 6 months.

Management

Acute urticaria usually resolves spontaneously within a few hours. If itchy, it can be treated with an antihistamine, e.g. chlorpheniramine maleate. Precipitating factors should be avoided.

In developed countries, congenital heart disease (CHD) accounts for the majority of cardiovascular problems in infants and children. With improved cardiac surgery, 80–85% of children with congenital cardiac disease survive into adulthood. In contrast to its incidence in adults, ischaemic heart disease is rare in children although it can occur in Kawasaki disease. Arrhythmias are very rare, with the exception of supraventricular tachycardias (SVTs). Important infections that affect the cardiovascular system (CVS) are infective endocarditis and viral myocarditis.

CONGENITAL HEART DISEASE (CHD)

CHD comprises the most common group of structural malformations, affecting 6–8 out of 1000 live-born infants. A number of important causative factors are recognized (Fig. 13.1) but, in the majority of cases, the cause is unknown. CHD presents or might be diagnosed in a limited number of ways. These include:

• Antenatal diagnosis by ultrasound.
• Heart murmur.
• Cyanosis.
• Shock: low cardiac output.
• Cardiac failure (see Chapter 2).

Although there are over 100 different cardiac malformations, a small number account for the majority of cases (Fig. 13.2). These are conveniently classified into:

• Acyanotic forms.
• Cyanotic forms.

Initial evaluation should include a chest X-ray (CXR) and electrocardiogram (ECG), although these investigations do not usually provide a lesion diagnosis. Diagnosis is usually achieved by a combination of echocardiography and Doppler ultrasound. Common investigations are shown in Fig. 13.3.

Acyanotic congenital heart disease

These conditions are caused by lesions that allow blood to shunt from the left to the right side of the circulation, or which obstruct the flow of blood by narrowing a valve or vessel.

Left to right shunts (L to R)

Atrial septal defect (ASD)

There are two types of ASD:

• The most common ASD (6 in 10 000 live births) is an ostium secundum defect, high in the atrial septum. It is more common in girls (F : M = 2 : 1) and accounts for 6% of all cases of CHD.
• Much less common is the ostium primum type, which occurs lower in the atrial septum (often associated with mitral regurgitation), and is a common defect in Down syndrome.

Secundum defects are usually asymptomatic in childhood. The left to right shunt develops very slowly and pulmonary hypertension is extremely uncommon. It is important to distinguish ASDs from patent foramen ovale (PFO), which is present in one-third of all children. The patent foramen opens only in conditions of raised atrial pressure or volumes, whereas ASDs are large and always open.

Clinical features   The clinical features include:

- Abnormal right ventricular impulse.
- Widely split and fixed second sound (S2).
- Tricuspid flow murmur: rumbling mid-diastolic murmur at the left sternal edge.
- Pulmonary flow murmur: soft, ejection systolic murmur in the pulmonary area.

No murmur is generated by the low velocity flow across the ASD. A significant left to right shunt generates flow murmurs at the tricuspid and pulmonary valves.

Diagnosis   The CXR shows pulmonary plethora and the ECG shows right ventricular hypertrophy with incomplete right bundle branch block. Echocardiography is diagnostic without cardiac catheterization.

Management   Treatment is surgical and aims to prevent cardiac failure and arrythmias in later life. This is best done at 3–5 years of age and 30% can be done in the cardiac catheter laboratory. Endocarditis prophylaxis is not required for children with isolated secundum ASD.

Ventricular septal defect (VSD)

Most are single, although multiple defects do occur and other heart defects coexist in about one-third of children. The natural history and prognosis depends on the:

Causes of congenital heart disease
Genetic chromosomal disorders
Down syndrome, e.g. atrioventricular septal defect
Turner syndrome, e.g. aortic stenosis, coarctation of aorta
chromosome 22 deletions
Williams syndrome, e.g. supravalvular aortic stenosis
Teratogens
Congenital rubella, e.g. PDA, pulmonary stenosis
Alcohol, e.g. ASD, VSD

Fig. 13.1 Causes of congenital heart disease.

Fig. 13.2 Common forms of CHD.

Common forms of congenital heart disease			
Type	**Name**	**Abbreviation**	**% of CHD**
Acyanotic	Ventricular septal defect	VSD	32
	Patent ductus arteriosus	PDA	12
	Pulmonary stenosis	PS	8
	Atrial septal defect	ASD	6
	Coarctation of the aorta	COA	6
	Aortic stenosis	AS	5
Cyanotic	Tetralogy of Fallot	—	6
	Transposition of the great arteries	TGA	5

Fig. 13.3 Investigations in CHD.

Investigations in congenital heart disease	
Investigation	**Demonstrates**
CXR	Cardiac shadow—may be enlarged or abnormal Lung fields—pulmonary vascular markings may be: Increased (plethora): Signifiant L to R shunt, e.g. VSD Decreased (oligaemia): Reduced pulmonary blood flow, e.g. pulmonary stenosis
ECG	Rate and rhythm of heart Mean QRS axis Hypertrophy of either ventricle
Echocardiogram	Precise anatomical abnormality
Cardiac catheter	Physiological/haemodynamic status rather than anatomy

- Size and position of the defect.
- Development of changes due to blood shunting from left to right through the defect. This includes narrowing of the right ventricular outflow tract and progressive pulmonary hypertension, both of which reduce the size of the shunt.

> A ventricular septal defect is the most common variety of congenital heart disease. It accounts for one-third of all cases.

The clinical features, treatment and outcome are best considered separately for the different sizes of defect.

Small VSD (maladie de Roger)
The child is asymptomatic and the murmur is often first noted on routine examination. The only abnormality is a pansystolic murmur (sometimes with a palpable thrill) at the lower left sternal border.

Antibiotic prophylaxis against bacterial endocarditis is necessary for dental extractions but no other treatment is required. Spontaneous closure might occur.

Medium VSD
These usually present with symptoms during infancy including slow weight gain, difficulty with feeding and recurrent chest infections. In time, symptoms might actually disappear due to relative or actual closure of the defect.

On examination, there may be:

- An increased cardiac impulse.
- Palpable thrill.
- Harsh pansystolic murmur, loudest in the third and fourth left intercostal spaces.

If the pulmonary blood flow is high, a mid-diastolic murmur occurs due to blood flow across the normal mitral valve.

A CXR will show moderate cardiac enlargement, a prominent pulmonary artery and increased vascularity of the lungs. Echocardiography will show the position of the defect. The shunt is measured by Doppler studies.

Heart failure, if present, should be treated with diuretics and angiotensin-converting enzyme (ACE) inhibitors. Spontaneous improvement occurs in many childhood cases and surgical correction can be avoided. However, if there is still evidence of a significant shunt at 4 years, closure should be considered before the child starts school.

Large VSD
Heart failure develops early on, especially if a chest infection occurs. The cardiac signs are similar to those of a medium VSD but it is worth noting that the systolic murmur might be soft in a very large defect. The defect tends to be larger than the cross-sectional area of the aortic valve.

Initial medical treatment of the heart failure is required and surgical closure under cardiopulmonary bypass is usually necessary. In young infants with multiple defects, banding of the pulmonary artery allows a temporary respite until the child is big enough for definitive correction. An example of a VSD is shown in Fig. 13.4.

Patent ductus arteriosus (PDA)
The ductus arteriosus connects the aorta to the left pulmonary artery and usually closes by the fourth day of life. A PDA is diagnosed if the duct does not close after 1 month of life. Risk factors include preterm infants, Down syndrome and high altitudes. PDA seen in preterm infants is a distinct clinical entity from congenital PDA in term infants.

> The risk of developing pulmonary vascular disease or infective endocarditis is higher in PDA than VSD and surgical closure is recommended for all PDAs. This can be achieved by division, ligation, or transvenous umbrella occlusion.

Clinical features   A shunt develops between the aorta and pulmonary artery. The clinical features include:

- 'Bounding' pulses: wide pulse pressure.
- Murmur: initially 'systolic'. As pulmonary vascular resistance falls a continuous run-off from the aorta to the pulmonary artery occurs with a continuous 'machinery' murmur.

Fig. 13.4 Ventricular septal defect and chest X-ray changes.

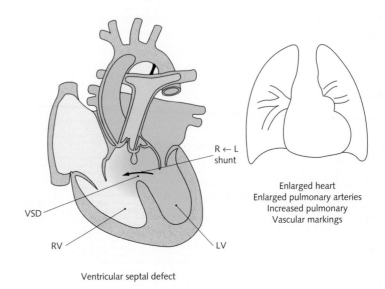

R ← L
shunt

Enlarged heart
Enlarged pulmonary arteries
Increased pulmonary
Vascular markings

VSD

RV

LV

Ventricular septal defect

The PDA is commonly asymptomatic. If the duct is large, a significant left to right shunt develops as pulmonary vascular resistance falls and cardiac failure occurs.

Diagnosis CXR and ECG changes with a large symptomatic PDA are similar to those seen in a patient with a large VSD. The CXR is usually normal but in large PDAs increased pulmonary markings are seen.

A PDA can be directly visualized by two-dimensional echocardiography and the ductal shunt can be confirmed by Doppler ultrasound.

Management The duct can be closed in the cardiac catheter laboratory at 1 year of age but, if large, it might need surgical closure at 1–3 months.

Obstructive lesions

Coarctation of the aorta (COA)

This accounts for about 6% of CHDs and has a male preponderance (M : F = 2 : 1). There is a narrowing of the aorta, which can be preductal or postductal. The site and severity of the coarctation determines the clinical features, which range from a severely ill newborn to an asymptomatic child, or adult, with hypertension.

The key to clinical diagnosis of coarctation of the aorta is weak or absent femoral pulses.

Preductal coarctation: symptomatic infants

The abnormal circulation is often diagnosed antenatally but after birth it presents as a sick neonate with absent femoral pulses. While the ductus arteriosus is open the right ventricle can maintain adequate cardiac output to the systemic circulation. There is usually no murmur and cardiac failure occurs when the duct closes.

On diagnosis, prostaglandin infusion to maintain ductal patency and transfer to a cardiac centre for surgery is indicated.

Postductal coarctation: asymptomatic children

Although usually asymptomatic, there might be leg pains or headache. On examination, there is hypertension in the arm and weak or absent femoral pulses. There might be an ejection click (due to an associated bicuspid aortic valve) and a systolic ejection murmur audible in the left interscapular area.

Surgical correction is required. Options include:

- Balloon dilatation.
- Resection of the coarcted segment with end-to-end anastomosis.

Aortic stenosis (AS)

This accounts for 5% of all CHDs and has a male preponderance (M : F = 4 : 1). Symptoms and signs depend on the severity of the stenosis:

- Children with mild or moderate stenosis present with an asymptomatic murmur and a thrill often conducted to the aorta and the suprasternal notch.
- Severe stenosis can present with heart failure in the infant or with chest pain on exertion and syncope in older children.

Sustained, strenuous exercise should be avoided in children with moderate to severe AS. Surgical treatment depends on the severity and site of the stenosis. Options include balloon or surgical valvotomy. Aortic valve replacement is often required for neonates and children with a significant stenosis requiring early treatment.

Pulmonary stenosis (PS)

This accounts for about 8% of CHD and might be valvular (90%), subvalvular (infundibular) or supravalvular. Infundibular PS occurs in association with a large VSD as part of the tetralogy of Fallot.

Most cases are mild and asymptomatic. The clinical features include:

- Widely split S2, with soft pulmonary component (P2).
- Systolic ejection click (valvular PS).
- A systolic ejection murmur maximal at the upper left sternal border, radiating to the back.

Treatment options include transvenous balloon dilatation or pulmonary valvotomy.

Cyanotic congenital heart disease

There are two principal pathophysiological mechanisms for cyanosis in congenital heart disease:

- Decreased pulmonary blood flow with shunting of deoxygenated blood from the right side of the circulation to the left (systemic circulation), e.g. tetralogy of Fallot.
- Abnormal mixing of systemic and pulmonary venous return, usually associated with an increased pulmonary blood flow, e.g. transposition of great arteries (TGA).

The four cardinal anatomical features of the tetralogy of Fallot

- A large VSD
- Right ventricular outflow tract (RVOT) obstruction:
  Infundibular stenosis (50%)
  Pulmonary valve stenosis (10%)
  Combination of above (30%)
- Aorta over-riding the ventricular septum
- Right ventricular hypertrophy

Fig. 13.5 The four cardinal anatomical features of tetralogy of Fallot.

Tetralogy of Fallot

This represents 6–10% of all CHDs and is the most common cause of cyanotic CHDs presenting beyond infancy. The four cardinal anatomical features are shown in Fig. 13.5.

Clinical features

Most patients present with cyanosis in the first 1–2 months of life. Hypoxic (hypercyanotic) spells are a characteristic feature, as is squatting on exercise which develops in late infancy.

Clinical signs include:

- Cyanosis with or without clubbing.
- Loud and single S2.
- Loud ejection systolic murmur maximal at the third, left intercostal space.

Diagnosis

The ECG shows right axis deviation and right ventricular hypertrophy but normal at birth. The CXR shows a characteristic 'boot-shaped' heart caused by right ventricular hypertrophy and a concavity on the left heart border where the main pulmonary artery and RV outflow tract normally create a convexity (Fig. 13.6). Pulmonary vascular markings are diminished. Congestive cardiac failure does not occur in tetralogy of Fallot.

Management

Prolonged hypercyanotic spells require treatment with:

- Morphine—relieves pain and abolishes hyperpnoea.
- Sodium bicarbonate (IV) to correct acidosis.
- Propranolol to cause peripheral vasoconstriction and relieve infundibular spasm. Oral propranolol can prevent hypoxic spells.

Fig. 13.6 Tetralogy of Fallot and CXR changes.

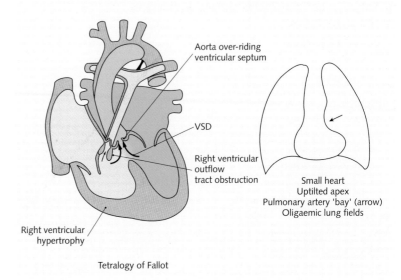

Aorta over-riding ventricular septum

VSD

Right ventricular outflow tract obstruction

Small heart
Uptilted apex
Pulmonary artery 'bay' (arrow)
Oligaemic lung fields

Right ventricular hypertrophy

Tetralogy of Fallot

Definitive treatment is surgical. Palliative procedures might be required in infants with severe cyanosis or uncontrollable hypoxic spells. Pulmonary blood flow is increased by creating a shunt between the subclavian and the pulmonary arteries. Corrective total repair can now be carried out from 4–6 months of age. This involves patch closure of the VSD and widening of the right ventricular outflow tract.

Transposition of the great arteries

This accounts for about 5% of CHDs and is more common in males (M:F = 3:1). In complete or D-transposition:

- The aorta arises anteriorly from the right ventricle.
- The pulmonary artery arises posteriorly from the left ventricle (Fig. 13.7).

Clearly, if completely separate, two such parallel circulations would be incompatible with life, but defects allowing mixing of the two circulations coexist. These include ASD, VSD or PDA.

Clinical features

Most cases present with severe cyanosis, often within the first day or two of life. Spontaneous closure of the ductus arteriosus reduces mixing of the systemic and pulmonary circulations. Arterial hypoxaemia is often profound (PaO_2 1–3 kPa) and unresponsive to O_2 inhalation.

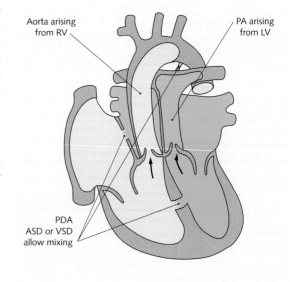

Aorta arising from RV

PA arising from LV

PDA
ASD or VSD allow mixing

Fig. 13.7 Transposition of the great arteries.

The second sound is single and loud. If the ventricular septum is intact, no heart murmur is audible. The systolic murmur of a VSD or PDA might be present.

Management

The immediate aim is to improve mixing of saturated and unsaturated blood. In the sick, cyanosed newborn, an infusion of prostaglandin (PG) E_1 is started to reopen the ductus arteriosus. Emergency cardiac catheterization and therapeutic balloon atrial septostomy (Rashkind procedure) is a life-saving palliative procedure. Definitive repair is usually achieved with an arterial switch procedure, which can be performed at a few weeks of age. The pulmonary artery and aorta are transected and switched over.

> Mixing of blood from left and right sides in cyanotic congenital cardiac disease is essential and might be done through a patent ductus arteriosus. A prostaglandin infusion can open the ductus, allowing mixing.

RHEUMATIC FEVER

Acute rheumatic fever is a sequela of group A β-haemolytic streptococcal infection, usually a tonsillopharyngitis. It is caused by an abnormal immune response that occurs in less than 1% of patients with streptococcal infection. Although the disease has largely been eradicated in developed countries with improved sanitation and the use of antibiotics for tonsillitis, it remains the most common cause of cardiac valvular disease worldwide. It mainly affects children aged between 5 and 15 years.

Clinical features

Polyarthritis, fever and malaise develop 2–6 weeks after the pharyngeal infection. The arthritis is 'fleeting', lasting less than a week in individual joints and commonly affects the large joints such as the knees and ankles.

There is a pancarditis in 50% of patients:

- Pericarditis can cause a friction rub and pericardial effusion.
- Myocarditis can cause heart failure.
- Endocarditis commonly affects the left-sided valves leading to murmurs, e.g. of mitral incompetence.

Erythema marginatum—pink macules on the trunk and limbs—is an uncommon painless, early mani-

festation. Hard subcutaneous nodules occur on the extensor surfaces in a minority of cases.

Sydenham's chorea is a late manifestation occurring 2–6 months after streptococcal infection in 10% of patients. There is emotional lability followed by involuntary, random, jerky movements lasting 2–3 months. Recovery is usually complete.

Diagnosis

The diagnosis is clinical and is based on a modified version of the Duckett Jones criteria (Fig. 13.8).

Diagnosis requires evidence of a preceding streptococcal infection together with two major criteria or one major and two minor criteria. The former is usually done serologically by finding an increase in antibodies to various streptococcal antigens, e.g. antistreptolysin O titre. Throat swab is often negative at the time of presentation.

Laboratory investigations in a suspected case include:

- ESR, C-reactive protein (CRP): elevated.
- Antistreptolysin O titre: might be elevated.
- Throat swab: usually negative at time of presentation.
- ECG: prolonged P-R interval.
- Echocardiography: might show evidence of carditis.

Management

The acute episode is treated by:

- Bed rest.
- High-dose aspirin to suppress fever and arthritis.

Modified Duckett Jones criteria (2 major or 1 major and 2 minor)	
Major	Minor
Carditis	Fever
Polyarthritis	Arthralgia
Chorea	Previous rheumatic fever
Erythema marginatum	Positive acute-phase reactant (ESR, CRP) Leucocytosis
Subcutaneous nodules	Prolonged P-R interval on ECG

Fig. 13.8 Modified Duckett Jones criteria for diagnosis of rheumatic fever.

- Steroids for severe carditis.
- Diuretics and ACE inhibitors for heart failure.
- Antibiotics if there is evidence of persisting streptococcal infection.

Recurrent attacks should be prevented by prophylactic penicillin (given either orally or as monthly intramuscular injections of benzathine penicillin). Lifelong prophylaxis has been advocated.

Complications

Rheumatic valvular disease is the most common form of long-term damage, its severity increasing with the number of acute episodes. There is scarring and fibrosis of valve tissue, most commonly affecting the mitral valve.

CARDIAC INFECTIONS

These are uncommon and include:

- Infective endocarditis.
- Myocarditis.

Infective endocarditis

This may be defined as infection of the endocardium or endothelium of the great vessels. It is a cause of great morbidity and prevention in high-risk groups by using prophylactic antibiotics is essential.

All children with congenital heart disease are at risk of bacterial endocarditis.

Clinical features

Endocarditis should be suspected in any child with fever and a significant cardiac murmur. The clinical features are caused by:

- Bacteraemia: fever, malaise.
- Valvulitis: cardiac failure and murmurs.
- Immunological causes: glomerulonephritis.
- Embolic causes: CNS abscess, splinter haemorrhages.

Non-cardiac manifestations are less common in children than in adults.

Diagnosis

It is important to stress that endocarditis is a clinical and laboratory diagnosis.

- Blood cultures: at least three should be obtained in the first 24 hours of hospitalization. The causative organism—most commonly *Streptococcus viridans* (α-haemolytic streptococcus)—is identified in 90% of cases.
- Cross-sectional echocardiography: although this might confirm the diagnosis by the identification of vegetations, it cannot exclude it. Vegetations might persist after successful antibiotic treatment has been completed.
- Acute-phase reactants: elevated.

Management

Treatment comprises 4–6 weeks of intravenous antibiotics, e.g. high-dose ampicillin with an aminoglycoside. Surgical removal of infected prosthetic material might be required.

Antibiotic prophylaxis against infective endocarditis is essential for dental or surgical treatment in all children with congenital heart disease except osteum secundum defects.

Parents should be given adequate information about endocarditis prophylaxis at the time of diagnosis of the heart lesion, so that this does not get missed when the child has to undergo a minor procedure.

Myocarditis

This uncommon disease primarily affects infants and neonates. Coxsackie and echoviruses, as well as rubella, have been associated with myocarditis. It can present acutely with cardiovascular collapse or slowly with a gradual onset of congestive cardiac failure.

Treatment is supportive. Most children recover but some develop a chronic dilated cardiomyopathy.

CARDIAC ARRHYTHMIAS

Sinus arrhythmia is more pronounced in children and shows as an increase in heart rate during inspiration and slowing during expiration. Normal sinus rhythm can be up to 210 beats/min and premature atrial and ventricular contractions are common and benign.

Supraventricular tachycardia

The child has a heart rate >220/min and often is asymptomatic, although infants can develop cardiac failure. An accessory connection can be present in up to 95% of all young children and infants.

Clinical features

Most children are asymptomatic but infants might present with signs of cardiac failure, such as poor feeding, sweating and irritability. Older children might describe palpitations.

Diagnosis

The ECG usually shows a narrow complex tachycardia with P waves discernible after the QRS complex.

In sinus rhythm, the Wolff–Parkinson–White syndrome might be evident if there is an accessory bundle allowing premature activation of the ventricles. The PR interval is short and there is a wide QRS with slurred upstroke (delta wave).

Management

An acute episode can be terminated and sinus rhythm restored by:

- Vagal stimulation: applying an ice-cold compress to the face or carotid sinus massage.
- Intravenous adenosine: safe and effective.
- Synchronized DC cardioversion: if the above fail.

The prognosis is good in the majority of cases. Ninety per cent of children will have no further episodes after infancy (over 1 year old). Radiofrequency ablation of the bypass tract has been used for those with persistent, frequently recurring paroxysms.

Further reading

Ferrieri P et al. Unique features of endocarditis in childhood. *Pediatrics* 2002; **109**(5):931–944.

Johnson Jr WH, Moller JH. *Pediatric Cardiology*. Philadelphia: Lippincott Williams & Wilkins, 2001.

Disorders of the respiratory system

Objectives

At the end of this chapter, you should be able to

- Understand the common upper respiratory tract infections in children.
- Understand the aetiology, clinical features and management of pneumonia in children.
- Identify the clinical features of bronchiolitis.
- Understand the aetiology, clinical features and management of chronic asthma.
- Outline the management of acute severe asthma in children.
- Understand the aetiology and clinical features of cystic fibrosis in children.

Respiratory tract infections are the most common infections of childhood and range from trivial to life-threatening illnesses; 90% of these infections are caused by viruses. They are classified into upper respiratory tract infections (URTIs) and lower respiratory tract infections (LRTIs). The other common and important diseases of this system are asthma and cystic fibrosis.

Children are more susceptible to respiratory tract infections than adults for many reasons:

- Chest wall is more compliant than that of an adult.
- Fatiguability of respiratory muscles.
- Increased mucous gland concentration.
- Poor collateral ventilation.
- Low chest wall elastic recoil.

Parental smoking should be discouraged because passive smoking worsens symptoms of all respiratory disease.

UPPER RESPIRATORY TRACT INFECTIONS

The upper respiratory tract comprises the ears, nose, throat, tonsils, pharynx and sinuses, together with the extrathoracic airways.

The common cold (acute nasopharyngitis)

This is a viral infection causing a clear or mucopurulent nasal discharge (coryza), cough, fever and malaise. Although over 200 viral types are known, 25–40% of colds are caused by rhinoviruses. Symptomatic treatment (e.g. paracetamol) is all that is required for this self-limiting illness as no known treatment affects clinical outcome. Young infants, who are obligate nose-breathers, might experience feeding difficulties.

Sore throat (pharyngitis and tonsillitis)

These are commonly viral, especially in the under 3 year olds, but might also be caused by group A β-haemolytic streptococci. Children present with a sore throat, fever and constitutional upset. It is very difficult to distinguish viral and bacterial infection clinically. However, a purulent exudate, lymphadenopathy and severe pain suggest a bacterial cause.

Treatment

Most treatment is symptomatic as there is no evidence that antibiotics prevent complications.

Complications

These include:

- Retropharyngeal abscess.
- Peritonsillar abscess (quinsy).

- Post-streptococcal glomerulonephritis or rheumatic fever.

Tonsillectomy is now less commonly performed than it used to be. Indications include recurrent tonsillitis, quinsy or obstructive sleep apnoea.

Acute otitis media

The cause of this can be viral—e.g. respiratory syncytial virus (RSV) influenza—or bacterial (*Pneumococcus* species, *Haemophilus influenzae*, group B streptococci, *Moraxella catarrhalis*). It is very common in preschool children, who present with fever, vomiting and distress. It is important to examine the eardrums in any ill and febrile toddler, as only older children will localize the pain to the ear.

Clinical features

Examination reveals a red eardrum with loss of the light reflex. The eardrum might bulge and perforation might occur, with a purulent discharge.

Management

Symptomatic treatment is usually all that is needed; amoxicillin can reduce symptoms but not complications.

Recurrent infections are associated with otitis media with effusion. Mastoiditis and meningitis are now uncommon complications of acute otitis media.

Otitis media with effusion (OME, secretory otitis media, glue ear)

In young children who are prone to recurrent upper respiratory tract infections, it is common for the middle ear fluid to persist (an effusion), causing a conductive hearing loss and an increased susceptibility to re-infection. An effusion can also occur without a history of acute infections and is probably due to poor Eustachian tube ventilation due to enlarged adenoids or allergy. The effusion and resulting hearing impairment is often transient but, if it is persistent, it can be an indication for surgical drainage of the middle ear with grommet insertion. A grommet is a hollow plastic tube that ventilates the middle ear and remains effective only while patent. Ultimately it is extruded from the tympanic membrane. Decongestants and antibiotics are widely used but have unproven value. A low-power hearing aid might be required.

Obstructive sleep apnoea (OSA)

This is increasingly recognized in children. There is usually a history of snoring and associated apnoea. It can be associated with failure to thrive, daytime somnolence, behavioural problems and poor school performance. Long-term complications include cor pulmonale. Gold standard diagnosis is by polysomnography. Children at high risk of OSA include those with craniofacial abnormalities. Treatment is by adenotonsillectomy with nocturnal continuous positive airway pressure (CPAP) if there is no improvement with surgery.

Croup

Croup, or viral laryngotracheobronchitis, is most commonly caused by the parainfluenza virus. It has a peak incidence in winter in the second year of life.

Clinical features

Symptoms of upper respiratory tract infection (coryza, fever) are usually present for a day or two before the onset of a characteristic barking ('sea lion') cough and stridor (which is caused by subglottic inflammation and oedema). Symptoms typically start, and are worse, at night.

Management

Most children are mildly affected and improve spontaneously within 24 hours. Management at home is symptomatic and duration of symptoms 3 days. About 1 in 10 children require hospitalization because of:

- More severe illness.
- Young age (under 12 months).
- Signs of dehydration and fatigue or respiratory failure.

There is evidence that a single dose of dexamethasone 0.15 mg/kg or nebulized budesonide 2 mg has a beneficial effect in croup. This should be used if stridor is present. Humidifiers and steam therapy are ineffective.

Nebulized adrenaline provides transient improvement by constricting local blood vessels and reducing swelling and oedema. It should be given only under close supervision in hospital where it can provide rapid, if transient, relief of airway obstruction, allowing time for transfer to the intensive therapy unit (ITU) and intubation in a child with severe airways obstruction.

Diphtheria

This potentially fatal and highly infectious disease is caused by a toxin produced by *Corynebacterium diphtheriae*. In the UK, this scourge of childhood has been eliminated by an effective immunization programme, but it remains endemic in some countries and imported cases occur.

Acute epiglottitis

Acute bacterial epiglottitis is an uncommon life-threatening emergency caused by infection with *Haemophilus influenzae* type B. It has become rare since the introduction of Hib immunization. It is most common in children aged 1–6 years.

Clinical features

The onset is rapid over a few hours with the development of an intensely painful throat. The characteristic picture is of an ill, toxic, febrile child who is unable to speak or swallow, with a muffled voice and soft inspiratory stridor. The child tends to sit upright with an open mouth to maximize the airway, and might drool saliva.

Management

It is vital to distinguish this illness from viral croup because the management is different:

- Minutes count if death is to be avoided.
- Urgent hospital admission should be arranged.
- No attempt should be made to lie the child down, to examine the throat with a spatula or to take blood, as these manoeuvres can precipitate total airway obstruction and death.

Examination under anaesthetic should be arranged without delay (preferably in the presence of a senior anaesthetist, paediatrician and ENT surgeon) to allow confirmation of the diagnosis, followed by intubation. Once the airway is secured, blood should be taken for culture and intravenous antibiotics started using a third-generation cephalosporin, e.g.

cefuroxime. Intubation is not usually required for longer than 48 hours.

Do not examine the throat if epiglottitis is suspected: complete airway obstruction might be provoked.

LOWER RESPIRATORY TRACT INFECTIONS

A minority of infections involve the lower respiratory tract, but these are more likely to be serious than infections of the upper respiratory tract and are more common in infants. Causative agents include viruses and bacteria. They vary with the child's age and the site of infection. Infection can occur by direct spread from airway epithelium or via the bloodstream.

A number of well-defined clinical syndromes (determined by the predominant anatomical site of inflammation) are recognized (e.g. bronchiolitis and pneumonia) and often provide a clue to the likely pathogen. The term 'chest infection' should be avoided. The hallmarks of a lower respiratory tract infection are apparent on inspection (Fig. 14.1).

Pneumonia

Pneumonia is characterized by inflammation of the lung parenchyma with consolidation of alveoli. It can be caused by a wide range of pathogens and different organisms affect different age groups (Fig. 14.2).

Clinical features

Usually, following an URTI the patient develops worsening fever, cough and breathlessness. Tachypnoea is a key sign. The classic signs of consolidation (dullness to percussion, decreased breath sounds and bronchial breathing) might be present but they are difficult to detect in infants; crackles might also be present. In bacterial pneumonia, pleural inflammation causing chest (or abdominal pain) and an effusion more commonly develops.

Fig. 14.1 Signs of lower respiratory tract infection in the infant.

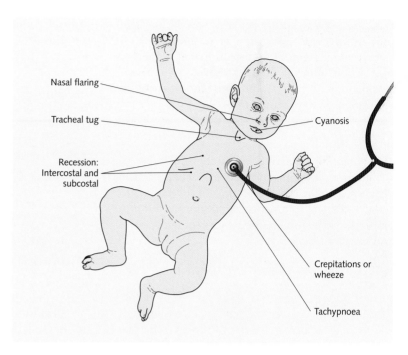

Nasal flaring

Tracheal tug

Cyanosis

Recession:
Intercostal and
subcostal

Crepitations or
wheeze

Tachypnoea

Pathogens causing pneumonia in infants and children	
Age	**Pathogens**
Neonates (<1 month)	Group B streptococci *E. coli* *Chlamydia trachomatis*
Infants	Respiratory viruses, e.g. RSV, adenovirus *Streptococcus pneumoniae* *Haemophilus influenzae* *Bordetella pertussis*
Children	*Streptococcus pneumoniae* *Haemophilus influenzae* Group A streptococci *Mycoplasma pneumonia*

Fig. 14.2 Pathogens causing pneumonia in infants and children.

Diagnosis

Diagnosis is largely clinical but a chest X-ray (CXR) is indicated if severe or complications suspected. A full blood count (FBC), C-reactive protein, blood culture and nasopharyngeal aspirate for viral isolation and PCR should be carried out in hospitalized children. Blood cultures positive in just 10% of cases; addition of NPA for culture and PCR increase yield of causative organisms up to 30%.

It is often difficult to distinguish between viral and bacterial infections clinically. Young children and babies are not good providers of sputum and definitive diagnosis of bacterial infection remains difficult. However, the following all suggest bacterial pneumonia:

- Polymorphonuclear leucocytosis.
- Lobar consolidation (Fig. 14.3).
- Pleural effusion.

Mycoplasma infection can be diagnosed reliably by acute and convalescent serology or by demonstration of cold agglutinins.

Management

Antibiotics are usually given if a diagnosis of bacterial pneumonia is made, the choice is dictated by the child's age and the severity of illness (e.g. toxic or requires O_2):

- Penicillin is first line in most children.
- Cefuroxime and flucloxacillin is indicated in severe illness.
- If mycoplasma is suspected, a macrolide antibiotic should be given.

Rarely, pneumonia can be complicated by empyema, this should be evaluated by ultrasound and initially needs drainage via a small bore chest drain or if

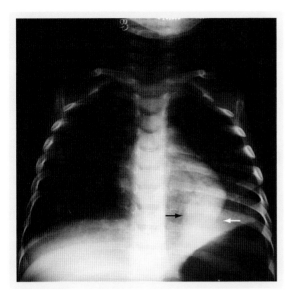

Fig. 14.3 CXR of lobar pneumonia. Consolidation is seen in the lower left lobe obscuring the left hemidiaphragm.

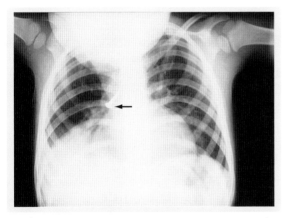

Fig. 14.4 CXR of an inhaled foreign object. Nail seen in the right intermediate bronchus with distal collapse of right middle and lower lobes.

necessary may require surgery. Recurrent or persistent pneumonia should raise the possibility of an inhaled foreign object (Fig. 14.4), or congenital abnormality of the lung, cystic fibrosis or tuberculosis.

Bronchiolitis

This common condition is caused by a viral infection mainly RSV. Annual winter epidemics occur in babies aged 1–9 months and many will be hospitalized. The infection causes an inflammatory response, predominantly in the bronchioles, hence the name.

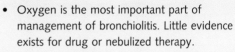

- Bronchiolitis is a common and severe infection in infants in the winter months.
- Oxygen is the most important part of management of bronchiolitis. Little evidence exists for drug or nebulized therapy.

Clinical features

Coryzal symptoms are followed by a cough with increasing breathlessness and associated difficulty in breathing. Small infants might develop apnoeic episodes. Ex-preterm infants with chronic lung disease and infants with congenital heart disease are at particular risk of being severely affected. Examination reveals:

- Tachypnoea.
- Subcostal and intercostal recession.
- Chest hyperinflation.
- Bilateral fine crackles.
- Wheeze on auscultation.

Infants at high risk of developing severe disease complicated by apnoeic episodes or respiratory failure include:

- Preterm infants.
- Infants under 6 weeks of age.
- Infants with chronic lung disease (e.g. cystic fibrosis, bronchopulmonary dysplasia).
- Infants with congenital heart disease.

Diagnosis

The CXR, if taken, usually shows hyperinflation of the lungs. The virus can be detected by immunofluorescence and cultured on a nasopharyngeal aspirate.

Management

Management is supportive with attention to treating hypoxia and maintaining hydration (Fig. 14.5). Breathing (apnoea monitor), heart rate and oxygen saturation (pulse oximeter) are monitored. Oxygen is the mainstay of treatment and is given via nasal cannulae or humidified via a head-box. Some infants might be well enough to continue oral feeds but most require fluids to be given either by

Management of bronchiolitis	
Mild	Feeding well Respiratory rate <40/min Minimal intercostal recession S_pO_2 >92% in air Manage at home—regular review
Moderate	Difficulty feeding Moderate tachypnoea—rate >40/min Marked intercostal recession S_pO_2 <92% in air Admit to hospital O_2 via nasal cannulae or head box Fluids intravenously or nasogastrically
Severe	Tachypnoea—rate >60/min Recurrent apnoea Severe recession Hypoxia in air—saturation <92% Admit to ICU or high-dependency area High inspired O_2 Intubation and assistive ventilation for Respiratory failure or recurrent severe apnoea IV fluids

Fig. 14.5 Management of bronchiolitis.

nasogastric tube or intravenously. A minority of hospitalized infants require assisted ventilation (only 1–2%). Secondary bacterial infection might occur (<1%), in which case antibiotic therapy is appropriate.

For high-risk infants, a monoclonal antibody (Palivizumab) can be given in the winter months to reduce severity.

Complications

Although most infants make a full recovery within 2 weeks, some—especially those hospitalized—have recurrent episodes of cough and wheeze over the subsequent few years. It is known that a subset of these infants will develop asthma.

Whooping cough (pertussis)

Whooping cough or pertussis is a highly contagious clinical syndrome caused by a number of pathogens, most commonly *Bordetella pertussis*. It is endemic, with epidemics occurring every 4 years. An effective vaccine exists and is a component of the routine triple vaccine containing diphtheria, tetanus and pertussis (DTP).

Whooping cough is spread by droplet infection and has an incubation period of 7–10 days. A case is infectious from 7 days after exposure to 3 weeks after the onset of the paroxysmal cough.

- Whooping cough is most dangerous to very young infants.
- Vaccination is given early to confer protection on this vulnerable group.

Clinical features

The clinical course can be divided into catarrhal, paroxysmal and convalescent stages.

During a paroxysm of coughing (which are often worse at night) the child might go blue and vomit. The inspiratory whoop can be absent in infants. Nosebleeds and subconjunctival haemorrhage can occur after vigorous coughing. Symptoms can persist for 3 months (the '100-day' cough).

Complications

Complications, including pneumonia, convulsions, apnoea, bronchiectasis and death, are more common in infants under 6 months of age.

Diagnosis

A marked lymphocytosis (>15.0 × 10^9/L) is characteristic and the organism can be cultured from a pernasal swab or PCR early in the disease.

Treatment

Erythromycin given early in the disease eradicates the organism and reduces infectivity but does not shorten the duration of the disease.

ASTHMA

Asthma is a chronic inflammatory disorder of the airways associated with widespread variable airflow obstruction and an increase in airways resistance in response to a variety of stimuli. The symptoms are reversible spontaneously or with treatment.

Asthma is the most common chronic respiratory disorder of childhood with a prevalence of 15% in the UK. It has increased in prevalence in the last decade and is twice as common in boys as girls.

Aetiology

Asthma is associated with a number of risk factors.

- Family history or co-existent atopy.
- Male sex.
- Parental smoking.
- Hospitalized for bronchiolitis in infancy.
- Preterm birth.

Pathophysiology

The pathophysiology of airway narrowing in asthma includes chronic inflammation of the bronchial mucosa associated with mucosal oedema, secretions, and the constriction of airway smooth muscle (Fig. 14.6).

In children there are many different patterns of asthma. In the infant age group there are many infants that have recurrent wheeze due to having underlying small airways, their symptoms improving as the airway grows. There is an association of small airways with exposure to antenatal smoking. These infants may not have the typical inflammatory changes we associate with asthma and often wheeze just with viral infections.

Diagnosis

A working practical definition is a child with recurrent cough and wheeze in a clinical setting where asthma is likely (e.g. atopy, family history of asthma) and in whom other—rarer—causes (e.g. suppurative lung disease) have been excluded.

In most children, a careful history and examination should distinguish those with asthma. Evidence of bronchial hyperreactivity by pulmonary function testing is difficult in young children, although children over 7 years might be able to perform spirometry, which can support a diagnosis of asthma. In younger children a response to treatment with recurrence of symptoms on discontinuing treatment supports the diagnosis.

Conditions that need to be distinguished from asthma are shown in Fig. 14.7.

History

Enquiry should be made concerning the pattern of symptoms (episodic or persistent), a family history

Fig. 14.6 Factors in the pathogenesis of asthma.

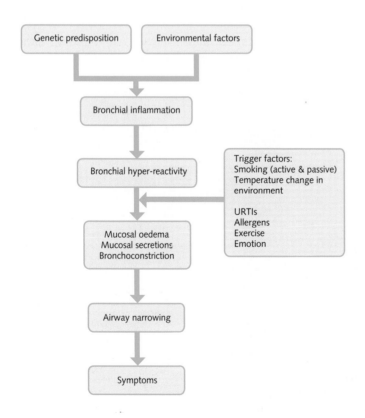

of asthma, trigger factors and those features that allow the clinical evaluation of severity (exercise tolerance, night-time disturbance, school absence). A full history should cover the differential diagnosis, e.g. growth, infections, gastrointestinal symptoms.

There are distinct patterns of asthma in childhood (Fig. 14.8).

Examination

Auscultation of the chest is usually normal between attacks. Chronic, severe asthma is associated with thoracic deformity:

- Hyperexpansion.
- Pigeon chest (pectus carinatum).
- Harrison sulcus.

Differential diagnosis of asthma	
	Clues
Cystic fibrosis	Failure to thrive, productive cough and finger clubbing
Gastro-oesophageal reflux	Excessive vomiting
Central airways disease	Inspiratory stridor with wheeze
Laryngeal problems	Abnormal voice
Inhaled foreign body	Sudden onset
Postviral wheeze	Recent respiratory infection in 2 years age

Fig. 14.7 Differential diagnosis of asthma.

Investigations

A plain CXR can be useful at initial presentation. In children aged over 5 years, the peak expiratory flow rate (PEFR) can aid diagnosis if the child can carry this out reliably. Significant diurnal variability or decrease after exercise suggests bronchial hyperreactivity. Spirometry in older children might demonstrate reversible airways obstruction. However, in the majority of children a diagnosis is made without lung function testing because this is too difficult to measure in young children; instead, an assessment of the child's response to a treatment is performed.

Allergy tests might indicate evidence of atopy, which is associated with asthma, but 50% of asthmatics are non-atopic.

Differential diagnosis

The differential diagnosis includes several important acute and chronic conditions. It must be remembered that 'all that wheezes is not asthma'. Alternative diagnoses are listed in Fig. 14.7.

Management

The aim of asthma treatment is to control symptoms and prevent exacerbations, optimize lung function and keep the side-effects of medication to a minimum. Important ways of achieving these goals are:

Asthma: patterns			
	Infrequent episodic	Frequent episodic	Persistent episodic
Proportion affected	Most common: 75% of all asthmatics	20%	5%
Clinical features	Triggered by viral URTIs Normal lung function and examination	Exacerbations more severe but mild interval symptoms, especially exercise induced Abnormal lung function when symptomatic	Daily symptoms and use of bronchodilators Abnormal lung function
Management step	Treat with intermittent bronchodilators and short course of oral steroids for severe exacerbations Step I	Treat with inhaled steroids ± add on therapy Step 2–3	Treat with inhaled steroid with add on therapy Need specialist advice (Step 4–5)
Prognosis	40% will remain symptomatic in adulthood	70% remain symptomatic in adulthood	90% remain symptomatic in adulthood

Fig. 14.8 Asthma: patterns.

- An education and management plan for child and carers (The Asthma UK is a useful source of information).
- Establishing the minimal effective dose of preventer medication, especially steroids.
- An age-appropriate delivery device.
- Accurate diagnosis and assessment of severity, with regular review.
- Avoiding triggers.

There is a colour code for asthma drug inhaler devices:
- 'Preventers' are mostly brown, e.g. inhaled steroid. Other colours are purple, red, green and orange.
- 'Relievers' are blue, e.g. inhaled salbutamol.

Triggers of asthma

Although the evidence for allergy avoidance is poor, skin-prick testing or specific IgE might identify allergens and a trial of avoidance may be indicated

Parents and the child must be advised to avoid exposures that might worsen the asthma. Simple measures include frequent vacuuming, damp dusting and foam filling for duvets and pillows to remove house dust mite, removing pets from home and discouraging parental smoking inside the house. Food allergy is uncommon as a trigger in asthma.

Medication

The drugs used in the management of asthma in children can be classified into 'preventers' and 'relievers'.

A stepwise approach to treatment has been devised (British Guidelines for Asthma Management) and is summarized in Fig. 14.9. Patients should start treatment at the step most appropriate to the initial severity. Once control is achieved, treatment can be stepped down. A rescue course of oral

prednisolone might be needed at any step (under 1 year old: 1–2 mg/kg/day; 1–5 years: 20 mg/day; maximum dose 40 mg/day). In children with marked seasonal variation in asthma severity, the treatment should be varied according to the season.

Inhalation therapy is central to most asthma treatment. The basic systems available are considered in Figs 14.10 and 14.11.

The mode of action, indications for use and side effects of the most commonly used bronchodilator drugs are outlined in Fig. 14.12.

Steroid therapy in asthma

Glucocorticoids are key drugs in the management of asthma, both in prophylaxis and the treatment of acute attacks. They can be given:

- By inhalation.
- Orally.
- Intravenously: in acute asthma.

Which inhaler device for which patient?
- MDI: suitable only for competent older children (breath-activated MDIs are available and do not require such a high level of coordination).
- MDI and spacer: beneficial in all children and as effective as nebulizers if used correctly.
- DPI: children from age 5 years.

Stepwise management of chronic asthma in children	
Step 1	All asthmatic children should have an inhaled β₂ bronchodilator
Step 2 If requiring 2–3 times daily inhaled β₂ agonists	Add low-dose inhaled steroids
Step 3	Try adding on long-acting β agonists or leukotriene receptor antagonists before increasing steroid dose
Step 4 If increasing steroid dose ineffective	Consider: • Leukotriene receptor antagonists • Oral theophylline • High-dose inhaled steroids
Step 5	Alternate day oral steroids

Fig. 14.9 Stepwise management of chronic asthma in children.

Fig. 14.10 Administration of medication by inhalation.

Administration of medication by inhalation		
	Advantages	Disadvantages
Metered dose inhaler with spacer	Coordination not required Usable at all ages	Bulky
Dry powder inhaler (DPI)	Coordination unimportant Small and portable Easy to operate	Requires rapid inspiration Unsuitable for children <5 years
Nebulizer	Coordination unimportant Usable at all ages Effective in severe attack	Expensive, noisy, cumbersome Treatment takes a long time, >5 min Frightens some infants

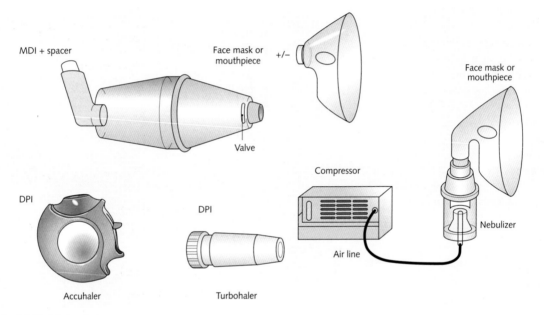

MDI + spacer

Face mask or mouthpiece +/–

Valve

DPI

Accuhaler

DPI

Turbohaler

Compressor

Air line

Face mask or mouthpiece

Nebulizer

Fig. 14.11 Inhaler devices.

Asthma drug therapy: mode of action, indications, and side effects of bronchodilators			
Relievers (bronchodilators)	Mode of action	Use	Side effects
Short-acting β_2 agonists, e.g. salbutamol, terbutaline	Smooth muscle relaxation	Relief of bronchospasm	Tachycardia Hypokalaemia Restlessness
Long-acting β_2 agonists, e.g. salmeterol	Smooth muscle relaxation	Nocturnal asthma, exercise-induced asthma Trial alternative to high-dose inhaled steroids	
Theophylline	Phosphodiesterase inhibition	Oral theophylline for nocturnal asthma IV aminophylline in acute severe asthma	Restlessness Diuresis Cardiac arrhythmias
Anticholinergics, e.g. ipratropium bromide	Inhibit cholinergic bronchoconstriction; add on to β_2 agonists in acute attack	First-line bronchodilator in infants	Dry mouth Urinary retention

Fig. 14.12 Asthma drug therapy: mode of action, indications and side effects of bronchodilators.

Inhaled steroids

Inhaled steroids are now the 'preventers' of choice in the management of childhood asthma. The lowest dose that achieves control should be used. They are indicated in frequent interval symptoms, nocturnal asthma, poor lung function tests and if using bronchodilator more than 3 times a week as rescue treatment. Inhaled steroids:

- Inhibit synthesis of inflammatory mediators (cytokines, leukotrienes and prostaglandins).
- Reduce airway hyperresponsiveness.
- Reduce both the symptoms and frequency of attacks.
- Prevent irreversible airway narrowing.

Local side effects, such as oral thrush or dysphonia, are uncommon. Ninety per cent of the dose is deposited in the mouth and pharynx, but this can be reduced by the use of a spacer (with metered-dose inhalers; MDIs) and mouth washing (with dry powder inhalers; DPIs). High doses (>800 µg) are associated with decreased growth and adrenal suppression, and children taking inhaled steroids must have their height monitored closely.

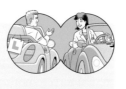

Parents and sometimes children are anxious about the adverse effects of long-term inhaled steroids. Since the dose is low and is targeted at the lungs, systemic absorption is less and therefore systemic adverse effects are rare. While transient growth failure can occur, there is good evidence that the final height is not affected. In any case, asthma itself can lead to growth failure, which is probably worse than that due to steroids. Steroids can cause adrenal failure, but this is again rare unless high doses are used.

Long-acting β₂ agonists

This class of inhaled drug can be used as an add-on therapy in children over 4 years if control is poor with low-dose inhaled steroids. New combination inhaled steroid and long-acting β₂ agonists are available.

Leucotriene receptor antagonists

This is a new class of oral drug and can be used as an add-on therapy from 6 months.

Theophylline

This oral drug can be used in difficult to treat asthma but its use is limited by side effects.

Oral steroids

Prednisolone as a single daily dose is the drug of choice. Short courses (3 days) are indicated for acute exacerbations. Regular oral steroids are indicated only for the most severe asthma that cannot be controlled with high-dose inhaled steroids and regular bronchodilators. Alternative day dosage is preferred to reduce systemic side effects.

Acute severe asthma

This is considered in more detail in Chapter 26. Features of acute severe asthma include:

- Respiratory rate >50 breaths/min.
- Pulse >140 beats/min.
- Use of accessory muscles.
- Too breathless to talk.

Life-threatening features include:

- Cyanosis.
- Silent chest (insufficient airflow to generate wheeze).
- Exhaustion, poor respiratory effort.
- Agitation, diminished consciousness (indicate hypoxia).

Immediate management

- High-flow O_2 via facemask.
- Salbutamol (2.5–5.0 mg) or terbutaline (5.0–10.0 mg) via an oxygen-driven nebulizer.
- Prednisolone orally or IV hydrocortisone.
- Pulse oximetry: O_2 saturation <92% in air indicates need for hospitalization.

If life-threatening features (or poor response):

- Intravenous aminophylline or intravenous salbutamol.
- Intravenous hydrocortisone.
- Add ipratropium bromide to nebulized β₂-agonist.

Prognosis of asthma

Most children with asthma improve as they get older (Fig. 14.8). Prognosis is better with earlier age at diagnosis. Children with poor pulmonary function testing and frequent wheezy episodes are associated with recurrent wheeze in adulthood.

CYSTIC FIBROSIS

Incidence and aetiology

Cystic fibrosis (CF) is the most common lethal genetic disease in Caucasian people. It has a carrier rate of 1 : 25 and incidence of 1 : 2500 live births. CF is an autosomal recessive disease arising from mutations in a gene on chromosome 7 that encodes an ATP-binding cassette (ABC) transporter, the cystic fibrosis transmembrane regulator (CFTR) protein. The most common mutation is a three base-pair deletion that removes the phenylalanine at position 508 (ΔF508). This is found in 90% of disease chromosomes, but 1200 mutations have now been identified so far.

The mutations in the CFTR result in defective chloride ion transport across epithelial cells and increased viscosity of secretions, especially in the respiratory tract and exocrine pancreas. This predisposes to recurrent chest infections and pancreatic insufficiency. In addition, abnormal transport in sweat gland epithelium results in high concentrations of sodium and chloride in sweat, which form the basis of the most useful diagnostic test, the sweat test.

Clinical features

Cystic fibrosis should be considered in any child with recurrent chest infection and failure to thrive. Viscid mucus in the small airways predisposes to infection with *Staphylococcus aureus*, *Haemophilus influenzae* and *Pseudomonas* species. Repeated infection leads to bronchial wall damage with bronchiectasis and abscess formation.

There is a cough productive of purulent sputum and on examination there might be:

- Hyperinflation.
- Crepitations.
- Wheeze.
- Finger clubbing.

An example of typical chest X-ray changes is shown in Fig. 14.13.

In most children, deficiency of pancreatic enzymes (protease, amylase and lipase) results in malabsorption, steatorrhoea and failure to thrive. Stools are pale, greasy and offensive. About 10% of infants with CF present with 'meconium ileus' in the

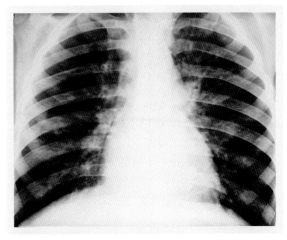

Fig. 14.13 Typical CXR of a child with cystic fibrosis, showing bilateral severe lung pathology: hyperinflated lungs with bronchial wall thickening.

neonatal period, in which inspissated meconium causes internal obstruction.

Diagnosis

The gold-standard diagnostic test is the sweat test, using pilocarpine iontophoresis. Failure of the normal reabsorption of sodium and chloride by the sweat duct epithelium leads to abnormally salty sweat: chloride concentrations of 60–125 mmol/L are found (the normal value is <15 mmol/L). Two sweat tests showing a chloride of >60 mmol/L confirm CF.

A CF genotype using DNA analysis is also available for the more common mutations and can help confirm a diagnosis.

Management

Cystic fibrosis is a multisystem disease (Fig. 14.14) and management requires a multidisciplinary approach, which is delivered most effectively by a specialist centre. The main aims are to:

- Prevent progression of lung disease.
- Promote adequate nutrition and growth.

A team approach is required, involving paediatricians with an interest in CF, physiotherapists, dieticians, CF nurses, community nurses, the primary care team and last—but not least—the child's parents or carers. The Cystic Fibrosis Trust plays an extremely important role in supporting families.

Multisystem aspects of cystic fibrosis	
Non-Pulmonary aspects of CF	
Airway Gastrointestinal	Nasal polyps Distal ileal obstruction syndrome
Pancreas/endocrine	Cystic fibrosis and diabetes Poor growth Osteoporosis
Reproductive	Infertility in males from absent vas deferens
Joints	Arthropathy
Vascular	Vasculitis
Hepatic Psychological	Portal hypertension

Fig. 14.14 Multisystem aspects of cystic fibrosis.

Cornerstones of CF treatment are:
- Aggressive treatment and prevention of infection.
- Effective mucociliary clearance.
- Nutritional support.
- Exercise.

Respiratory management

Physiotherapy (chest percussion with postural drainage, breathing exercises, positive expiratory pressure (PEP) masks and flutter devices) is the mainstay of respiratory management. Many centres recommend continuous prophylactic antibiotics with oral flucloxacillin in the first 2 years of life and, if children are colonized with *Pseudomonas*, antipseudomonal nebulized antibiotics. Acute exacerbations require vigorous treatment, with oral or if needed IV antibiotics directed against the common bacterial pathogens (*Haemophilus influenzae*, *Staphylococcus aureus* and *Pseudomonas aeruginosa*) and guided by recent sputum culture results if available. Use of indwelling vascular devices (e.g. Port-A-Cath) aid regular intravenous antibiotic courses.

Mucolytics such as nebulized DNase or hypertonic saline to reduce sputum viscosity can help mucociliary clearance.

Nutritional management

The combined threats of malabsorption due to pancreatic insufficiency, poor appetite, increased metabolism due to chronic infection and increased respiratory work render nutritional management of vital importance in CF. The following supplements can be given:

- A high-calorie diet with vitamin supplements, especially fat-soluble vitamins A, D, E and K. Oral high calorie diet alone may be inadequate in many children and enteral feeding via a gastrostomy is often needed in older patients.
- Pancreatic enzyme supplementation using enteric-coated microspheres in gelatin-coated capsules (e.g. Creon), which contain amylase, lipase and protease. This usually has a marked effect on steatorrhoea and allows 'catch-up' growth.

Prognosis

The median survival in the UK in the 1990s was 40 years, and this will hopefully improve further. Lung transplantation for some patients is an option but lack of donors mean its role is limited.

Genetic screening

Isolation of the CF gene and identification of the common mutations has made it technically possible to screen newborns for CF. Newborn screening is now UK wide using a method measuring immunoreactive trypsin (IRT), DNA analysis and, if needed, a second IRT. The aim of screening in CF is to pick up children severely affected, limit identifying those mildly affected and avoid picking up carriers. Early treatment benefits the prognosis of CF patients and aids reproductive decision making for the parents.

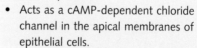

The CFTR protein:
- Acts as a cAMP-dependent chloride channel in the apical membranes of epithelial cells.
- Is composed of 1480 amino acid residues.
- Contains functional domains including membrane-spanning regions, ATP-binding domains, and a regulatory domain.
- Is an ATP-binding cassette (ABC) transporter.

Mutations in the CFTR gene:
- The ΔF508 mutation is found on 90% of CF chromosomes in the UK.
- A three base-pair deletion causes the loss of the phenylalanine (F) at residue number 508.
- 1200 mutations have now been reported in the CFTR gene, but few of these occur at a worldwide frequency of more than 1%.

Further reading

British Guideline on the Management Of Asthma. *Thorax* 2003; **58**:Suppl 1.

British Thoracic Guideline on Childhood Community Acquired Pneumonia. *Thorax* 2002; **57**:1–24.

Cystic Fibrosis UK Screening programme: www.ich.ucl.uk/newborn/cf/index/htm

King VJ et al. Pharmacologic treatment of bronchiolitis in infants and children: a systematic review. *Archives of Pediatric and Adolescent Medicine* 2004; **158**:127–137.

Spencer H, Jaffe A. Newer therapies for cystic fibrosis. *Current Paediatrics* 2003; **13**:259–263.

Disorders of the gastrointestinal system

Objectives

At the end of this chapter, you should be able to

- Identify the common causes of vomiting in children.
- Recognize dehydration in a child with diarrhoeal illness and calculate the fluid requirements.
- Understand some of the common surgical conditions involving the gastrointestinal tract.
- Understand the pathology and clinical features of inflammatory bowel disease.

Both medical and surgical disorders of the gastrointestinal tract are common in paediatric practice. At least 5 million young children die each year from diarrhoeal diseases.

The range of pathological processes affecting the gastrointestinal tract is broad. It includes:

- Congenital abnormalities.
- Infection.
- Immune-mediated allergy or inflammation.

Inconsolable crying in an infant, consider:

- Colic.
- Otitis media.
- Incarcerated hernia.
- Urinary tract infection.
- Anal fissure.
- Intussusception.

INFANTILE COLIC

This is a common syndrome characterized by recurrent inconsolable crying or screaming accompanied by drawing up of the legs during the first few months of life, usually beginning around 2 weeks and resolving by 4 months of age. It can occur several times a day, particularly in the evening.

Diagnosis

The differential diagnosis of inconsolable screaming includes some important conditions. Occasionally 'colic' may be due to cow's milk protein intolerance or gastro-oesophageal reflux.

Treatment and prognosis

The condition is benign and has a good prognosis, although it might provoke non-accidental injury in infants at risk. Sympathetic counselling is important. There is no evidence that any medical intervention is effective.

GASTRO-OESOPHAGEAL REFLUX

The involuntary passage of gastric contents into the oesophagus is a common problem, especially in babies during the first year of life. Functional immaturity of the lower oesophageal sphincter, liquid milk rather than solid feeds and a supine posture are all contributory factors. It is a physiological finding in infancy.

Clinical features

Symptoms are usually mild (regurgitation/posseting) and no treatment is required. In a minority, however, symptoms are severe and complications such as failure to thrive, oesophagitis or recurrent aspiration pneumonia might occur.

Infants at risk of severe gastro-oesophageal reflux include:

- Preterm infants: especially those with chronic lung disease (bronchopulmonary dysplasia).
- Children with cerebral palsy.
- Infants with congenital oesophageal anomalies, e.g. after repair of a tracheo-oesophageal fistula.

The main symptom is recurrent regurgitation or vomiting. About 10% of infants with symptomatic reflux develop complications. Oesophagitis might be manifested by:

- Irritability.
- Features of pain after feeding.
- Blood in the vomit.
- Iron-deficiency anaemia.

Reflux can cause recurrent aspiration pneumonia, failure to thrive, cough, bronchospasm (with wheezing) and exacerbation of chronic lung conditions such as cystic fibrosis or bronchopulmonary dysplasia.

Diagnosis

Most reflux can be diagnosed clinically but several techniques are available for confirming the diagnosis and assessing the severity:

- 24-hour ambulatory oesophageal pH monitoring: gold standard in older children but less useful in infants and neonates.
- Barium studies: might be required to exclude underlying anatomical abnormalities.
- Endoscopy: indicated in patients with suspected oesophagitis.
- Nuclear medicine milk scan.

In the majority of mildly affected infants, reassurance and the early introduction of solids at 3 months are all that is required and 95% will resolve by the age of 18 months. Nursing the baby in a 30° prone position after feeds can help. More troublesome reflux might respond to an alginate and antacid combination (e.g. Gaviscon Infant) or thickening the feed with inert carob-based agents.

The following drugs can be used in more severe reflux:

- Prokinetic drugs such as domperidone: these speed gastric emptying and increase lower oesophageal sphincter pressure.
- Drugs to reduce gastric acid secretion (H_2 antagonists or proton pump inhibitors): especially if there is evidence of oesophagitis.

Surgery is required for very severe cases with complications. The most commonly used procedure is Nissen fundoplication in which the fundus of the stomach is wrapped around the lower oesophagus. This is commonly combined with a gastrostomy for feeding.

GASTROENTERITIS

Gastroenteritis is an infection of the gastrointestinal tract, usually viral, which presents with a combination of diarrhoea and vomiting (D&V).

Incidence and aetiology

In developed countries it is usually mild and self-limiting (affecting 1 in 10 children under the age of 2 years) but in the developing world approximately 5 million children under 5 years old die from gastroenteritis each year.

Rotavirus is the most common pathogen in the UK but gastroenteritis can also be caused by:

- Bacteria, including *Shigellae*, *Salmonellae* and *Campylobacter* species and *Escherichia coli*.
- Three parasites: *Entamoeba histolytica*, *Giardia lamblia* and *Cryptosporidium* species.

Clinical features

Viral infection can cause a prodromal illness followed by vomiting and diarrhoea:

- The vomiting might precede diarrhoea and is not usually stained with bile or blood.
- Abdominal pain and blood or mucus in the stool suggests an invasive bacterial pathogen.

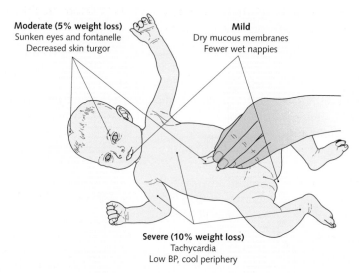

Fig. 15.1 Clinical features of dehydration.

Moderate (5% weight loss)
Sunken eyes and fontanelle
Decreased skin turgor

Mild
Dry mucous membranes
Fewer wet nappies

Severe (10% weight loss)
Tachycardia
Low BP, cool periphery

- The severity of diarrhoea can be underestimated if it pools in the large bowel or if very watery stool is mistaken for urine in the nappy.

On examination, the most important physical signs relate to the presence and severity of dehydration (Fig. 15.1). The high surface area to bodyweight ratio in babies and infants renders them susceptible to rapid derangement of fluid and electrolyte balance.

Diagnosis

The differential diagnosis includes at least two important surgical conditions:

- In young infants, especially boys (aged 2–12 weeks), vomiting might be due to pyloric stenosis. Stool output is reduced and visible peristalsis with a palpable pyloric mass might be evident.
- In older infants and toddlers (aged 1–2 years) intussusception presents with vomiting. Paroxysmal abdominal pain and the eventual passage of 'redcurrant jelly' stools should raise suspicion of this condition, which is lethal if overlooked.

Investigations should include:

- Measurement of the plasma urea and electrolytes if dehydrated.
- Stool culture and microscopy.
- Stool viral antigen detection.

Gastroenteritis, by definition, includes diarrhoea. It is important to look for other causes when a child presents with vomiting alone.

Dehydration can be further classified according to whether the plasma sodium concentration is normal, low (hyponatraemia) or high (hypernatraemia). This has a bearing on the fluids used for rehydration (see below).

Management

Rehydration

The key to management is rehydration with correction of the fluid and electrolyte imbalance. The strategy depends on the severity of dehydration.

It is important to emphasize the importance of oral rehydration. Unless the child has persistent vomiting, oral fluids is the best means for rehydration. Smaller, more frequent sips may be better tolerated and should be encouraged.

Mild dehydration

Oral rehydration solutions (ORS; e.g. Dioralyte, Rehidrat) are used. These contain dextrose to stimulate sodium and water reabsorption across the bowel wall.

Moderate to severe dehydration

Oral rehydration is still indicated if tolerated. IV rehydration should be reserved for those with vomiting or severe dehydration.

Early refeeding reduces duration of diarrhoeal illness caused by gastrointestinal infections. IV therapy is over-used.

If there are signs of circulatory failure, immediate resuscitation is achieved by intravenous administration of 10–20 mL/kg of 0.9% NaCl (normal saline). Further rehydration can usually be achieved satisfactorily with 5% dextrose/0.45% saline with KCl added at a concentration of 20–40 mmol/L.

The volume required in 24 hours is calculated from estimated deficit + maintenance + ongoing losses:

Deficit Deficit = % dehydration ÷ bodyweight in kg (1 kg = 1000 mL).

Maintenance Allow:

- 100 mL/kg/24 h for 0–10 kg bodyweight.
- 50 mL/kg/24 h for 10–20 kg bodyweight.
- 20 mL/kg/24 h for >20 kg bodyweight.

Ongoing losses

Estimate the volume of vomit and diarrhoea. Calculate the volume required as shown in the following example of a child weighing 10 kg with estimated 10% dehydration:

- Deficit = 10% of 10 kg = 1 kg = 1000 mL.
- Maintenance in 24 h = 100 mL/kg = 1000 mL.
- Total required in 24 h = 2000 mL.

1. Give IV 0.9% NaCl 20 mL/kg over 30 min = 200 mL.
2. Give 1800 mL 4% dextrose/0.18% NaCl over 24 h, i.e. IV infusion at 75 mL/h.

Medication

There is no role for antiemetic or antidiarrhoeal medication in gastroenteritis. Antibiotics are rarely indicated except for specific bacterial infections, such as invasive salmonellosis or severe *Campylobacter* infection, and amoebiasis or giardiasis.

PYLORIC STENOSIS

Pyloric stenosis is due to hypertrophy of the smooth muscle of the pylorus and is an important cause of vomiting in babies.

Incidence

Pyloric stenosis is five times more common in boys and is familial with multifactorial inheritance.

The incidence of pyloric stenosis is 1–5 per 1000 live births:

- It is more common in boys.
- It causes a metabolic alkalosis.
- Surgical treatment is by Ramstedt's procedure.

Clinical features

It presents with persistent, projectile non-bilious vomiting between 2 and 6 weeks of age (it does not occur in the newborn or beyond 3 months of age). The infant remains hungry and eager to feed after vomiting. Weight loss, constipation, mild jaundice and dehydration develop after a few days (Fig. 15.2).

Diagnosis

Diagnosis is clinical and made by palpation of the hypertrophied pylorus during a test feed. Peristaltic waves might be visible.

Ultrasound of the abdomen can confirm diagnosis, demonstrating the hypertrophied pylorus. In addition, a characteristic electrolyte disturbance develops with a hypochloraemic metabolic alkalosis (serum HCO_3^- elevated to 25–35 mEq/L). This is due to the loss of acidic gastric contents and the kidneys excreting hydrogen ions to maintain potassium.

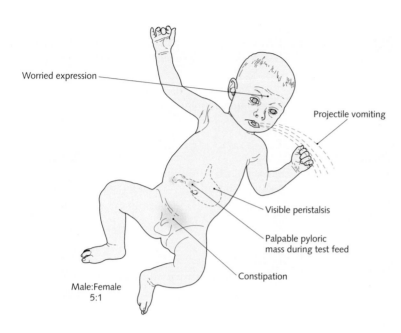

Fig. 15.2 Clinical features of pyloric stenosis.

Worried expression

Projectile vomiting

Visible peristalsis

Palpable pyloric
mass during test feed

Constipation

Male:Female
5:1

Management

Medical

Correction of fluid and electrolyte abnormalities is vital. In the presence of severe dehydration, a fluid bolus is needed. For maintenance, a fluid containing adequate chloride (such as half normal saline with 5% dextrose) is used, which will gradually correct the hypochloremic alkalosis.

Surgical

The definitive treatment is the Ramstedt's procedure, in which the hypertrophied pyloric musculature is divided.

INTUSSUSCEPTION

Intussusception is a condition in which one segment of bowel telescopes into an adjacent distal part of the bowel. It most commonly begins just proximal to the ileocaecal valve (ileum invaginates into caecum-ileocolic). The peak age is between 6 and 9 months, when the lead point is believed to be Peyer's patches that have been enlarged by a preceding viral infection. An anatomical lead point, such as a Meckel's diverticulum or polyp, is more likely to be present in an older child.

Clinical features

The classical presenting 'triad' is:

- Colicky abdominal pain.
- Vomiting.
- An abdominal mass.

The typical history is of episodes of screaming during which the infant draws up the legs and becomes pale. Vomiting occurs and the vomit might be bile-stained. As the blood supply to the bowel becomes progressively compromised, the characteristic 'redcurrant jelly' stool will be passed; this is a late sign.

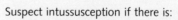

Suspect intussusception if there is:
- An infant aged 6–9 months.
- Paroxysmal colicky abdominal pain.
- Vomiting.
- 'Redcurrant jelly' stool.
- A 'sausage-shaped' mass in right upper quadrant.

Examination might reveal a 'sausage-shaped' mass formed by the intussusceptum, which is usually palpable in the right upper quadrant. Signs of intestinal obstruction and shock develop over 24–48 hours. Ultrasound is the imaging modality of choice.

Management

Intussusception is a life-threatening condition and can easily be misdiagnosed as gastroenteritis or colic by the unwary. If suspected, an immediate diagnostic enema using air or contrast material (barium or gastrograffin) should be carried out.

In most cases, reduction by air enema is possible, however if this is unsuccessful, operative reduction is necessary.

Enema and attempts at hydrostatic reduction are contraindicated if the history is long (24–48 hours) or if there are signs of intestinal obstruction, peritonitis, or shock.

MECKEL'S DIVERTICULUM

This remnant of the fetal vitello-intestinal duct occurs in 2% of the population. It is usually 2 inches (5 cm) long and found 2 feet (60 cm) proximal to the ileocaecal valve (the rule of 2's). It contains ectopic gastric mucosa. Diagnosis is by a technetium scan. The majority are asymptomatic but the most typical presentation is painless, severe rectal bleeding due to peptic ulceration. Treatment is surgical.

ACUTE APPENDICITIS

This important cause of acute abdominal pain occurs when the appendix becomes obstructed (usually by a faecolith) or inflamed by lymphatic hyperplasia. It occurs at any age, although it is rare in infants when the lumen of the appendix is wider and well drained.

Clinical features

The classic symptoms are a central abdominal pain that moves to the right iliac fossa (RIF) over a period of hours. The pain is of increasing severity and aggravated by movement (as the peritoneum is exquisitely pain sensitive).

Atypical presentations with poorly localized pain are common in young children (<5 years) or when the inflamed appendix is retrocaecal or pelvic.

Anorexia is usual and often associated with nausea and vomiting. Constipation might be a feature. Clinical signs include:

- Mild fever.
- Tachycardia.
- Dehydration.
- RIF tenderness.
- Guarding in a toxic child.

The differential diagnosis is shown in Fig. 15.3.

Diagnosis

The diagnosis is usually made clinically. If there is diagnostic uncertainty, useful investigations include:

- Urine: microscopy and culture.
- Full blood count (FBC).
- Chest X-ray (CXR): pneumonia can mimic appendicitis.
- Abdominal ultrasound.

Management

A short period of observation can be undertaken before appendicectomy when there is uncertainty, although progression to peritonitis can occur within a few hours in young children.

The differential diagnosis of acute abdominal pain	
Surgical	**Medical**
Appendicitis	Mesenteric adenitis
Intussusception	Gastroenteritis
Volvulus	Constipation
Meckel's diverticulum	UTI
Strangulated hernia	Lower lobe pneumonia
Ovarian torsion	Diabetic ketoacidosis
	Henoch–Schönlein purpura
	Sickle cell crisis

Fig. 15.3 The differential diagnosis of acute abdominal pain.

Other complications include septicaemia, appendix abscess and appendix mass. An abscess requires surgical drainage. Conservative management is given for an appendix mass with elective appendectomy carried out 6 weeks later.

MESENTERIC ADENITIS

This non-specific inflammation of mesenteric lymph nodes is thought to provoke a peritoneal reaction causing acute abdominal pain that mimics appendicitis.

Clinical features

It occurs commonly in children and is often associated with other systemic symptoms and signs including fever, headache, pharyngitis and cervical lymphadenopathy. It is likely to be viral in origin.

Diagnosis and management

Observation in hospital is often required due to the difficult diagnosis. Management is conservative, as the symptoms are self-limiting, although persisting right iliac fossa tenderness warrants surgical exploration to identify appendicitis.

COELIAC DISEASE

Incidence and aetiology

Coeliac disease arises from malabsorption caused by gluten-mediated immunological damage to the mucosa of the proximal small intestine with subsequent atrophy of the villi and loss of the absorptive surface. The incidence varies between 1 in 250 and 1 in 4000 live births, and appears to be increasing in some areas of the world.

There is a familial predisposition with 10% of first-degree relatives affected. There appear to be associations with HLA DQ2.

Clinical features

A few children present with failure to thrive following weaning when gluten-containing foods are introduced to the diet. Malabsorption of fat (steatorrhoea) occurs first, with bulky, light-coloured, offensive stools. On examination, there is:

- Poor weight gain.
- Abdominal distension.
- Buttock wasting.

The majority of cases present with more subtle problems such as:

- Diarrhoea.
- Transient poor weight gain.
- Irritability.
- Growth failure.
- Ataxia.
- Anaemia due to iron or folate deficiency: this is the most common symptom.

Diagnosis

Specific IgA antigliadin or antiendomysial antibodies are useful as a screening test. Definitive diagnosis requires the demonstration of a flat mucosa on jejunal biopsy followed by clinical improvement on dietary gluten withdrawal. A third biopsy on gluten challenge should be then taken to confirm the diagnosis.

Management

A diet free of gluten-containing products should be adhered to for life. Dietary supervision is required. Manufacturers use a special sign on packaging to indicate that food is gluten free.

Coeliac disease is associated with a variety of autoimmune disorders, including thyroid disease and pernicious anaemia, and the risk of small bowel malignancy (especially lymphoma) is increased 20-fold. A strict gluten-free diet might protect against this risk of malignancy and decrease the risk of autoimmune disease.

FOOD INTOLERANCE

Adverse reactions to specific foods or food ingredients are not uncommon and can be transitory or permanent. The majority are immune-mediated reactions, usually to proteins, and are properly referred to as food allergies. However, non-immune-mediated intolerance also occurs, e.g. lactose intolerance due to intestinal disaccharidase deficiency.

Transient dietary protein intolerances

These are more common in infants with a strong family history of atopy or IgA deficiency. They are most commonly manifested by protracted diarrhoea with or without vomiting and failure to thrive. However, allergy to specific proteins might also play a role in eczema and migraine and, occasionally, can cause acute anaphylaxis.

Intolerance to the following foods has been described:

- Cow's milk.
- Soya.
- Wheat.
- Fish, egg, chicken and rice.
- Nuts.

Diagnosis

Diagnosis is made when the symptoms are relieved by removal of specific foods or food constituents, and recur on reintroduction.

Management

Cow's milk protein intolerance, if severe, can cause a protein-losing enteropathy and blood loss. It is best managed with a casein-hydrolysate-based formula as up to 30% of infants will also be, or will become, intolerant to soya. Most patients grow out of their intolerance by the age of 2 years, which is therefore an appropriate time to conduct a dietary challenge.

Lactose intolerance

Lactose is the predominant disaccharide in milk and requires the intestinal brush-border enzyme lactase for its digestion. Lactase deficiency is most commonly encountered as a secondary and transient phenomenon after gastroenteritis. Congenital lactase deficiency is rare; hereditary late-onset lactose intolerance is predominantly seen in Afro-Carribean and oriental people.

Clinical features

Accumulation of intestinal sugar results in watery diarrhoea and bacterial production of organic acids, which lowers stool pH and causes excoriation of the perianal region.

Diagnosis

Lactose is a reducing sugar and may therefore be detected in the stool by the Clinitest method.

Treatment

Treatment is with a diet free of products containing lactose and milk.

INFLAMMATORY BOWEL DISEASE

Up to one-quarter of cases of inflammatory bowel disease have their onset during childhood or adolescence (Fig. 15.4).

Comparison of Crohn's disease with ulcerative colitis		
Feature	Crohn's disease	Ulcerative colitis
Colonic disease	50–75%	100%
Transmural involvement	Common	Unusual
Skip lesions	Common	Not present
Rectal bleeding	Sometimes	Common
Abdominal pain	Common	Variable
Abdominal mass	Common	Not present
Growth failure	Common	Variable
Perianal disease	Occasional	Unusual
Mouth ulceration	Common	Unusual
Toxic megacolon	Not present	Present

Fig. 15.4 Comparison of Crohn's disease with ulcerative colitis.

Crohn's disease

Crohn's disease, or regional enteritis, is a transmural and focal inflammatory process that can affect any portion of the gastrointestinal tract from the mouth to the anus; the distal ileum or the colon are most frequently involved. The cause is unknown, although there is a clear genetic predisposition. Affected intestine is thickened and non-caseating epithelioid cell granulomata are found on histology.

Ulcerative colitis

Ulcerative colitis is a chronic, recurrent inflammatory disease involving the mucous membrane of the colon. The disease process is restricted to the mucosa and begins in the rectum, extending proximally.

Clinical features of inflammatory bowel disease

It presents with:

- Cramping lower abdominal pain.
- Bloody diarrhoea.
- Weight loss/failure to thrive.

Extra intestinal features might be present, including growth retardation, delayed puberty, arthritis, spondylitis and erythema nodosum.

Management

Crohn's disease is managed initially by dietary measures with steroids for active relapse. Elemental diets are as effective as steroids but without the side effects. Immunosuppressives are the next line and new therapies such as anti-TNF antibodies are under evaluation. Surgery remains an option for failure of medical treatment.

Ulcerative colitis is treated with the aminosalicylates with steroids reserved for active disease. Surgery is curative but requires a colectomy. The role of probiotics is under study.

HIRSCHSPRUNG'S DISEASE (CONGENITAL AGANGLIONIC MEGACOLON)

This is a rare genetic disorder of bowel innervation. There is an absence of ganglion cells in the myenteric and submucosal plexuses for a variable segment of bowel extending from the anus to the colon. The aganglionic segment is narrow and contracted. It ends proximally in a normally innervated and dilated colon. It is more common in males.

Clinical features

Infants with the disease usually present in the neonatal period with:

- Delayed passage of meconium (>48 h of life).
- Subsequent intestinal obstruction with bilious vomiting and abdominal distension.

Enterocolitis is a severe, life-threatening complication.

Older children present with:

- Chronic, severe constipation present from birth.
- Abdominal distension.
- An absence of faeces in the narrow rectum.

Diagnosis and management

An unprepped barium enema might demonstrate a transition zone where the bowel lumen changes in diameter. Confirmation of the diagnosis is made by demonstrating the absence of ganglion cells on a suction biopsy of the rectum. Surgical resection of the involved colon is required. An initial colostomy is usually followed by a definitive pull-through procedure to anastomose normally innervated bowel to the anus.

BILE DUCT OBSTRUCTION

Obstruction of bile flow due to biliary atresia or a choledochal cyst are rare, but treatable, causes of persistent neonatal jaundice. Early recognition and diagnosis of these liver diseases is important.

Biliary atresia

This is a rare disorder of unknown aetiology in which there is either destruction or absence of the extrahepatic biliary tree. It represents a rare but important cause of persistent neonatal jaundice (Fig. 15.5).

Clinical features

The jaundice persists from the second day after birth and is distinguished by being due to a predominantly conjugated hyperbilirubinaemia

Liver disease presenting in the newborn period: causes of conjugated hyperbilirubinaemia	
Bile duct obstruction	Biliary atresia Choledochal cyst
Neonatal hepatitis	Congenital infection Inborn errors: α_1 antitrypsin deficiency Galactosaemia

Fig. 15.5 Liver disease presenting in the newborn period: causes of conjugated hyperbilirubinaemia.

accompanied by dark urine and pale stools. As the disease progresses there is failure to thrive due to:

- Malabsorption.
- Enlargement of the liver and spleen.

A bleeding tendency might develop due to vitamin K deficiency.

Diagnosis

Abdominal ultrasound, liver biopsy and intraoperative cholangiography might be required to clarify the diagnosis.

Treatment

Treatment consists of the Kasai procedure (hepatoportoenterostomy), which should ideally be carried out before the age of 6 weeks. Liver transplantation is needed if this fails or if presentation is late. Even with treatment, prognosis is poor.

Constipation

Functional constipation is an increasingly common condition and presents as infrequency in stooling, difficulty in bowel movements and stool retention. It is important to distinguish this from Hirschsprung's disease in that vomiting is unusual, it occurs during toilet training, stool palpable in rectal vault and soiling commonly occurring.

Note that functional constipation is not associated with abdominal pain and treatment is often prolonged with stool softeners and stimulant laxatives. Psychological help is often sought for difficult cases.

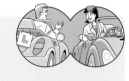

Constipation often leads to a vicious cycle—it leads to the development of megarectum which in turn worsens the constipation. It is vital to stress the importance of long-term treatment with laxatives even if the child's constipation improves—this is so that the rectum returns to its normal size and function.

Further reading

King AL, Ciclitira PJ. Celiac disease. *Current Opinion in Gastroenterology* 2000; **16**:102–106.

Renal and genitourinary disorders

16

Objectives

At the end of this chapter, you should be able to

- Know the common developmental anomalies of the urinary tract.
- Recognize common inguinoscrotal conditions like undescended testes and inguinal hernia.
- Know the pathogenesis and clinical features of UTI in children.
- Outline the investigations for a child with UTI.
- Distinguish between acute nephritis and nephrotic syndrome.

Structural abnormalities of the kidney and urinary tract are common and many are now identified on antenatal ultrasound screening. The most common disease encountered in this system is urinary tract infection, which has special significance because of its potential to damage the growing kidneys, leading to hypertension and chronic renal failure.

Presentation of urinary tract anomalies:
- Urinary tract infection.
- Recurrent abdominal pain.
- Palpable mass.
- Haematuria.
- Failure to thrive.

URINARY TRACT ANOMALIES

Congenital abnormalities of the kidneys and urinary tract can be identified in about 1 in 400 fetuses. They might be detected on antenatal ultrasound screening or present with a variety of symptoms and signs in infancy or later childhood.

Congenital anomalies of the urinary tract include:

- Renal anomalies.
- Obstructive lesions of the urinary tract.
- Vesicoureteric reflux.

Renal anomalies

Absence of both kidneys (renal agenesis) results in Potter syndrome in which oligohydramnios (caused by lack of fetal urine) is associated with lung hypoplasia and postural deformities. Other anomalies include:

- Abnormalities of ascent and rotation.
- Duplex kidney (Fig. 16.1).
- Horseshoe kidney (Fig. 16.1).
- Cystic disease of the kidney.
- Renal dysplasia.

Ectopia of the kidney is common and pain arising from an ectopic kidney can be misleading on account of its site.

Duplex systems are commonly associated with other abnormalities such as renal dysplasia and vesicoureteric reflux. The upper pole ureter might be ectopic (draining into the urethra or vagina) and the lower pole ureter often refluxes.

There are many conditions associated with cystic kidneys including:

- Autosomal recessive infantile polycystic kidney disease.
- Autosomal dominant adult-type polycystic kidney disease.
- Tuberous sclerosis.

Obstructive lesions of the urinary tract

The site of obstruction may be at the pelviureteric (PU) junction, the vesicoureteric (VU) junction, the

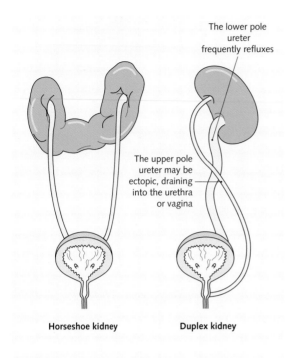

The lower pole ureter frequently refluxes

The upper pole ureter may be ectopic, draining into the urethra or vagina

Horseshoe kidney   **Duplex kidney**

Fig. 16.1 Urinary tract anomalies.

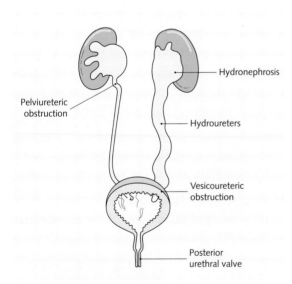

Pelviureteric obstruction

Hydronephrosis

Hydroureters

Vesicoureteric obstruction

Posterior urethral valve

Fig. 16.2 Sites of urinary tract obstruction and dilatation.

bladder, or the urethra (Fig. 16.2). If undetected before birth, the patient can present with:

- A urinary tract infection.
- Abdominal or loin pain.
- Haematuria.
- A palpable bladder or kidney.

128

Pelviureteric obstruction (congenital hydronephrosis)

Obstruction is caused by a narrow lumen or compression by a fibrous band or blood vessel, and can vary in degree from partial to almost complete obstruction (with gross hydronephrosis and minimal remaining renal tissue).

Mild degrees of obstruction can resolve spontaneously but severe obstruction requires surgical treatment with conservation of renal tissue wherever possible.

> Antenatal hydronephrosis is commonly seen and often resolves after birth but urgent investigation is indicated if hydronephrosis is bilateral because it might indicate urethral obstruction.

Vesicoureteric obstruction

Obstruction can be due to stenosis, kinking or dilatation of the lower part of the ureter (ureterocele) and can be unilateral or bilateral. There is a combination of hydroureter and hydronephrosis.

Posterior urethral valves

These are abnormal folds of the urethral mucous membrane, which occur in males in the region of the verumontanum. They impede the flow of urine with back-pressure on the bladder, ureters and kidneys. The degree of obstruction varies from the very severe (with death *in utero* from renal failure or after birth from Potter syndrome) to the less severe (which usually presents with urinary tract infection, poor urinary stream and renal insufficiency in a male).

Vesicoureteric reflux

Primary vesicoureteric reflux (VUR) is caused by a developmental anomaly of the vesicoureteric junction. The ureters enter directly into the bladder, rather than at an angle and the segment of ureter within the bladder wall is abnormally short. Urine refluxes up the ureter during voiding, predisposing to infection and exposing the kidneys to bacteria

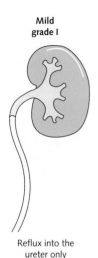
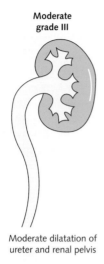
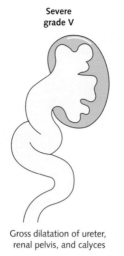

Mild grade I	Moderate grade III	Severe grade V
Reflux into the ureter only	Moderate dilatation of ureter and renal pelvis	Gross dilatation of ureter, renal pelvis, and calyces

Fig. 16.3 Grades of vesicoureteric reflux.

and high pressure. There is a spectrum of severity which is graded I–V (Fig. 16.3).

Clinical features

VUR is often associated with other genitourinary anomalies and may be secondary to bladder pathology, e.g. neuropathic bladder. The important consequences of VUR include:

- Predisposition to urinary tract infection.
- Urinary tract infection and pyelonephritis.
- Reflux nephropathy: this is destruction of renal tissue with scarring due to infection and back-pressure. If severe, it may result in high blood pressure and chronic renal failure.

Diagnosis

VUR is diagnosed by a micturating cystourethrogram (MCUG).

Management

Mild VUR resolves spontaneously (10% each year) but prophylactic antibiotics (e.g. trimethoprim) are given to prevent infection until the child:

- Is free of infection.
- Has regained normal bladder control.
- Is older than 5 years.

Surgery is indicated if prophylaxis fails and the VUR is in grades IV or V. The siblings of children should be investigated.

GENITALIA

Inguinoscrotal disorders

Inguinoscrotal disorders include:

- Undescended testis.
- Inguinal hernia and hydrocele.
- The acute scrotum.

Undescended testis

The testes develop intra-abdominally and migrate through the inguinal canal to the scrotum in the third trimester. The testes are therefore normally in the scrotum in term newborns, but are frequently undescended in preterm infants.

Clinical features and examination

A testis that has not reached the scrotum (undescended testis) might be:

- Incompletely descended: lying along normal pathway (the minority, 20%).
- Maldescended or ectopic: deviated from the normal path after emerging from the superficial inguinal ring (the majority, 80%).

An undescended testis must be distinguished from a 'retractile' testis that can be coaxed down into the scrotum. (Examination should be undertaken in a warm room with warm hands.)

The testes are examined during routine surveillance in the newborn, at 6 weeks and at 18 months. Referral to a surgeon should be made if either testis is impalpable or an ectopic testis is found at the 6-week check.

Further investigations are helpful if one or both testes are impalpable to determine their existence and location. These can include:

- Ultrasound.
- Magnetic resonance imaging.
- Laparoscopy.
- Endocrine investigations.

The testes might be absent in cases of intersex.

Management

Treatment is by orchidopexy and this is best performed between the age of 1 and 2 years. Potential, but unproven, benefits include:

- A reduced risk of torsion.
- Psychological and cosmetic benefits.
- Reduced risk of malignancy.
- Improved fertility.

Orchidectomy is indicated for a unilateral intra-abdominal testis that is not amenable to orchidopexy.

In many children, the testes may descend to its normal position in the first year of life even if it was high up in the scrotum at birth. So parents should be informed that a surgical referral will usually be made only after a year and this should not cause any harm to the child.

Inguinal hernias and hydroceles

The testis descends into the scrotum, taking with it a connecting fold of peritoneum (the processus vaginalis), which normally becomes obliterated at or around birth. Failure of the processus vaginalis to close results in an inguinal hernia or a hydrocele (Fig. 16.4).

Inguinal hernias

Inguinal hernias are more common in boys, premature babies, and infants, with a positive family history. A minority are bilateral. The parents notice an intermittent swelling in the groin or scrotum.

The main concern is the risk of strangulation, which is higher in young infants. Referral for prompt

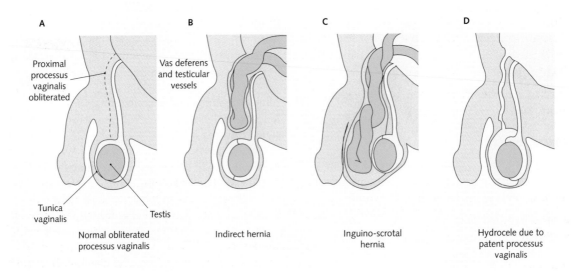

Fig. 16.4 (A) The normal testis. Following normal testicular descent, the processus vaginalis, an evagination of the parietal peritoneum between the internal inguinal ring and testis, disappears leaving only the tunica vaginalis around the testis. Persistence of the processus vaginalis results in an inguinal hernia (B, C), or a hydrocele (D).

surgery is indicated. Danger signs in the initially irreducible hernia are:

- Hardness.
- Tenderness.
- Vomiting.

These suggest entrapment of bowel within the sac and compromise of its vascular supply (strangulation). Urgent referral is imperative.

Sedation, analgesia and expert manipulation allow reduction, which is followed by surgical repair.

Hydroceles

If the connection with the processus vaginalis is small, a hydrocele forms rather than an inguinal hernia. The swelling is painless and, being full of fluid, it transilluminates. It is possible to get above the swelling, which cannot be reduced.

Spontaneous resolution by the age of 12 months is common and treatment during infancy is not required unless the hydrocele is extremely large.

The acute scrotum

Acute pain and swelling of the scrotum is an emergency because of the possibility of testicular torsion. It occurs most frequently in the neonatal period and at puberty, but can occur at any age.

Inadequate fixation to the tunica vaginalis allows the testis to rotate and occlude its vascular supply. Doppler studies can assist in diagnosis.

Surgical exploration must not be delayed, as the testis might become non-viable. The defect is often bilateral, so the contralateral testis should also be fixed at surgery.

The differential diagnosis includes:

- Torsion of the testicular appendix (hydatid of Morgagni).
- Epididymo-orchitis.
- Idiopathic scrotal oedema.

Penile abnormalities

Penile abnormalities include:

- Hypospadias.
- Phimosis.

Hypospadias

A spectrum of congenital abnormalities of the position of the urethral meatus occurs. Severe forms are associated with chordee, a ventral curvature of the penis.

Phimosis

This refers to adhesion of the foreskin to the glans penis after the age of 3 years. Mild degrees can be managed with periodic, gentle retraction. Paraphimosis is irreducible retraction of the foreskin beyond the coronal sulcus.

Circumcision

Non-retractility of the foreskin and preputial adhesions are normal in small boys and forcible attempts to retract the foreskin are ill-advised because this might result in scarring and phimosis.

Ballooning of the prepuce during urination is not uncommon and this usually resolves as the prepuce becomes more retractile.

Balanitis xerotica obliterans (lichen sclerosus) causes a thickened, scarred, white prepuce that is fixed to the glans. This, recurrent balanitis (infection of the glans) and sometimes recurrent urinary tract infection (UTI), are the only medical indications for circumcision. Most circumcisions are performed for religious reasons.

Complications of circumcision

- Haemorrhage.
- Infection.
- Damage to the glans.

The procedure should not be undertaken lightly.

An infant with hypospadias must *not* be circumcised because the foreskin is used at surgical correction.

Vulvovaginitis

Inflammation of the vulva and vaginal discharge is a common gynaecological complaint in prepubertal girls. Poor hygiene and tight fitting clothes have *not* been shown to be predisposing factors. A vulval swab might detect a yeast or streptococcal infection, which can be treated with the appropriate topical or oral therapy. It is important to think of foreign bodies if a persistent discharge is seen. Rarely, vulvovaginitis results from sexual abuse.

URINARY TRACT INFECTION

Infection of the urinary tract is common in children. About 3–5% of girls and 1–2% of boys will have a symptomatic UTI during childhood; boys outnumber girls until 3 months of age.

In children, most infections are caused by *Escherichia coli* originating from the bowel flora. Other pathogens include *Proteus* (especially in boys), *Klebsiella*, *Pseudomonas* and *Enterococcus* species. The most common host factor predisposing to UTI is urinary stasis. Important causes of urinary stasis include:

- Vesicoureteric reflux (VUR).
- Obstructive uropathy, e.g. ureterocoele, urethral valves.
- Neuropathic bladder, e.g. spina bifida.
- Habitual infrequent voiding and constipation.

UTIs occur:
- Predominantly in boys up to age 3 months.
- Equally in boys and girls from 3 to 12 months.
- Increasingly in girls rather than boys after age 1 year.
- UTI presents with non-specific features in infants.
- UTI must be suspected in any febrile infant with no obvious clinical source.

Clinical features

The clinical features vary markedly with age:

- In neonates and very young infants: jaundice might occur and septicaemia can develop, rapidly leading to shock and hypotension.
- In infants: UTI can occur, with or without fever, and symptoms are non-specific; vomiting, diarrhoea, irritability, failure to thrive.
- Between 1 and 5 years of age: fever, malaise, abdominal discomfort, urinary frequency and nocturnal enuresis are the presenting features. In this age group, dysuria might also be due to balanitis or vulvovaginitis.
- Over 5 years of age: the classic presenting features of cystitis (frequency, dysuria, fever and

enuresis) or pyelonephritis (fever and loin pain) occur. Asymptomatic bacteriuria is common in school-age girls. This does not need treatment.

Diagnosis

Confirmation of diagnosis requires culture of a pure growth of a single pathogen of at least 10^8 colony-forming units per litre of urine. However, obtaining an uncontaminated urine sample from infants and children is not always easy (Fig. 16.5). Specimens should be chilled without delay to 4°C (i.e. refrigerate) to prevent bacterial multiplication.

A positive nitrite and leucocyte esterase stick test is a reliable test for coliform infection, but false negatives occur if the urine has been in the bladder for less than an hour or the organism does not convert nitrate (e.g. enterococci).

A urine sample should be cultured from:
- An infant with a fever and no obvious clinical source.
- Any child with recurrent or prolonged fever.
- Any child with unexplained abdominal pain.
- Any child with dysuria or frequency, enuresis or haematuria.

Treatment of the acute infection

Prompt treatment with antibiotics is indicated to reduce the risk of renal scarring. This should be initiated as soon as a urine sample has been taken for culture. Treatment can be modified when urine culture results are available and stopped if the culture is negative.

Collecting a urine sample	
Method	**Indication**
Suprapubic aspirate	All babies under 6 months if an urgent or reliable sample required
Bag or pad sample	Non-urgent samples or outpatient use
Clean catch	Older, more cooperative children
Catheter	Only fresh samples valid for infection

Fig. 16.5 Collecting a urine sample.

Antibiotic choice

- Oral trimethoprim is a suitable initial choice for uncomplicated UTI in an older child but increasing microbial resistance is becoming a problem.
- Parenteral antibiotics, e.g. ampicillin plus gentamicin or cefuroxime, should be given to neonates, any systemically unwell older child and to children with signs of acute pyelonephritis or a known urinary tract abnormality.
- Prophylactic antibiotics should be given in low dose after treatment of the acute infection, until investigation of the urinary tract is complete.

Further investigation

All children require further imaging of their urinary tract after a first confirmed UTI. The aim of this is to identify:

- Any predisposing underlying anatomical or functional abnormality of the urinary tract such as vesicoureteric reflux.
- Renal scars.

Although the outcome for the majority of infants and children with UTI is benign, a small minority are at risk of renal damage, especially those with recurrent infection associated with vesicoureteric reflux.

The exact scheme depends on the age of the child. No single imaging investigation provides a full assessment.

An initial ultrasound of the kidneys and urinary tract is performed on all infants and young children. A renal ultrasound scan is valuable for:

- Demonstrating the presence of two kidneys.
- Identifying obstruction with urinary tract dilatation.

It is not reliable for detecting renal scars or vesico-ureteric reflux.

Infants aged under 1 year

In addition to ultrasonography, recommendations include:

- Micturating cystourethrogram (MCUG), to identify vesicoureteric reflux.
- Static radioisotope scan (DMSA), to identify renal scars.

These investigations are deferred until 3 months after the acute infection to avoid detecting transient abnormalities. Prophylactic antibiotics should be given in the interim.

Children aged between 1 and 5 years

Ultrasonography and a radioisotope scan are recommended. MCUG can be reserved for:

- Children in whom the radioisotope scan shows an abnormality.
- Children with recurrent infection.
- Children with a family history of reflux or reflux nephropathy.

The risk of developing renal scarring becomes less with increasing age and is uncommon with infection in children over 5 years of age.

Simple advice should be given concerning measures, which can reduce recurrence risk, i.e.

- High fluid intake.
- Regular unhurried voiding.
- Lactobacilli, cranberry juice.
- Good perineal hygiene.

Children with recurrent UTI or scarring require regular follow-up with a repeat urine culture, blood pressure monitoring and further renal imaging to check for new scar formation and resolution of vesicoureteric reflux.

ACUTE NEPHRITIS

Acute nephritis is a clinical condition caused by inflammatory changes in the glomeruli. It is characterized by:

- Fluid retention (oedema, facial puffiness).
- Hypertension.
- Haematuria.
- Proteinuria.

The majority of cases are postinfectious and follow a streptococcal throat or skin infection with Group A β-haemolytic streptococci. Less common causes include:

- Henoch–Schönlein purpura.
- IgA nephropathy.
- Systemic lupus erythematosus (SLE).
- Mesangiocapillary glomerulonephritis.

Clinical features

The presenting history will be of discoloured 'smoky' urine. Physical examination reveals signs of fluid overload such as oedema and raised blood pressure.

Diagnosis

The urine is positive for blood and protein, and microscopy might reveal red cells and casts. Renal function should be evaluated by measuring plasma urea, electrolytes and creatinine.

An abdominal X-ray and ultrasound might be required to exclude other causes of haematuria.

The aetiology is pursued with a throat swab, anti-DNAase B, complement C3 levels and biopsy if severe.

Management

Management centres around:

- Control of fluid and electrolyte balance by monitoring intake and output.
- Use of diuretics and antihypertensives as required.

The prognosis of poststreptococcal nephritis is good. However, rarely, a rapidly progressive glomerulonephritis with renal failure occurs, especially in nephritis from other causes. No evidence that treatment of the preceding infection prevents renal complications.

NEPHROTIC SYNDROME

The nephrotic syndrome is a clinical condition characterized by heavy proteinuria, oedema and a low plasma albumin (Fig. 16.6).

It is best classified into steroid sensitive (90%) or steroid resistant (10%) as this is predictor of outcome.

Clinical features

The usual presenting feature is oedema, which manifests as:

- Puffiness around the eyes.
- Swelling of the feet and legs.
- In severe cases, gross scrotal oedema, ascites and pleural effusions.

Diagnosis

Diagnosis is confirmed by documentation of proteinuria and hypoalbuminaemia, usually less than 25 g/L (normal range 35–40 g/L). Additional investigations should include biochemical renal function tests (urea, electrolytes, creatinine), urine microscopy, C3, C4, antiDNAse B and hepatitis serology.

The following features should prompt consideration of renal biopsy to identify rarer causes such as focal segmental glomerulosclerosis or membranoproliferative glomerulonephritis, which are usually steroid resistant:

Comparison of acute glomerulonephritis and nephrotic syndrome		
Feature	Acute glomerulonephritis	Nephrotic syndrome
Aetiology	Most often poststreptococcal	Usually idiopathic
Gross haematuria	Very common	Unusual
Hypertension	Common	Less common
Oedema	Less prominent	Prominent, generalized oedema
Urinalysis	Red cell casts, proteinuria +	Proteinuria +++
Serum C3 and C4	Usually decreased	Usually normal
Anti DNase B/ASOT	May be positive	Negative
Treatment	Supportive	Steroids

Fig. 16.6 Comparison of acute glomerulonephritis and nephrotic syndrome.

- Age: <1 year or >12 years.
- Presence of macroscopic haematuria.
- Low C3.
- Failure to respond to 4 weeks of steroid therapy.
- Persistent hypertension.
- Evidence of renal failure.

Management

If the clinical features are consistent with classic steroid-sensitive nephrotic syndrome, treatment is begun with oral steroids (prednisolone, 60 mg/m^2/day). Remission usually occurs within 10 days and the doses tapered. Steroid resistance is defined as no remission after 4 weeks. These cases are often resistant to other drugs and associated with chronic renal failure.

Fluid balance must be closely monitored with daily weighing and salt restriction.

Several serious complications may occur including:

- Hypovolaemia (manifested by a high PCV, hypotension and peripheral vasoconstriction).
- Thrombosis.
- Secondary infection.
- Hyperlipidaemia is not usually problematic in children.

Penicillin prophylaxis is given in the acute phase to prevent secondary infection.

Subsequent relapses might occur which are treated with steroids, but if frequent, use of additional immunosuppressive agents such as cyclophosphamide, levamisole or cyclosporin A may be needed.

HAEMOLYTIC URAEMIC SYNDROME

This is the most common cause of paediatric acute renal failure and is associated with diarrhoea from *E. coli* O157:H7, which produces a verocytotoxin. This toxin is released from the gastrointestinal tract and results in fragmentation of the red blood cells, microangiopathic haemolytic anaemia and thrombocytopenia. The kidney vasculature becomes thrombosed and infarcted.

Management is supportive and most (90%) children recover full renal function. Antibiotics are contraindicated.

Further reading

Eddy AA, Symons JM. Nephrotic syndrome in childhood. *Lancet* 2003; **362**:629–639.

Larcombe J. Clinical evidence: Urinary tract infection in children. *British Medical Journal* 1999; **319**: 1173–1175.

Neurological disorders

The developing nervous system is susceptible to damage by a host of diverse pathological processes: inherited and acquired. Malformations, infections, trauma, genetic diseases and tumours all affect the nervous system. Several important conditions affecting the nervous system are considered elsewhere:

- Neonatal hypoxia–ischaemia (see Chapter 25).
- Head injury (see Chapter 26).
- Coma (see Chapter 26).
- Brain tumours (see Chapter 20).
- Neural tube defects (see Chapter 9).

MALFORMATIONS OF THE CENTRAL NERVOUS SYSTEM

If severe, these cause fetal loss or early death. They encompass such important conditions as:

- Hydrocephalus.
- Craniosynostosis.
- Neural tube defects.

Hydrocephalus

Hydrocephalus is enlargement of the cerebral ventricles due to excessive accumulation of cerebrospinal fluid (CSF). This condition is the most frequent cause of an enlarged and rapidly expanding head in newborn infants.

Suspect hydrocephalus in an infant with a rapidly enlarging head circumference.

The causes include a variety of acquired pathological mechanisms as well as malformations (Fig. 17.1). Hydrocephalus is classified according to whether or not the ventricles communicate with the subarachnoid space:

- In non-communicating hydrocephalus the obstruction is intraventricular.
- In communicating hydrocephalus the obstruction is extraventricular.

Clinical features

The presenting clinical features vary with age. Dilated ventricles can be detected on antenatal ultrasound. In infants:

- The head circumference is disproportionately large and its rate of growth is excessive.
- The pressure on the anterior fontanelle is increased, sutures become separated and scalp veins are prominent. If untreated, the eyes deviate downward (setting-sun sign).

Causes of hydrocephalus
Non-communicating (intraventricular obstruction)
Congenital malformation:
• Aqueduct stenosis
• Dandy–Walker syndrome
Intraventricular haemorrhage
Ventriculitis
Brain tumour
Communicating (extraventricular obstruction)
Subarachnoid haemorrhage
Tuberculous meningitis
Arnold–Chiari malformation

Fig. 17.1 Causes of hydrocephalus.

In older children, the clinical features are those of raised intracranial pressure:

• Headache.
• Vomiting.
• Lethargy.
• Irritability.
• Papilloedema.

Signs of increased intracranial pressure:
• Altered sensorium.
• Headache.
• Vomiting.
• Decerebrate/decorticate posturing.
• Abnormalities of pupillary size and reaction.
• Papilloedema.
• Respiratory abnormalities.

Diagnosis

Diagnosis is confirmed by imaging. If the anterior fontanelle is still open, ultrasound can be used to assess ventricular dilatation. A computed tomography scan (CT) or magnetic resonance imaging (MRI) will establish the diagnosis, evaluate the cause and is useful for monitoring treatment and detecting complications.

Treatment

The mainstay of treatment is insertion of a ventriculoperitoneal shunt. Complications of shunts include obstruction and infection.

Craniosynostosis

This is premature fusion of the cranial sutures. Most affected infants present soon after birth with an abnormal skull; the shape of this depends on which sutures have fused. The sagittal suture is most commonly involved, causing a long, narrow skull.

Generalized craniosynostosis is a cause of microcephaly.

In the presence of increased intracranial pressure, a craniectomy is performed.

Neural tube defects

These used to be the most common congenital defects of the CNS and are considered in detail in Chapter 9. In the UK, the birth prevalence has fallen because of antenatal screening. There has also been a natural decline, the cause of which is uncertain. A range of lesions occur:

• Spina bifida occulta: the vertebral arch fails to fuse; seen in 5% of all children.
• Meningocele: meninges herniate through a vertebral defect. Usually minimal neurological defects.
• Myelomeningocele: meninges and spinal cord herniated—the most severe form of spinal dysraphism.
• Encephalocoele: extrusion of the brain and meninges through a midline skull defect.
• Anencephaly: the cranium and brain fail to develop (detected on antenatal ultrasound and termination of pregnancy is usually performed).

INFECTIONS OF THE CNS

Meningitis

A range of bacteria and viruses (Fig. 17.2) can cause acute meningitis. Rare causes include tuberculosis, fungal infections and malignant infiltration. The serious and potentially lethal nature of bacterial meningitis renders it most important. Although more common, viral meningitis is a relatively benign and self-limiting disease.

Acute meningitis: common pathogens

Bacterial
Neisseria meningitidis
Streptococcus pneumoniae
Haemophilus influenzae type B
During the neonatal period:
- Group B streptococci
- *E. coli*
- *Listeria monocytogenes*
Viral
Mumps
Enteroviruses
Epstein–Barr virus

Fig. 17.2 Meningitis: common pathogens.

Early signs of meningitis in infants are non-specific. Immediate treatment with parenteral penicillin is indicated for suspected meningococcal septicaemia.

Bacterial meningitis

The peak age of incidence is younger than 5 years old and 80% of all cases occur in children under 16 years. Meningococcal meningitis accounts for over half of all cases and in the UK; group B is the most common variety. Pneumococcal meningitis is uncommon but affects younger children and is associated with higher fatality and neurological sequelae. Since the introduction of Hib vaccination (in 1992 in the UK) and Men C vaccination, meningitis due to *H. influenzae* type B and meningococcus C has become rare.

The pathogens are carried in the nasal passages and invade the meninges via the bloodstream. In the early stages, symptoms and signs are non-specific, making diagnosis difficult, especially in infants.

Clinical features
There might be irritability, poor feeding, vomiting, fever and drowsiness. More specific signs develop later, including:

- A bulging fontanelle in infants.
- Neck stiffness and photophobia in the older child.

- Seizures: beware the child diagnosed with benign febrile convulsions.

Meningococcal infection can present with a characteristic non-blanching purpuric rash if septicaemia is present.

Diagnosis
Lumbar puncture (LP) and examination of the cerebrospinal fluid (CSF) is diagnostic. A high index of suspicion is necessary in young children in whom signs and symptoms of meningitis are non-specific.

Treatment should be started and LP performed if there is no contraindication. Contraindications to LP include signs of raised intracranial pressure (depressed conscious state, papilloedema and or focal neurological signs), coagulopathy and septic shock. A CT scan does not exclude raised intracranial pressure.

Rapid diagnostic tests are available (see Chapter 30). Blood cultures should also be taken prior to antibiotic therapy.

Treatment
Broad-spectrum intravenous antibiotic treatment is initiated using a third-generation cephalosporin, e.g. ceftriaxone. A febrile child with a purpuric rash (i.e. suspected meningococcal sepsis) should be treated immediately with benzylpenicillin (IM or IV) and transferred urgently to hospital. Meningococcal septicaemia can kill within hours and early antibiotic treatment significantly reduces fatality rates.

There is evidence that a component of the tissue damage in meningitis is caused by the host's inflammatory response. Attempts have been made to suppress this with steroids: dexamethasone has been shown to reduce the incidence of some neurological sequelae, e.g. hearing loss, in non-neonatal meningitis caused by *H. influenzae* and *S. pneumoniae*.

Complications
Acute complications of meningitis include:

- Subdural effusion.
- Cerebral oedema.
- Convulsions.
- SIADH.

Neurological sequelae include sensorineural deafness: all children should have their hearing tested following meningitis. Rifampicin, ciprofloxacin or ceftriaxone should be given to all household contacts following infection with meningococcus to eradicate nasopharyngeal carriage.

Encephalitis

In encephalitis there is inflammation of the brain substance. Acute encephalitis is usually viral. The most common causes in the UK are:

- Herpes simplex virus 1 and 2.
- Enteroviruses.
- Varicella.

The common viral exanthems (measles, rubella, mumps and varicella) can all cause encephalitis by direct viral invasion of the brain or can be complicated by an immune-mediated postinfectious encephalomyelitis (see below).

Clinical features

The clinical features include early non-specific symptoms and signs such as fever, headache, and vomiting, followed by the abrupt development of an encephalopathic illness characterized by altered consciousness and personality and seizures.

Diagnosis and management

High-dose aciclovir should be given in all cases to cover herpes simplex until results of investigations are available.

Diagnosis is difficult acutely, but EEG and MRI might show evidence of the characteristic temporal lobe abnormalities.

Supportive management for severe encephalitis requires:

- Admission to an intensive care unit if there are concerns about airway, breathing or circulation.
- Seizure control and monitoring for raised intracranial pressure.

Postinfectious syndromes

These can affect the brain or peripheral nervous system:

- Postinfectious encephalomyelitis: delayed brain swelling caused by an immune-mediated inflammatory reaction to viral infection. It may follow any of the common viral exanthems.
- Varicella zoster typically causes an acute cerebellitis.

Acute postinfectious polyneuropathy (Guillain–Barré syndrome)

This demyelinating polyneuropathy follows 2–3 weeks after a viral infection with, for example, cytomegalovirus or Epstein–Barr virus, or infection with *Mycoplasma pneumoniae* or *Campylobacter jejuni*.

Clinical features

Guillain–Barré syndrome usually begins with fleeting sensory symptoms in the toes and fingers and progresses to a symmetrical, ascending paralysis with early loss of tendon reflexes. Autonomic involvement might occur, with dysrhythmias, and bulbar involvement can cause respiratory failure. The disease can progress over several weeks. The CSF protein is characteristically markedly raised without an increase in white cell count.

Management

Supportive care including assisted ventilation might be required. Respiratory function must be monitored closely. Specific therapy includes immunoglobulin infusion and plasma exchange. There might be residual neurological problems but in children a full recovery is expected.

CEREBRAL PALSY

Cerebral palsy (CP) is defined as a disorder of motor function due to a non-progressive (static) lesion of the developing brain. It is useful to remember that:

- Although the lesion is non-progressive, the clinical manifestations evolve as the nervous system develops.
- Children with cerebral palsy often have problems in addition to disorders of movement and posture, reflecting more widespread damage to the brain.

The cause is unknown in many patients but identified risk factors can be categorized into antenatal, intrapartum and postnatal (Fig. 17.3). It is important to be aware that perinatal asphyxia is an uncommon cause (3–21%) of CP.

Clinical features

There might be a history of risk factors and motor delay. CP can present with:

Causes of cerebral palsy

Antenatal (80%)
Cerebral dysgenesis
Congenital infections:
- Rubella
- CMV
- Toxoplasmosis

Intrapartum (10%)
Birth asphyxia

Postnatal (10%)
Preterm birth:
- Hypoxic–ischaemic encephalopathy
- Intraventricular haemorrhage

Hyperbilirubinaemia
Hypoglycaemia
Head injury
Intracranial infection:
- Meningitis
- Encephalitis

Fig. 17.3 Causes of cerebral palsy.

- Delayed motor milestones.
- Abnormal tone and posturing in infancy.
- Feeding difficulties due to lack of oromotor coordination.
- Speech and language delay.

Diagnosis

The diagnosis is made on clinical examination, which might show abnormalities of:

- Tone, e.g. hypertonia or hypotonia.
- Power, e.g. hemiparesis.
- Reflexes, e.g. brisk tendon reflexes or abnormal absence (or persistence) of primitive reflexes.
- Abnormal movements, e.g. athetosis or chorea.
- Abnormal posture or gait.

Classification

Cerebral palsy is classified according to the anatomical distribution of the lesion and the main functional abnormalities (Fig. 17.4).

Spastic cerebral palsy

Damage to the pyramidal pathways causes increased limb tone (spasticity) with brisk deep-tendon reflexes and extensor plantar responses. Hypotonia might precede spasticity. The distribution of affected limbs allows further classification:

- Hemiparesis: an arm might be affected more than leg or vice versa.

Classification of cerebral palsy

Spastic (70%)
Hemiplegic
Diplegic
Quadriplegic
Dyskinetic (10%)
Athetoid
Dystonic
Ataxic (10%)
Hypotonic
Mixed (10%)

Fig. 17.4 Classification of cerebral palsy.

- Diplegia: all four limbs are affected, but legs more than arms. This is the characteristic CP of the preterm infant.
- Quadriplegia: all four limbs are affected, but arms worse than legs. There is often truncal involvement, with seizures and intellectual impairment. This is the most severe form and is the characteristic CP of severe birth asphyxia.

Ataxic cerebral palsy

Caused by damage to the cerebellum or its pathways. Features include early hypotonia with poor balance, uncoordinated movements and delayed motor development.

Dyskinetic cerebral palsy

Caused by damage to the basal ganglia or extrapyramidal pathways (e.g. in kernicterus). The clinical presentation is often with hypotonia and delayed motor development. Abnormal involuntary movements, which include chorea (abrupt, jerky movements), athetosis (slow writhing continuous movements) or dystonia (sustained abnormal postures) might appear later.

Management

Management of CP requires a multidisciplinary approach involving the paediatrician, often a community paediatrician, GP, paediatric neurologist health visitor, community nursing team, speech and language therapist, physiotherapists and occupational therapists. Accurate diagnosis and prognosis must be given to the parents. Prognosis in early infancy can be uncertain. Motor function may be worsened by hypertonia, which is treated by physiotherapy, muscle relaxants (e.g. diazepam,

Problems associated with cerebral palsy

Mental retardation and learning difficulty
Ophthalmic and auditory abnormalities
Seizures
Gastro-oesophageal reflux
Feeding problems and failure to thrive
Recurrent pneumonia

Fig. 17.5 Problems associated with cerebral palsy.

baclofen), botulinum toxin injections to specific muscle groups or surgical intervention. A programme of physiotherapy might be indicated and orthopaedic intervention is often beneficial (braces, surgery, special shoes). Attention must be paid to associated problems such as sensory deficits, learning difficulties and epilepsy (25–50% of all children experience seizures) which are often difficult to control (Fig. 17.5).

EPILEPSY

Epilepsy is common, affecting 5 out of 1000 school-age children. It is useful to distinguish between an 'epileptic seizure', which is a transient event, and epilepsy, which is a disease or syndrome:

- An epileptic seizure is a transient episode of abnormal and excessive neuronal activity in the brain that is apparent either to the subject or an observer.
- Epilepsy is a chronic disorder of the brain characterized by recurrent, unprovoked epileptic seizures.

Several important features of these definitions require emphasis. With epileptic seizures:

- The abnormal neuronal activity during an epileptic seizure can be manifested as a motor, sensory, autonomic, cognitive or psychic disturbance. The neurophysiological basis is inferred on clinical grounds.
- A convulsion is a subtype of seizure in which motor activity occurs.
- An electrophysiological disturbance unaccompanied by any clinical change is *not* classified as an epileptic seizure.
- Many paroxysmal disturbances ('funny turns') mimic epileptic seizures (see Chapter 5).

In epilepsy, a diagnosis is made in a patient in whom epileptic seizures recur spontaneously. However, it is important to recognize that an 'epileptic seizure' can be provoked in individuals who do *not* have epilepsy (examples of provoking insults include fever, hypoglycaemia, trauma and hypoxia).

Diagnosis of epilepsy rests in a good history from a witness, not on investigations.

- Epilepsy affects 5 per 1000 school-age children.
- Up to 75% of childhood epilepsy will have no identifiable cause.
- Children with partial seizures require brain imaging.

Classification and terminology

The International League Against Epilepsy has devised a useful classification system for epileptic seizures and for epilepsies and epilepsy syndromes. In any patient, an attempt should be made to:

- Identify the types of seizure occurring.
- Diagnose the epilepsy or epilepsy syndrome present.

Terms such as grand mal and petit mal are outdated and should be avoided.

Classification of epileptic seizures

The initial division is into (Fig. 17.6):

- Generalized seizures: in which the first clinical change indicates initial involvement of both cerebral hemispheres.
- Partial seizures: in which there is initial activation of part of one cerebral hemisphere.

Partial seizures are further classified into:

- Simple, in which consciousness is retained.
- Complex, in which consciousness is impaired or lost.

A partial seizure can become secondarily generalized.

Classification of epilepsies and epilepsy syndromes

The recent trend is to classify epilepsy into syndromes. Most epilepsy syndromes have a typical prognosis and respond to specific anticonvulsants.

The initial division is according to the seizure type (Fig. 17.7) into:

- Generalized epilepsies and syndromes.
- Localization: related epilepsies and syndromes.

Classification of epileptic seizures

Generalized
- Absence seizures
- Myoclonic seizures
- Clonic seizures
- Tonic seizures
- Tonic–clonic seizures
- Atonic seizures

Partial
Simple (consciousness not impaired)
- With motor symptoms (Jacksonian)
- With somatosensory or special sensory symptoms
- With autonomic symptoms
- With psychic symptoms

Complex (with impairment of consciousness)
- Beginning as simple partial seizure
- With only impairment of consciousness
- With automatisms

Partial seizure with secondary generalization

Fig. 17.6 Classification of epileptic seizures.

An additional category is provided for those in which it is undetermined whether seizures are focal or generalized, either because the seizure type is uncertain or because both focal and generalized seizures occur.

Further subdivision is according to aetiology into:

- Idiopathic (or primary): in which there is no apparent cause except perhaps for genetic predisposition.
- Symptomatic: in which the cause is known or suspected.

Causes of epilepsy

Epilepsy can result from a very diverse group of pathological processes but it is important to realize that in about 50% of children no cause will be identified, even after extensive evaluation. It can be assumed that the aetiology in these cases of so-called idiopathic or primary epilepsy is genetic. A specific cause (Fig. 17.8) is more likely to be identifiable in patients with partial or intractable epilepsy.

Diagnosis

A careful and complete history is the mainstay of diagnosis. A detailed description is required of the events before, during and after a suspected seizure (a video recording is a potentially useful adjunct). The first aim is to distinguish true epileptic seizures

Fig. 17.7 Classification of epilepsy.

Classification of epilepsy

Generalized epilepsies and epilepsy syndromes
Idiopathic generalized epilepsy (IGE), defined syndromes include:
- Benign familial neonatal convulsions
- Childhood absence epilepsy (CAE)
- Juvenile absence epilepsy (JAE)
- Juvenile myoclonic epilepsy (JME)

Symptomatic generalized epilepsy, defined syndromes include:
- Infantile spasms (West syndrome)
- Lennox–Gastaut syndrome
- Cerebral malformations
- Progressive myoclonic epilepsies including:
    Inborn errors of metabolism
    Neurodegenerative diseases

Localization-related epilepsies and epilepsy syndromes
Idiopathic partial epilepsy, defined syndromes include:
- Benign childhood epilepsy with centrotemporal spikes (benign rolandic epilepsy)

Symptomatic partial epilepsy, defined syndromes include:
- Epilepsy caused by focal lesions of the brain associated with:
    Cortical dysgenesis
    CNS infection
    Head injury
    AV malformations
    Brain tumours

Causes of 'symptomatic' epilepsy
Cortical dysgenesis
Cerebral malformations
Genetic diseases:
• Neurocutaneous syndromes
• Down syndrome
• Fragile X syndrome
• Neurodegenerative disorders
• Inborn errors of metabolism
Cerebral tumours
Cerebral damage due to:
• Head trauma
• Birth asphyxia, hypoxia–ischaemia
• Intracranial infection (meningitis, encephalitis)

Fig. 17.8 Causes of 'symptomatic' epilepsy.

from the many paroxysmal disturbances (see Chapter 5) that can mimic them:

- Breath-holding attacks.
- Reflex anoxic seizures.
- Vasovagal syncope (simple faints).
- Cardiac dysrhythmias.

Enquiry should be made concerning possible predisposing events (head injury, intracranial infection) and any family history of epilepsy.

Physical examination in a child with uncomplicated epilepsy is frequently normal. Careful attention should be paid to the skin to identify the stigmata of neurocutaneous syndromes (including Wood's light examination) and to the fundi because retinal changes can provide a clue to aetiology.

Always examine the skin completely in children with recurrent seizures.

Investigations

EEG

This might be useful as an aid to diagnosis, in identifying a particular epilepsy syndrome or in identifying an underlying anatomical lesion or neurodegenerative disorder. However, it must be borne in mind that a single interictal EEG will be normal in up to 50% of children with epilepsy, and

non-specific or even so-called 'epileptiform' abnormalities can be found in 2–3% of normal asymptomatic children. A routine interictal EEG does not therefore prove or disprove a diagnosis of epilepsy. Additional information can be obtained from ambulatory EEG monitoring, telemetry with simultaneous video recording or recordings during sleep or after sleep deprivation.

Neuroimaging

Not all children with epilepsy require a brain scan. Indications for neuroimaging include:

- Partial seizures.
- Intractable, difficult to control seizures.
- A focal neurological deficit.
- Evidence of a neurocutaneous syndrome or of neurodegeneration.
- Children less than 2 years old with nonfebrile convulsions.

CT is more readily available and quicker to perform. However, new modalities of MRI offer greater sensitivity in the detection of small lesions, e.g. in temporal lobe or subtle cortical dysgeneses.

Other investigations

Additional specific investigations, which might be appropriate if there is clinical suspicion of an underlying neurometabolic disorder, include:

- Plasma and urine amino acids.
- Biopsy of skin or muscle.
- Measurement of white blood cell enzymes.
- DNA analysis.

Some important epilepsy syndromes

Infantile spasms (West syndrome)

This is a sinister but happily uncommon variety of epilepsy with peak onset between 4 and 6 months of age. Myoclonic seizures occur, often as 'salaam attacks'—violent flexor spasms of head, trunk and limbs followed by extension of the arms. They are often multiple and can be misdiagnosed as colic. The EEG shows hypsarrhythmia, a chaotic pattern of large-amplitude slow waves with spikes and sharp waves. Seventy per cent of the patients have the symptomatic form, and important causes include

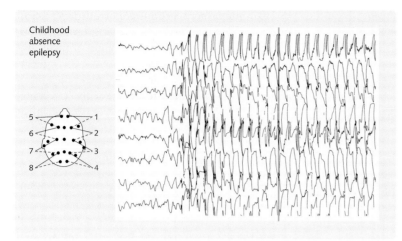

Childhood absence epilepsy

Fig. 17.9 EEG in a typical absence seizure. There is 3/s spike and wave discharge, which is bilaterally synchronous.

tuberous sclerosis and perinatal hypoxic–ischaemic encephalopathy. The prognosis is poor but can be improved by early treatment. Treatment is with adrenocorticotrophic hormone (ACTH) or vigabatrin, the latter is particularly effective if associated with tuberous sclerosis.

Childhood absence epilepsy

This relatively common variety of epilepsy has a peak onset at 6–7 years (range 4–12 years). The absence seizures comprise transient unawareness (blank spells), but without loss of body tone. They typically last for 5–15 seconds but can be very frequent, with up to several hundred daily. Episodes can be induced by hyperventilation. The ictal EEG is characteristic with generalized, bilaterally synchronous three-per-second spike-wave discharges (Fig. 17.9). The prognosis is good with spontaneous remission in adolescence in the majority of children. Sodium valproate is the drug of first choice, although medication is not required for infrequent absences.

Management of epilepsy

Effective management of a child with epilepsy involves far more than the prescription of anti-epilepsy drugs (AEDs). Both the child and parents need to be educated about the condition, the prognosis and the nature of the particular epilepsy or epilepsy syndrome.

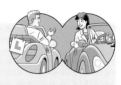

Children with epilepsy should be encouraged to participate in and enjoy a full social life. Certain activities however, do require special precautions:

- Swimming: a competent adult swimmer should be present to provide supervision.
- Domestic bathing: patients should be supervised in the bath, older children should be advised not to lock the door.
- Cycling: a helmet must be worn and traffic avoided.
- Climbing: climbing trees and rocks is best avoided.

It is important to consider the psychological and educational implications. Overprotection by the parents should be sympathetically discouraged. Behavioural and emotional difficulties can occur in the teenage years, with loss of self-esteem, anxiety or depression. The diagnosis should be discussed with school staff. Learning difficulties are present in a proportion of children with epilepsy, but only a minority require special schooling.

Anti-epilepsy drugs (AEDs)

Not all children with epilepsy require drug treatment. Many clinicians would not start treatment after a single brief generalized tonic-clonic seizure or for infrequent myoclonic or absence seizures. Commonly used AEDs are sodium valproate and carbamazepine, though newer antiepileptics like lamotrigine, topiramate, vigabatrin etc. are being increasingly used. The currently recommended first line treatment is:

- Sodium valproate for generalized epilepsy.
- Carbamazepine for partial epilepsy.

Monotherapy will achieve total seizure control in 70% of children. Blood level monitoring reflects compliance and not efficacy. Identifying the epilepsy syndrome may help to choose the right drug, e.g. vigabatrin is particularly effective in treating infantile spasms but is associated with permanent visual field defects.

FEBRILE SEIZURES

A febrile seizure is a seizure associated with fever in a child between 6 months and 6 years of age in the absence of intracranial infection or an identifiable neurological disorder.

Febrile seizures are the most common cause of seizures in childhood and occur in about 3% of children. There might be a familial predisposition. The seizures usually occur when body temperature rises rapidly. They are typically brief (1–2 min), generalized, tonic-clonic seizures.

The underlying infection causing the fever might be a viral illness or a bacterial infection such as otitis media, tonsillitis, pneumonia or urinary tract infection.

Clinical features

Most children are well after the seizure but meningitis can present with seizures and fever, so it is very important to exclude this diagnosis. This often requires a lumbar puncture in young children (under 18 months) presenting with a first febrile seizure in whom specific signs of meningitis might be absent. Prognosis is very good and, despite a 30% chance of recurrence, a normal neurological outcome is expected.

Management

Management includes:

- Identification and treatment of underlying infection: this might be apparent on clinical examination but additional investigations to consider include CXR, FBC, blood culture, urine microscopy and culture, and lumbar puncture.
- Keeping the patient cool with regular antipyretics and tepid sponging.
- Termination of a prolonged convulsion (i.e. for longer than 5–10 min) with rectal diazepam.
- Parental education (Fig. 17.10).

Information for parents about febrile seizures	
Will it happen again?	About one third of children have recurrent febrile seizures Recurrence is more likely if the first seizure occurs under the age of 18 months or if there is a family history
Can I prevent further episodes?	During febrile illnesses, the child should be kept cool with antipyretics, removal of clothing, and tepid sponging
What should I do if a convulsion occurs?	Place child in recovery position Parents of children at risk of frequent or prolonged seizures can be supplied with rectal diazepam to administer if a seizure lasts longer than 5 minutes
Is it epilepsy?	Febrile seizures are not classified as epilepsy About 3% of children with febrile seizures go on to develop afebrile recurrent seizures, i.e. epilepsy, in later childhood Risk factors for epilepsy include: • Seizures that are focal, prolonged (>15 minutes) or recur in the same illness • First-degree relative with epilepsy • Neurological abnormality

Fig. 17.10 Information for parents about febrile seizures.

NEUROCUTANEOUS SYNDROMES

It is no surprise that skin and CNS disease are associated as both organs develop from the endoderm.

Neurofibromatosis type 1 (von Recklinghausen disease)

This is an autosomal dominant disorder affecting about 1 in 4000 live births. About 50% of cases result from new mutations and have no family history. The important clinical features include:

- Café-au-lait patches on the skin: at least six must be present because 50% of normal individuals have at least one.
- Lisch nodule (pigmented hamartomas on the eye): usually seen after 5 years of age.
- Neurofibromas, which might be palpable, on the peripheral nerves: these manifest after 8 years of age.

Neurofibromatosis type 2 (NF2)

Also known as central neurofibromatosis, NF2 is a distinct disease due to mutations in a different gene on chromosome 22. It is much rarer than type 1 (affecting 1 in 40 000 people) and is characterized by bilateral acoustic neuromata and other CNS tumours (Fig. 17.11).

Tuberous sclerosis

This is an autosomal dominant disorder affecting 1 in 7000 live births. Up to 75% of cases represent new mutations. It is genetically heterogeneous with one disease gene on chromosome 9 and a second gene on chromosome 16.

Classically it presents with seizures, mental retardation and facial angiofibromas (adenoma sebaceum). Examination reveals hypopigmented macules, which are better seen on examination with a Wood's light.

It is a multisystem disease affecting not only the skin and brain but also the heart, kidneys and lungs.

Sturge–Weber syndrome

This sporadic disorder is characterized by:

- Unilateral facial naevus (port-wine stain) in the distribution of the trigeminal nerve.
- Angiomas involving the leptomeningeal vessels in the brain leading to seizures.
- Haemangiomas in the spinal cord.

There are abnormal blood vessels over the surface of the brain, which might be associated with seizures, hemiplegia and learning difficulties. Ocular involvement can result in glaucoma.

A CT scan of the brain typically shows unilateral intracranial calcification with a double contour like a railway line and cortical atrophy.

NEURODEGENERATIVE DISORDERS OF CHILDHOOD

A large number of individually rare but important inherited diseases are associated with progressive

Differences between NF1 and NF2		
Feature	NF1	NF2
Incidence	About 1/4000	About 1/50 000
Inheritance	Autosomal dominant; chromosome 17	Autosomal dominant; chromosome 22
Café-au-lait spots	Characteristic	Uncommon
Skin neurofibromas	Common	Uncommon
Lisch nodules	Characteristic	Uncommon
Family history	About 50% are inherited	Mostly new mutations
Acoustic neuromas	Uncommon	Characteristic, often bilateral
Risk of CNS tumours	Common	Common

Fig. 17.11 Differences between NF1 and NF2.

neurodegeneration in childhood. Most are autosomal recessively inherited and genetic and biochemical defects have been established at a molecular level in many cases. Acquired forms do occur, such as prion disease and subacute sclerosing panencephalitis. Loss of acquired skills is the hallmark of a neurodegenerative disorder

Clinical features

The clinical hallmark is a progressive, worsening deficit. It is important to distinguish between developmental delay and developmental regression—in delayed development, milestones are not achieved in time, but once attained, they are not lost. In regression, there is a gradual loss of milestones that have already been attained. The child may have a normal initial development, only to lose those skills later, indicating a progressive disorder of the brain.

Features of neurodegerative diseases include:

- Regression of milestones.
- Progressive dementia.
- Epilepsy.
- Visual loss.
- Ataxia.
- Alterations in tone and reflexes (depending on the precise pattern of nervous system involvement).

Parental consanguinity increases the risk of such disorders (Fig. 17.12).

NEUROMUSCULAR DISORDERS

These are best considered according to their anatomical site (Fig. 17.13) in the lower motor pathway. Genetic, infective, inflammatory and toxic factors can cause this group of diseases (Fig. 17.14).

Inherited neurodegenerative diseases--some examples
Lysosomal storage diseases
Sphingolipidosis, e.g. Tay–Sachs disease
Mucopolysaccharidosis, e.g. Hurler syndrome (MPS1)
Peroxisomal disorders
Adrenoleucodystrophy
Trace metal metabolism
Wilson's disease
Menke's syndrome

Fig. 17.12 Inherited neurodegenerative diseases—some examples.

Neuromuscular disorders
Anterior horn cell
Spinal muscular atrophy
Poliomyelitis
Peripheral nerve
Hereditary neuropathy
Guillain–Barré syndrome
Bell's palsy
Neuromuscular junction
Myasthenia gravis
Muscle
Muscular dystrophies
Myotonia
Congenital myopathies

Fig. 17.13 Neuromuscular disorders.

Pattern of inheritance of some of the conditions affecting the nervous system		
Condition	Inheritance	Locus
Duchenne/Becker muscular dystrophy	X-linked recessive	Xp21
Myotonic dystrophy	Autosomal dominant (genomic imprinting)	19q13
Neurofibromatosis type 1	Autosomal dominant	17q11.2
Neurofibromatosis type 2	Autosomal dominant	22q1.11
Tuberous sclerosis	Autosomal dominant	TSC 1–9q34 TSC 2–16p13

Fig. 17.14 Pattern of inheritance of some of the conditions affecting the nervous system.

Clinical features

The hallmark of these disorders is weakness. They can present with:

- Floppiness (hypotonia).
- Delayed motor milestones.
- Weakness, fatiguability.
- Abnormal gait.

Clinical features on examination include hypotonia, muscle weakness or wasting, abnormal gait and reduced tendon reflexes.

Diagnosis

Special investigations useful in the diagnosis of neuromuscular diseases include:

- Muscle enzymes: serum creatine kinase is elevated in Duchenne and Becker dystrophies.
- Electrophysiology: nerve conduction studies and electromyography.
- Biopsy: muscle or nerve may be biopsied.
- DNA analysis: direct mutational analysis of disease genes in certain disorders.
- Imaging: ultrasound, CT or MRI of muscle.
- Edrophonium test: for myasthenia gravis.

Muscular dystrophies

This group of inherited disorders is characterized by progressive degeneration of muscle and absence of abnormal storage material. The most common and important is Duchenne muscular dystrophy.

Duchenne muscular dystrophy

This X-linked recessive disease affects 1 in 4000 male infants. About one-third of cases are new mutations. The disease gene is very large (2 Mb) and encodes dystrophin, a sarcolemmal membrane protein.

Affected boys usually develop symptoms between 2 and 4 years of age. Independent walking tends to be delayed and affected children never run normally. Patients are wheelchair bound by 12 years of age and die from congestive heart failure or pneumonia by 25 years of age.

Clinical features
Associated clinical features include:

- Pseudohypertrophy of calf muscles and proximal muscle weakness.
- Positive Gower's sign (evident at 3–5 years): the hands are used to push up on the legs to achieve an upright posture, indicating weakness of the lower back and pelvic girdle muscles.
- Scoliosis and contractures.
- Dilated cardiomyopathy.
- Mild learning difficulties.

Diagnosis
Investigations to confirm the diagnosis include:

- Serum creatine kinase level (10–20 times normal).
- Muscle biopsy and EMG.
- DNA analysis (identification of mutations in the dystrophin gene): positive in 65%.

Management
Treatment is supportive. Walking can be prolonged by provision of orthoses and scoliosis can be helped by a truncal brace or moulded seat. Early diagnosis is important to allow identification of female carriers and genetic counselling. Respiratory symptoms can be helped with non-invasive respiratory ventilation in certain cases. Cardiomyopathy worsens with age and is often the cause of death.

Becker muscular dystrophy

This disease is milder than Duchenne muscular dystrophy but is caused by a mutation in the same gene. The average age of onset is much later (in the second decade of life) with prolonged survival.

Myotonic dystrophy

This is the second most common muscular dystrophy in Europe and acquired as an autosomal dominant trait. It is a multiorgan disorder affecting muscle, endocrine system, cardiac function, immunity and the central nervous system.

Clinical features
- Hypotonia.
- Progressive muscle wasting.
- Typical facial features with an inverted V-shaped upper lip, thin cheeks and high arched palate.

- Myotonia: a characteristic feature, usually seen beyond 5 years. This is a slow relaxation of muscle after contarction and may be demonstrated by asking the patient to make tight fists and then to quickly open the hands.
- Arrhythmias, endocrine abnromalities, cataracts and immunologic deficiencies can also occur.

Diagnosis

This is by DNA analysis to show the CTG repeat. Serum CK is usually normal.

Management

Treatment is supportive.

Spinal muscular atrophies

Spinal muscular atrophies (SMA) are progressive degenerative diseases of motor neurons, that may have its onset as early as foetal life. The more severe forms present in early infancy with severe hypotonia and weakness whereas the late onset forms present later during childhood. These disorders are characterised by hypotonia, generalized weakness and absent or weak tendon reflexes. Fasciculations seen in the tongue, deltoids or biceps are characteristic and indicate denervation of the muscle. Children with the severe early onset type rarely survive beyond 2 yrs while intermediate forms lead to severe motor disability. Diagnosis is by muscle biopsy and identifying the genetic marker for the SMN gene. Treatment is supportive.

Musculoskeletal disorders

DISORDERS OF THE HIP AND KNEE

Developmental dysplasia of the hip

This term has replaced the previous name of 'congenital dislocation' of the hip. Perinatal hip instability results in progressive malformation of the hip joint; it occurs in 1.5 in 1000 births.

Developmental dysplasia of the hip (DDH) represents a spectrum of hip instability ranging from a dislocated hip to hips with various degrees of acetabular dysplasia (in which the femoral head is in position but the acetabulum is shallow). It was previously thought to be entirely congenital, but is now known to also occur after birth in previously normal hips. There are two types:

1. Typical, which affects normal infants.
2. Teratological, which occurs in neurological and genetic conditions. Teratological DDH requires specialized management.

All babies are screened clinically but 40% will be missed and the use of national ultrasound screening remains controversial; 90% will spontaneously resolve without treatment.

Clinical features

The cause is unknown but risk factors for DDH include:

- Congenital muscular torticollis.
- Congenital foot abnormalities.
- Breech or caesarean delivery.
- Family history.
- Neuromuscular disorders.
- Female sex.

Babies are screened at birth and at the 6-week check using the Barlow and Ortolani manoeuvres. With increasing age, contractures form and these tests are then unhelpful. Warning signs might be:

- Delayed walking.
- A painless limp.
- A waddling gait.

Asymmetrical skin creases are found in 30% of all infants and are an unreliable guide; 10% of all babies have hip clicks and this is normal.

Diagnosis

Typically, on examination there is limited abduction (a supine child should be able to abduct fully the flexed hip up until the age of 2 years). The femur might be shortened (Allis sign). Ultrasound scanning is diagnostic. Hip X-rays are not useful until after 4–5 months of age when the femoral head has ossified (Fig. 18.1).

Management

Note that clinical examination will miss many hip dislocations and ultrasound of high-risk babies is indicated.

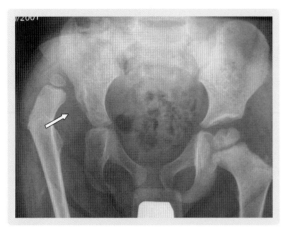

Fig. 18.1 X-ray of congenital dislocation of the right hip in an older child. (Reproduced with permission from Crash Course: Rheumatology and Orthopaedics, 2nd edn. by Marsland, Kapoor, Coote and Haslam, Elsevier Mosby, 2008.)

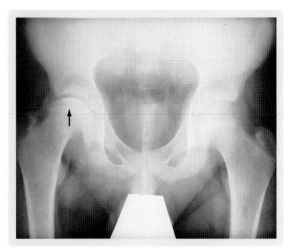

Fig. 18.2 Perthe's disease. Increased density in the right femoral head, which is reduced in height.

This involves:

- Fixing the hip in abduction with a Pavlik or Von Rosen harness. This is effective in children under 8 months of age.
- Important to note that the harness must be adjusted every 2 weeks for growth and be kept on at all times.

For children in whom the diagnosis has been delayed, open reduction and derotation femoral osteotomy needs to be performed. In these cases, accelerated degenerative changes might necessitate total hip replacement in early adult life.

Legg–Calvé–Perthes disease

This idiopathic disorder results in osteonecrosis of the femoral head prior to skeletal maturity. It results in growth disturbance associated with temporary ischaemia of the upper femoral epiphysis. This leads to a cycle of avascular necrosis with flattening and fragmentation of the femoral head. Revascularization and reossification occurs with the resumption of growth (which might not be normal); the whole cycle takes 3–4 years. Risk factors include:

- A previous family history.
- Male sex: it is five times more common in boys.

The incidence is 1 in 2000.

Clinical features

There is an insidious onset of limp between the ages of 3 and 12 years (the majority occur between 5 and 7 years). Pain, which might be intermittent, can be felt in the hip, thigh or knee. Between 10 and 20% of cases are bilateral. Abduction and rotation is limited on examination.

Diagnosis

Hip X-rays are diagnostic (Fig. 18.2). If there is doubt then serial films or MRI might be necessary.

Management

The prognosis in most children is good, especially in those under 6 years of age or if less than half of the femoral head is involved. In younger children only analgesia and mild activity restriction with bracing is needed.

In older children, and those in whom more than half of the epiphysis is involved, permanent deformity of the femoral head occurs in over 40%, resulting in earlier degenerative arthritis. In severe disease, the hip needs to be fixed in abduction allowing the femoral head to be covered and moulded by the acetabulum as it grows. Plaster, callipers or femoral or pelvic osteotomy may achieve fixation.

Transient synovitis (irritable hip)

This common self-limiting condition occurs in children between 2 and 12 years of age often following a viral infection. Typical features are:

- Sudden onset of hip pain.
- Limp.
- Refusal to bear weight on the affected side.

There is no pain at rest. Examination reveals limited passive abduction and rotation in an otherwise well and afebrile child. The critical differential diagnosis is septic arthritis, in which the child is febrile, unwell with pain at rest and refusal to move the affected joint.

Diagnosis

This is a diagnosis of exclusion and it is important to distinguish transient synovitis from septic arthritis:

- Acute-phase reactants: white blood cell count (WBC), C-reactive protein (CRP) and erythrocyte sedimentation rate (ESR).
- Blood cultures.

Hip X-ray does not enable differentiation and is therefore not useful. If there is doubt, antibiotics should be given and the joint aspirated for culture.

Irritable hip is a diagnosis of exclusion. Septic arthritis must always be considered.

Management

Treatment is supportive (bed rest and analgesia) because the condition spontaneously resolves in 2 weeks.

Slipped upper femoral epiphysis (SUFE)

In this relatively uncommon condition of unknown aetiology, there is progressive posterior and medial translation of the femoral head on the femoral neck through the epiphysis. SUFE occurs during the adolescent growth spurt and:

- Is most common in boys (obese white or tall thin black).
- Is associated with delayed skeletal maturation and endocrine disorders.
- Typically presents between 10 and 15 years of age.
- Presents with limp or with hip or referred knee pain.

Thirty per cent have a family history and 20% are bilateral, although not necessarily synchronous. Diagnosis is by plain radiographs and unstable hips are an orthopaedic emergency. Complications are avacsular necrosis and premature fusion of the epiphysis. Management is by pinning the femoral head or osteotomy. Non-surgical treatment is ineffective.

DISORDERS OF THE SPINE

Back pain

Back pain is uncommon before adolescence. In infants and young children it is usually associated with significant pathology such as connective tissue disorders. Referral is warranted.

In adolescence back pain may be caused by:

- Muscle spasm or soft tissue pain: this is usually a sports-related injury.
- Scheuermann's disease: this is osteochondritis (idiopathic avascular necrosis of an ossification centre) of the lower thoracic vertebrae causing localized pain, tenderness and kyphosis.
- Spondylolysis and spondylolisthesis: there is a defect in the pars interarticularis of (usually) L4 or L5 (spondylolysis). If there is anterior shift of the vertebral body—graded according to severity—there is lower back pain exacerbated by bending backwards (spondylolisthesis).
- Vertebral osteomyelitis or discitis: this presents with severe pain on weight bearing and walking associated with local tenderness.
- Tumours: these can be benign or malignant and might cause cord or root compression.
- Idiopathic: this is a diagnosis of exclusion but pain might be exacerbated by stress and poor posture.

Think of malignancy in bone pain. Suggestive features include:
- Non-articular bone pain.
- Back pain.
- Pain out of proportion to swelling or at night.

Scoliosis

This is lateral curvature of the spine associated with a rotational deformity and affects 4% of children. It is classified according to cause:

- Vertebral abnormalities, e.g. hemivertebra, osteogenesis imperfecta.
- Neuromuscular, e.g. polio, cerebral palsy.
- Miscellaneous, e.g. idiopathic (most common), dysmorphic syndromes.

Idiopathic scoliosis

As well as lateral curvature, there is rotation of the thoracic region, which can be demonstrated as the child bends forwards and a rib hump is noted (Fig. 18.3). More than 85% of cases occur in adolescence. It is more common in girls and often there is a family history. Pain is not a typical feature. The scoliosis is monitored clinically, radiologically and chronologically:

- Mild curves are not treated.
- Moderate curves are braced (23 hours a day until growing has stopped).
- Severe curves (>40°) require surgery that fuses the spine and therefore terminates further growth. Untreated severe curves result in later degenerative changes, pain and unwanted cosmetic appearance.

Torticollis

Acute torticollis (wry neck) is a relatively common and self-limiting condition in young children, often associated with an upper respiratory tract infection.

The most common cause of torticollis in infants is a sternomastoid tumour. A mobile non-tender nodule within the sternomastoid muscle is noticed in the first few weeks of life. The cause is unknown. It usually resolves by 1 year and is managed conservatively by passive stretching. Surgery is reserved for persistent cases.

BONE AND JOINT INFECTIONS

Osteomyelitis

Early recognition and aggressive treatment is essential for a favourable outcome in bone infections. The infection is usually haematogenous in origin or might be secondary to an infected wound. It typically starts in the metaphysis where there is relative stasis of blood. Two-thirds of cases occur in the femur and tibia. The peak incidence is bimodal, occurring in the neonatal period and in older children (9–11 years).

In all age groups, the most common pathogen is *Staphylococcus aureus*, although group B streptococci and *E. coli* occur in neonates.

Children with sickle-cell disease have increased susceptibility to salmonella osteomyelitis. *M. tuberculosis* should also be considered.

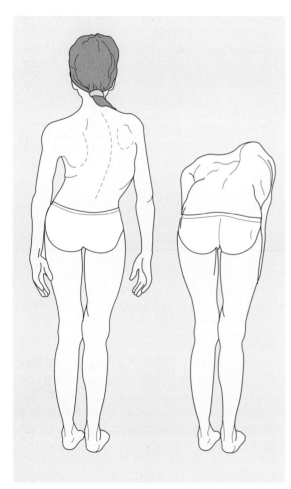

Fig. 18.3 Idiopathic adolescent scoliosis showing vertebral rotation (rib hump) when bending forward.

Bacterial bone and joint infections: *Staphylococcus aureus* is the most common pathogen in all age groups.

Clinical features

Infants present with fever and refusal to move the affected limb. Older children will localize the pain and are also systemically unwell. Examination reveals exquisite tenderness over the affected bone usually with warmth and erythema. Pain limits movement.

Diagnosis

The acute-phase reactants (WBC, CRP and ESR) are usually significantly elevated. Blood cultures are positive in more than half of the cases and aspiration of the bone is therefore necessary to identify the organism and its sensitivity. Bone scans are more sensitive in the early phase of the illness (24–48 hours) compared with X-rays, which tend to be normal in the first 10 days. Periosteal elevation or radiolucent necrotic areas can usually be demonstrated between 2 and 3 weeks.

Treatment

Early treatment with intravenous antibiotics is imperative until there is clinical improvement and normalizing of the acute-phase reactants. Several weeks of oral antibiotics follow. Failure to respond to medical treatment is an indication for surgical drainage.

Complications include:

- Chronic osteomyelitis.
- Septic arthritis.
- Growth disturbance and limb deformity (occurs if the infection affects the epiphyseal plate).

Septic arthritis

Purulent infection of a joint space is more common than osteomyelitis and can result in bone destruction and considerable disability. The incidence is highest in children younger than 3 years of age and is usually haematogenous in origin. Other causes include:

- Osteomyelitis.
- Infected skin lesions.
- Puncture wounds.

In infants, the hip is the most common site (the knee is the most common site in older children). *Staphylococcus aureus* is the most common pathogen

in all age groups. The organisms are similar to those found in osteomyelitis and the conditions might occur together.

Clinical features

The typical presentation is a painful joint with:

- Fever.
- Irritability.
- Refusal to bear weight.

Infants often hold the limb rigid (pseudoparalysis) and cry if it is moved. There is tenderness and a variable degree of warmth and swelling on examination.

Investigation

The acute-phase reactants are usually elevated. Aspiration of the joint space might reveal organisms and the presence of white cells. The aspirate can then be cultured.

Ultrasound can identify effusions but X-rays are often initially normal or show a non-specific, widened joint space.

Management

Early and prolonged intravenous antibiotics are necessary. Surgical drainage is indicated only if the infection is recurrent or if it affects the hip.

RHEUMATIC DISORDERS

These include:

- Juvenile idiopathic arthritis (JIA).
- Dermatomyositis.
- Systemic lupus erythematosus.

Juvenile idiopathic arthritis

Juvenile idiopathic arthritis has replaced the term 'juvenile chronic arthritis'. It is diagnosed after arthritis in one or more joints for 6 weeks after excluding other causes in a child. It occurs in 1 : 1000 children. There are eight groups and three are discussed in detail below; classification is by mode of onset over the first 6 months (Fig. 18.4). Blood investigations for antinuclear antibodies (ANA) and rheumatoid factor (RF) are helpful in classification but not diagnostic.

Fig. 18.4 Classification of juvenile idiopathic arthritis.

Classification of juvenile idiopathic arthritis			
	Systemic	Polyarticular	Oligoarticular
Number of joints involved	Variable	Greater than 4	4 or less
Joints involved	Knees Wrist Ankle and tarsal	Any joint	Knees Ankles Elbows Hips spared
Pattern	Symmetrical	Symmetrical	Asymmetrical
Rheumatoid factor	Negative	Positive or negative	Negative
Eye involvement	No	No	Yes in 30%
Clinical course	Poor in one-third	Good if rheumatoid factor negative	Good

Systemic (previously Still's disease)

This mainly affects children under 5 years. The arthritis primarily affects the knees, wrist, ankles and tarsal bones. Other features include:

- High daily spiking fever.
- A salmon-pink rash.
- Lymphadenopathy and hepatosplenomegaly.
- Arthralgia, malaise and myalgia.
- Inflammation of pleura and serosal membranes.

There is often no arthritis at presentation. One-third will have a progressive course and the worst prognosis occurs in the younger age.

Polyarticular

Rheumatoid factor (RF) negative

This affects all ages and all joints but spares metacarpophalangeal joints (MCPs). Limitation of the motion of the neck and temporomandibular joints is seen. It has a good prognosis but disease may be prolonged.

Rheumatoid factor (RF) positive

This mainly affects females over 8 years and causes arthritis of the small joints of the hand and feet. Hip and knee joints are affected early and rheumatoid nodules are seen over pressure points. There might be a systemic vasculitis; functional prognosis is poor.

Oligoarticular

Early onset is the most common subtype and typically occurs in young girls under 6 years with asym-
metric arthritis involving knees, ankle and elbows. Antinuclear antibodies are nearly always present and one-third will develop chronic iridocyclitis (inflammation of the iris and ciliary body, which comprise the anterior uveal tract: anterior uveitis). The definition 'oligoarticular' requires that the disease affects four or fewer joints and it has a good prognosis but eye involvement is independent of the joints. There is a subclass called 'extended oligoarticular' in which more than four joints are affected after 6 months; this has a poorer prognosis.

Ophthalmological screening with a slit lamp to detect anterior uveitis is especially important in children with oligoarticular JIA.

Diagnosis
Useful tests for the evaluation of JIA include:

- FBC: anaemia occurs in systemic disease.
- Acute-phase reactants: elevated.
- RF: negative in the majority.
- ANA.
- X-rays: soft tissue swelling in early stages. Bony erosion and loss of joint space later.

Management
A multidisciplinary team approach is required. This will encompass:

- Physiotherapy: to optimize joint mobility, prevent deformity and increase muscle strength.
- Medication: pain control and suppression of inflammation are provided by non-steroidal anti-inflammatory agents (NSAIDs), e.g. ibuprofen or aspirin. Systemic steroids are indicated for severe systemic disease or severe uveitis. The trend is towards early use of methotrexate, to reduce joint damage, and local steroid injections. Biologics, which target specific parts of the inflammatory pathway, have been used in severe cases.

GENETIC SKELETAL DYSPLASIAS

Achondroplasia

See Chapter 25.

Osteogenesis imperfecta (brittle bone disease)

Osteogenesis imperfecta is a heterogeneous group of disorders:

- Caused by mutations in type I collagen genes.
- Characterized by fragile bones and frequent fractures.

There are four forms:

- Type I (the most common form) is an autosomal dominant disorder. Affected children have recurrent fractures, blue sclerae and conductive hearing loss.
- Type II is a severe, lethal form with multiple fractures present before birth. Many affected infants are stillborn. Inheritance is usually autosomal recessive.
- Type III causes severe bone fragility but the sclera are not blue in later life. Survival to adulthood is uncommon. This is autosomal recessive.
- Type IV is mild with a variable age of onset and only bone fragility without the other features of type I.

Management is by aggressive orthopaedic treatment of fractures to correct deformities and genetic counselling of the parents.

Further reading

Kocher MS, Zurakowski D, Kasser JR. Differentiating between septic arthritis and transient synovitis of the hip in children: an evidence-based clinical prediction algorithm. *Journal of Bone and Joint Surgery* 1999; **81**(12):1662–1170.

Petty RE, Southwood TR, Baum J et al. Revision of the proposed classification criteria for juvenile idiopathic arthritis: Durban, 1997. *Journal of Rheumatology* 1998; **25**:1991–1994.

Haematological disorders

Objectives

At the end of this chapter, you should be able to

- Understand the normal development of the haematopoietic system.
- Identify the common causes of anaemia.
- Understand the clinical features and management of iron deficiency anaemia.
- Understand the common types of haemolytic anaemia.
- Identify the common disorders affecting haemostasis.

These encompass defects in the cellular elements of the blood or in those soluble elements involved in haemostasis. Neoplastic diseases of the white cells or lymphatic system are considered separately (see Chapter 20). The most common problem encountered is iron deficiency anaemia.

Normal developmental variations are important in the interpretation of changes in the blood in infancy and childhood.

HAEMATOPOIESIS

Early prenatal haematopoiesis occurs in the liver, spleen and lymph nodes. It commences in the bone marrow at about the fourth or fifth month of gestation. At birth, haematopoietic activity is present in most of the bones, especially long bones.

Cells in the peripheral blood have a relatively short life span. Continuous replenishment in massive amounts from the bone marrow is required to maintain adequate blood counts.

Normal developmental changes in haemoglobin

The haemoglobin (Hb) concentration and haematocrit are relatively high in the term newborn infant because of the low oxygen tension prevailing in utero. The wide range encountered, 14–20 g/dL, is accounted for by:

- Variation in how rapidly the umbilical cord is clamped.
- The infant's position after delivery.

If cord clamping is delayed and the baby is held lower than its placenta, haemoglobin and blood volume are both increased by a placental transfusion. These values subsequently decline, reaching a nadir at:

- About 7 weeks in preterm infants.
- 2–3 months for term infants.

The lower limit of normal for this 'physiological' anaemia is 9.0 g/dL. During this period, there is erythroid hypoplasia of the marrow and a change from fetal to adult haemoglobin.

Life span of peripheral blood cells:
- Red cells: 120 days.
- Platelets: 10 days.
- Neutrophils: 6–7 hours.

The haemoglobin concentration:
- Is high at birth: 14–20 g/dL.
- Falls to a nadir of 9–13 g/dl at 2–3 months in term infants.
- HbF values decline postnatally to 2% of total at 9–12 months.

ANAEMIA

Anaemia is a decrease of the haemoglobin concentration in the blood to below normal. Dietary iron deficiency is the most common cause but there are many others. In clinical practice, anaemia can be classified initially according to the red cell:

- Colour intensity (normochromic/hypochromic).
- Size (microcytic/normocytic/macrocytic).

Important causes based on this classification are shown in Fig. 19.1.

Iron deficiency anaemia (IDA)

This is the commonest cause of anaemia in childhood. It usually results from inadequate dietary intake rather than loss of iron through haemorrhage.

Iron requirements

The fetus absorbs iron from the mother across the placenta.

- Term infants have adequate reserves for the first 4 months of life.
- Preterm infants have limited iron stores and because of their higher rate of growth, they outstrip their reserves by 8 weeks of age.

Both breast milk and unmodified cow's milk are low in iron concentration (0.05–0.10 mg/100 mL). However, 50% of the iron is absorbed from breast milk, in comparison to just 10% from cow's milk. Most formula milks are fortified with iron and contain 10 times the concentration in breast milk (1.0 mg/100 mL); however, only 4% is absorbed.

Dietary sources of iron include red meat, fortified breakfast cereals, dark green vegetables and bread. About 10–15% of dietary iron is absorbed. Absorption is:

- Enhanced by ascorbic acid (vitamin C).
- Reduced by tannin in tea.

Iron requirements increase during adolescence, especially for girls who lose iron through menstruation.

Classification and causes of anaemia

Microcytic, hypochromic anaemia
Defects of haem synthesis
- Iron deficiency
- Chronic inflammation
Defects of globin synthesis
- Thalassaemia

Normocytic, normochromic anaemia
Haemolytic anaemias
- Intrinsic red cell defects
  Membrane defects: Spherocytosis
  Haemoglobinopathies: Sickle cell disease
  Enzymopathies: G6PD deficiency
- Extrinsic disorders
  Immune-mediated: Rh incompatibility
  Microangiopathy
  Hypersplenism
Haemorrhage (acute or chronic)
- Hookworm infestation
- Meckel's diverticulum
- Menstruation
Hypoproduction disorders
- Red cell aplasia, e.g. renal disease
- Pancytopenia, e.g. marrow aplasia, leukaemia

Macrocytic anaemia
Bone marrow megaloblastic
- Vitamin B_{12} deficiency
- Folic acid deficiency
Bone marrow not megaloblastic
- Hypothyroidism
- Fanconi anaemia

Fig. 19.1 Classification and causes of anaemia.

Concerning iron in milk:
- Breast and unmodified cow's milk are low in iron.
- Iron is better absorbed from breast milk (50%) than cow's milk (10%).
- Formula milks are fortified with iron.

Causes of iron deficiency

Nutritional deficiency is common in certain at-risk groups (Fig. 19.2). Malabsorption can be complicated by iron deficiency. Blood loss is a less common cause but might occur with:

- Menstruation.
- Hookworm infestation.
- Repeated venesection in babies.
- Meckel's diverticulum.
- Recurrent epistaxis.

Clinical features

Mild iron deficiency is asymptomatic. As it becomes more severe there might be:

Fig. 19.2 Dietary iron deficiency.

Dietary iron deficiency	
Infants	Preterm infants require iron supplements from 6–8 weeks Term infants will develop iron deficiency after 4 months if • Mixed feeding is unduly delayed • Unmodified cow's milk is introduced early
Children	Poor diet associated with low socio-economic status or strict vegetarian diets

- Irritability.
- Lethargy.
- Fatigue.
- Anorexia.

On examination, the only signs might be pallor of the skin and mucous membranes.

Severe anaemia can cause congestive cardiac failure. IDA in infancy and early childhood is associated with developmental delay and poor growth, which is reversible by long-term oral iron treatment.

Diagnosis

Diagnosis is confirmed by the blood count and film, supplemented by investigations of iron status.

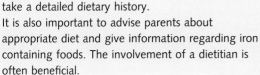

While taking history in suspected iron deficiency anaemia, it is important to take a detailed dietary history.
It is also important to advise parents about appropriate diet and give information regarding iron containing foods. The involvement of a dietitian is often beneficial.

Management

Primary prevention in infants can be achieved by the:

- Avoidance of unmodified cow's milk.
- Use of iron-supplemented formulae.

Mild to moderate anaemia is treated with dietary counselling and oral iron using, for example, sodium iron edetate. Therapy should be continued for another 3 months after the correction of anaemia to allow replenishment of tissue iron stores.

Severe anaemia with cardiac decompensation might require transfusion. Investigation for occult gastrointestinal tract bleeding is indicated if there is a failure of response to treatment or recurrence despite an adequate intake.

Reference nutrient intakes of iron are:
- 6 months: 4 mg/day.
- 12 months: 8 mg/day.
- Adult male: 9 mg/day.
- Adult female: 15 mg/day.

Thalassaemias

The thalassaemias are a group of hereditary anaemias caused by defects of globin chain synthesis. They are classified into:

- α-thalassaemia: reduced synthesis of α-globin chains.
- β-thalassaemia: reduced synthesis β-globin chains.

Mutations in the globin genes lead to a reduction or absence of the corresponding globin chains. Excess unpaired globin chains produce insoluble tetramers that precipitate causing membrane damage and either:

- Cell death within the bone marrow (ineffective erythropoiesis).

or

- Premature removal by the spleen (resulting in haemolytic anaemia).

β-thalassaemia

This occurs most frequently in people from the Mediterranean and Middle East. Over 150 million people carry β-thalassaemia mutations. There are two main types:

1. Homozygous β-thalassaemia (β-thalassaemia major, Cooley's anaemia).
2. Heterozygous β-thalassaemia (β-thalassaemia minor, (β-thalassaemia trait).

β-thalassaemia major

There is usually a complete absence of β-globin chain production (genotype β^o/β^o), although some mutations allow partial synthesis (genotype β^+/β^+); haemoglobin A (HbA) cannot be synthesized.

Clinical features

Affected infants usually present at 6 months with severe haemolytic anaemia, jaundice, failure to thrive and hepatosplenomegaly. If untreated, bone marrow hyperplasia occurs with development of the classical facies:

- Maxillary hypertrophy.
- Skull bossing.

Diagnosis

Haemoglobin electrophoresis reveals a markedly reduced or absent HbA with increased haemoglobin F (HbF) (30–90%) (see Chapter 30).

Treatment

The mainstay of treatment is regular blood transfusion, aiming to maintain the haemoglobin concentration above 10 g/dL. Unfortunately, chronic transfusion therapy is complicated by accumulation of iron in parenchymal organs including the heart, liver, pancreas, gonads and skin.

Chelation therapy with subcutaneous desferrioxamine, given regularly overnight, is used to promote iron removal but negative iron balance is rarely achieved. Many patients succumb to congestive heart failure due to cardiomyopathy in their second or third decade.

Splenectomy is useful in selected patients and bone marrow transplantation can restore haematopoietic function. In the future, the developments of bone marrow transplantation, oral chelating agents and gene therapy hold promise.

β-thalassaemia minor (β-thalassaemia trait)

The only abnormality is a mild, hypochromic, microcytic anaemia. Most are asymptomatic. β-thalassaemia trait can be misdiagnosed as iron deficiency anaemia. The important diagnostic feature is the raised HbA_2 and about 50% have a mild elevation of HbF (1–3%) on electrophoresis.

α-thalassaemia

This is caused by absence or reduced synthesis of α-globin genes. Most result from gene deletion. The manifestations and severity depend on the number of genes deleted (Fig. 19.3).

Fig. 19.3 Clinical manifestations of α-thalassaemia variants.

Clinical manifestations of α-thalassaemia variants			
Variant	Number of genes deleted	Hb pattern	Clinical features
α-thalassaemia major	Four	γ4 (Hb Bart)	Hydrops fetalis/death *in utero*
Haemoglobin H disease	Three	β4 (Hb H) (beyond early infancy)	Severe anaemia, persists through life
α-thalassaemia minor	Two	Normal	Mild anaemia
Silent carrier	One	Normal	No anaemia Normal RBC indices

Genetic counselling is important in all haemoglobinopathies. Folic acid supplements are usually given but iron supplementation should be avoided.

HAEMOLYTIC ANAEMIA

Haemolytic anaemia occurs when the life span of the red blood cell is shorter than the normal 120 days. Haemolytic anaemia can be caused by:

- Intrinsic red cell defects, e.g. spherocytosis, sickle-cell disease, glucose-6-phosphate dehydrogenase (G6PD) deficiency.
- Extrinsic defects, e.g. Rhesus (Rh) incompatibility, microangiopathy and hypersplenism.

It is characterized by:

- Anaemia.
- Reticulocytosis.
- Increased erythropoiesis in the bone marrow.
- Unconjugated hyperbilirubinaemia.

Hereditary spherocytosis

This is an autosomal dominant disorder caused by abnormalities in spectrin, a major supporting component of the red blood cell membrane. About 25% of cases are sporadic with no family history and are due to new mutations. As the name suggests the red cell shape is spherical and the life span is reduced by early destruction in the spleen.

Clinical features

The clinical features are highly variable and include:

- Mild anaemia: 9–11 g/dL.
- Jaundice: hyperbilirubinaemia.
- Splenomegaly: mild to moderate.

Complications

These include:

- Aplastic crises secondary to parvovirus B19 infection.
- Gallstones: caused by increased bilirubin excretion.

Diagnosis

Spherocytes are seen on peripheral blood film. Diagnosis is confirmed by the osmotic fragility test (spherocytes already have maximum surface area to volume and rupture more easily than biconcave red cells in hypotonic solutions), though this is being replaced by gel electrophoresis to identify the protein defect or by molecular genetic studies

Management

Mild disease requires no treatment other than folic acid to meet the increased demands of the marrow.

Splenectomy is indicated for more severe disease, but should be deferred until school age because of the subsequent risk of overwhelming infection. The child should receive:

- Hib, meningococcal and pneumococcal vaccines before splenectomy.
- Prophylactic penicillin for life afterwards.

Sickle-cell disease

This chronic haemolytic anaemia occurs in patients homozygous for a mutation in the β-globin gene (which causes substitution of valine for glutamine in the sixth amino acid position of the β-globin chain). This causes a solubility problem in the deoxygenated state: haemoglobin S (HbS) aggregates into long polymers that distort the red cells into a sickle shape.

The heterozygous state (sickle-cell trait) confers resistance to falciparum malaria; this 'heterozygote advantage' explains the high incidence of the mutation in populations originating in malarious areas such as tropical Africa, the Mediterranean, the Middle East and parts of India. Neonatal screening by Guthrie test has been recently expanded to include sickle cell diease.

Sickle-cell disease:
- HbS differs from HbA by the substitution of valine for glutamine at position 6 in the β-globin chain.
- HbS forms insoluble polymers in the deoxygenated state.
- The heterozygous state confers some protection against malaria.

Sickled red cells have a reduced life span and are trapped in the microcirculation, causing ischaemia.

Clinical features

The synthesis of HbF during the first few months affords protection until the age of 4–6 months. Progressive anaemia with jaundice and splenomegaly then develops, and the infant might present with an episode of dactylitis or overwhelming infection. The subsequent course of the disease is punctuated by crises of which 'vaso-occlusive' crises are by far the most common.

Vaso-occlusive crises

These episodes are often precipitated by infection, dehydration, chilling or vascular stasis. The clinical features depend on the tissue involved but episodes most commonly manifest as a 'painful' crisis, with pain in the long bones or spine. Cerebral or pulmonary infarction are less common but more serious. The latter might present as 'acute chest syndrome', which is characterized by:

- Fever.
- Crepitations.
- Chest pain.
- Pulmonary shadowing on chest X-ray arising from a combination of infarction and infection.

In infancy, patients with sickle-cell disease have a functional hyposplenism despite splenomegaly. Repeated vaso-occlusive episodes lead to infarction and fibrosis so that the spleen is no longer palpable from 5 years of age (so-called 'autosplenectomy'). These patients are, therefore, at risk of overwhelming infection with encapsulated organisms (*Haemophilus influenzae*, *Streptococcus pneumoniae*). There is an increased risk of osteomyelitis due to *Salmonella* and other organisms.

The long-term consequences of sickle-cell disease include:

- Myocardial damage and heart failure.
- Aseptic necrosis of long bones.
- Leg ulcers.
- Gallstones.
- Renal papillary necrosis.

Management

Antenatal and neonatal screening is available and this allows initiation of antibiotic prophylaxis early in life. Prophylactic penicillin should be taken to prevent pneumococcal infection. Daily folic acid supplements help to meet the demands of increased red cell breakdown. Pneumococcal and meningococcal vaccine should be given as well as the standard course of Hib vaccine. Hydroxyurea reduces vaso-occlusive crisis and is currently under clinical trials.

The treatment of a vaso-occlusive crisis includes:

- Analgesia: opioids for severe pain.
- Oxygenation.
- Hyperhydration with IV fluids.

Exchange transfusion, designed to reduce the proportion of sickle cells, is indicated for brain or lung infarction and priapism. Transfusion with packed red cells might be required if a sudden fall in haemoglobin occurs during an aplastic sequestration or haemolytic crisis.

Vasoocclusive crises can result in loss of function of the limb or organ if not treated early. It is important to give adequate information to parents about its symptoms and advise them to seek medical advice early in such an event.

Sickle-cell trait

The heterozygote with sickle-cell trait (HbAS) is asymptomatic unless subjected to hypoxic stress (e.g. general anaesthesia). Sickle cells are not seen on peripheral smear and diagnosis requires a solubility test (e.g. sodium metabisulfate slide test) or Hb electrophoresis. The trait is worth detecting to allow genetic counselling and precautions to be taken against hypoxaemia during flying and general anaesthesia.

The spleen in sickle-cell disease:
- In infancy, there is splenomegaly.
- Recurrent infarction and 'autosplenectomy' causes the spleen to regress and become impalpable after age 5 years.
- Splenic hypofunction renders patients susceptible to infections with encapsulated organisms.

Red cell enzyme deficiencies

These include glucose-6-phosphate dehydrogenase (G6PD) deficiency and the much rarer pyruvate kinase deficiency.

G6PD deficiency

This is an X-linked recessive disorder with variable clinical severity. Over 100 million people are affected worldwide, particularly in the Mediterranean, Middle Eastern, Oriental and Afro-Caribbean populations. G6PD-deficient red cells do not generate enough glutathione to protect the cell from oxidant agents. Males are more severely affected but females can manifest the phenotype.

Clinical features

G6PD deficiency can manifest with:

- Neonatal jaundice: worldwide it is the most common cause of neonatal jaundice requiring exchange transfusion.
- Haemolytic episode: induced by infection, oxidant drugs or fava beans. Intravascular haemolysis occurs with fever, malaise and the passage of dark urine (haemoglobinuria).

Pyruvate kinase deficiency

This is an autosomal recessive condition and is characterized by infection associated (parvovirus) haemolysis and tolerance of low haemoglobin levels. Management by splenectomy is sometimes useful.

BLEEDING DISORDERS

Normal haemostasis requires a complex interaction between three factors:

- Blood vessels.
- Platelets (thrombocytes).
- Coagulation factors.

A bleeding diathesis can result from a deficiency or disorder of any of these elements. Clinical presentation of a generalized bleeding diathesis might include:

It is unlikely that inherited bleeding disorders are present if the child has had a major haemostatic challenge, e.g. major surgery, without complications.

- Petechiae or purpura.
- Prolonged bleeding after dental extraction, surgery or trauma.
- Recurrent bleeding into muscles or joints.

Disorders of blood vessels

Injury to blood vessels provokes two responses that limit bleeding:

- Vasoconstriction.
- Activation of platelets and coagulation factors by subendothelial collagen.

Rare inherited disorders include Ehlers–Danlos syndrome associated with excessive capillary fragility and hereditary haemorrhagic telangiectasia.

Acquired disorders include vitamin C deficiency (scurvy) and Henoch–Schönlein purpura.

Henoch–Schönlein purpura

This is a multisystem vasculitis involving the small blood vessels. It commonly follows an upper respiratory tract infection or exposure to a drug or allergen, and is assumed to be immune-mediated with IgA playing a major role.

It is more common in boys and 75% of affected children are under 10 years old.

Clinical features

The condition affects skin, joints, gastrointestinal tract and kidneys. Clinical features are described in Fig. 19.4.

Diagnosis and management

Diagnosis is clinical. Normal platelet count and coagulation studies exclude other causes of purpura.

Treatment is symptomatic and supportive. Steroids may be of benefit in severe gastrointestinal disease. The prognosis is excellent. Most children

Fig. 19.4 Clinical features of Henoch–Schönlein purpura.

Clinical features of Henoch-Schönlein purpura	
Skin	A purpuric rash typically affects the legs and buttocks
GI tract	Colicky abdominal pain accompanied by gross or occult bleeding intussusception may occur
Joints	Pain and swelling of the large joints, e.g. knees and ankles
Kidneys	Glomerulonephritis manifested by microscopic haematuria rarely severe and progressive

Causes of thrombocytopenia
Decreased production Bone marrow failure • Aplastic anaemia • Leukaemia Wiskott–Aldrich syndrome **Reduced survival** Immune-mediated thrombocytopenia • Idiopathic thrombocytopenic purpura (most common) • Secondary to viral infection, drugs Hypersplenism Giant haemangioma Disseminated intravascular coagulation

Fig. 19.5 Causes of thrombocytopenia.

recover within 4–6 weeks, although, rarely, chronic renal disease can develop.

Disorders of platelets

These might be quantitative or qualitative, with the former (thrombocytopenia) being most common.

Thrombocytopenia

A decreased number of platelets (from the normal count of $150–450 \times 10^9/L$) is the most common cause of abnormal bleeding. Purpura usually occurs when the count is below $20 \times 10^9/L$. The cause might be decreased platelet production or reduced platelet survival (Fig. 19.5).

Idiopathic thrombocytopenic purpura (ITP)

This is the most common cause of thrombocytopenia in childhood and refers to an immune-mediated thrombocytopenia for which an exogenous cause is not apparent. The platelets are destroyed within the reticuloendothelial system, mainly in the spleen.

Clinical features

ITP mainly affects children between 2 and 10 years of age. Presentation is with purpura and superficial bleeding, which might be accompanied by bleeding from mucosal surfaces, e.g. epistaxis. The spleen is palpable in a minority of cases.

Diagnosis

The differential diagnosis includes:

- Acute leukaemia.
- Non-accidental injury.
- Henoch–Schönlein purpura.

A full blood count reveals thrombocytopenia but no pancytopenia. Bone marrow aspiration to exclude marrow infiltration, or aplasia, is advocated by some. This should be done if there is doubt about the diagnosis or steroid therapy is contemplated (see below). An increase in megakaryocytes (platelet precursors) is characteristic.

Treatment

In most children, the disease is acute, benign, and self-limiting, and no therapy is required. Even platelet levels $<10 \times 10^9$ are well tolerated. Serious bleeding is extremely rare as the platelets function more efficiently. Platelet infusions are rapidly destroyed and have no role except in life-threatening emergencies. Intravenous gammaglobulin infusions cause a rise in the platelet count and might be indicated in severe disease.

A short course of oral steroids is an alternative. These act by reducing capillary fragility and inhibiting platelet destruction. Bone marrow should be examined to exclude leukaemia before starting steroids.

Teenage girls have a higher risk of chronic disease (greater than 1 year) and splenectomy might have to be used if medical therapy fails.

COAGULATION DISORDERS

Haemophilia A and B and von Willebrand disease account for the majority of inherited coagulation disorders.

Haemophilia A (factor VIII deficiency)

This is an X-linked recessive disorder due to reduced or absent factor VIII. The incidence is 1 in 5000–10 000 males. It is the result of a new mutation in one third of cases. The factor VIII molecule is a complex of two proteins:

- VIII:C: small molecular weight unit, antihaemophiliac factor.
- VIII:R: large molecular weight unit, von Willebrand factor.

Clinical features

Haemophilia A results from deficiency of VIII:C. Clinical severity varies greatly and depends on the factor VIII levels (Fig. 19.6). The characteristic clinical feature is spontaneous or traumatic bleeding, which can be:

- Subcutaneous.
- Intramuscular.
- Intra-articular.

Mild haemophilia might remain undetected until excessive bleeding occurs, e.g. after dental extraction. Even severely affected boys often have few problems in the first year of life (unless circumcision is performed) but early bruising and abnormal bleeding is noted from the time they begin to walk and fall over.

In later life, recurrent soft tissue, muscle and joint bleeding are the main problems. Haemarthroses cause pain and swelling of the affected joint and repeated haemorrhage might result in chronic joint disease. Life-threatening internal haemorrhage (e.g. intracranial) can follow trauma.

Diagnosis

Diagnostic evaluation reveals a prolonged activated partial thromboplastin time (APTT), indicating a defect in the intrinsic pathway; factor VIII assay confirms the diagnosis.

Management

Bleeding is treated by replacement of the missing clotting factor with intravenous infusion of factor VIII concentrate. The amount required depends on the site and severity of the bleed. Prompt and adequate therapy is important to avoid chronic arthropathy; home therapy can avoid delay and minimize inconvenience.

Recombinant DNA technology is now used to produce factor VIII that is safer than the blood products previously used. In the past, infection with hepatitis B and C, and with HIV, occurred from contaminated blood products. Antibodies to factor VIII can develop.

Mild haemophilia can be managed with infusion of desmopressin that releases factor VIII from tissue stores.

Haemophilia B (factor IX deficiency, Christmas disease)

This is an X-linked recessive disorder caused by deficiency of factor IX. It is clinically similar to haemophilia A, but much less common. Investigation reveals a prolonged APTT and reduced factor IX activity. Treatment is with prothrombin complex concentrate.

von Willebrand disease

This is due to a deficiency of von Willebrand factor (VWF; VIII:R), which has two major roles:

- Carrier protein for factor VIII:C (preventing it from breakdown).
- Facilitates platelet adhesion.

Around 1% of the population is known to be affected. Inheritance is usually autosomal dominant with variable penetrance. The clinical hallmark is bleeding into the skin and mucous membranes (gums and nose).

Factor VIII levels in haemophilia A	
Mild	5–25% of normal
Moderate	1–4% of normal
Severe	No detectable factor VIII activity

Fig. 19.6 Factor VIII levels in haemophilia A.

Disseminated intravascular coagulation (DIC)

Intravascular activation of the coagulation cascade may be secondary to various disease processes:

- Damage to vascular endothelium: sepsis, renal disease.
- Thromboplastic substances in the circulation, e.g. in acute leukaemia.
- Impaired clearance of activated clotting factors, e.g. in liver disease.

There is fibrin deposition in small blood vessels with tissue ischaemia, consumption of labile clotting factors and activation of the fibrinolytic system.

Clinical features

Clinical features are:

- A diffuse bleeding diathesis, with oozing from venepuncture sites.
- Bleeding from the lungs.
- Bleeding from the gastrointestinal tract.

Diagnosis and treatment

Investigations reveal:

- Prolonged prothrombin type (INR), activated partial thromboplastin time (APTT) and thrombin time (TT).
- Thrombocytopenia and microangiopathic red cell morphology.

- Hypofibrinogenaemia.
- Elevated fibrinogen degradation products.

Supportive treatment includes treating the underlying cause and replacement of platelets and fresh frozen plasma.

THROMBOTIC DISORDERS IN CHILDHOOD

Recognition of thrombotic disorders in children is increasing. Although thrombosis is usually rare in children, certain genetic conditions predispose to it:

- Factor V Leiden: caused by an abnormal factor V protein that is resistant to activated protein C.
- Protein C deficiency: protein C inactivates the activated forms of factor V and VIII and stimulates fibrinolysis.
- Protein S deficiency: protein S is a cofactor to protein C.
- Antithrombin III deficiency.

Thromboembolic diseases are rare in children because thrombin is inhibited more than it is in adults and is generated less readily.

Malignant disease

Objectives

At the end of this chapter, you should be able to

- Understand the aetiology of childhood malignancy.
- Understand the types, clinical features and outline the management of childhood leukaemias.
- Outline the common types of brain tumours.
- Understand some of the commmon soft tissue tumours of childhood.

Cancer in childhood is uncommon. Approximately 1 out of 600 children between the ages of 1 and 15 years will develop cancer. Despite the dramatic increases in survival rate due to new treatments, it remains an important cause of death in childhood. The spectrum of cancer in childhood is very different from that in adults (Fig. 20.1). Leukaemia accounts for over one-third of cases.

The aetiology, clinical features, investigation and management of malignant disease in childhood are considered below, before the individual diseases are described.

Aetiology

Most childhood cancers are of uncertain cause and occur sporadically in otherwise healthy children. Risk is increased by a combination of:

- Genetic predisposition: genetic factors are often more evident in childhood than adult malignancy.
- Environmental factors.

Malignant cells proliferate and develop abnormally because they have escaped normal control mechanisms. In younger children in particular, the malignant cells might be immature precursor cells that fail to mature into normal, differentiated functional cells.

Important causative factors in childhood malignancy include:

- Genetic.
- Infections.
- Environmental.

Genetic causes of childhood cancer

During periods of rapid proliferation, a normal cell may undergo a genetic alteration that transforms it into a malignant cell. Two important mechanisms of transformation are:

- Activation of oncogenes.
- Loss of tumour suppressor genes.

Examples of childhood cancer with an identifiable genetic aetiology are shown in Fig. 20.2.

Infections

Two viruses that infect the cells of the human immune system are associated with malignancy:

- Epstein–Barr virus: the virus transforms human B cells. If not limited by an effective immune response, a translocation disrupts the *c-myc* oncogene on chromosome 8 leading to malignant change, e.g. Burkitt's lymphoma.
- Human immunodeficiency virus (HIV): this retrovirus targets the human helper T cells. Children who develop AIDS are susceptible to lymphoid malignancies.

Environmental

Carcinogens and toxins are less often a cause of childhood cancer. One important risk factor, sadly, is previous treatment of malignancy in a child.

Clinical features

Cancer in childhood presents in a limited number of ways, some of which are non-specific (Fig. 20.3).

Relative frequencies of childhood cancer

Type	% childhood cancer
Leukaemia	35
CNS tumours	23
Lymphomas	12
Wilms tumour	7
Neuroblastoma	7
Bone tumours	6
Other	10

Fig. 20.1 Relative frequencies of childhood cancer.

Genetic childhood cancer syndromes

Genetic cancer syndromes	Gene defect
Retinoblastoma	Chromosome 13-deletion of tumour suppressor gene
Li-Fraumeni	p53 mutation
Ataxia-telangiectasia	DNA repair defect
Down syndrome	Trisomy 21

Fig. 20.2 Genetic childhood cancer syndromes.

Childhood cancer-clinical features at presentation

Clinical feature	Type of cancer
Constitutional symptoms: fever, weight loss, night sweats	Lymphomas
A localized mass in: • Abdomen • Thorax • Soft tissue	Wilms tumour, neuroblastoma Non-Hodgkin lymphoma Rhabdomyosarcomas
Lymph node enlargement	Lymphomas
Bone marrow failure	Acute leukaemia
Bone pain	Leukaemia, bone tumours
Signs of raised ICP	Primary CNS tumours

Fig. 20.3 Childhood cancer—clinical features at presentation.

Classification systems employ numerical staging for solid tumours based on the extent of dissemination:

- Stage I: localized.
- Stages II and III: advanced, localized disease.
- Stage IV: disseminated disease with metastases.

Investigations

Histological confirmation is the cornerstone of diagnosis. This is provided by biopsy (although initial biopsy is not possible at some sites, e.g. brain tumours) or bone marrow aspiration.

Imaging is a vital aid and all modalities can be useful: ultrasound, X-ray, computed tomography (CT) and magnetic resonance imaging (MRI) scans. Tumour markers are useful in certain tumours, e.g. α-fetoprotein in liver tumours, urinary catecholamines in neuroblastoma.

Management

The main therapeutic strategies available are:

- Surgery: required for biopsy, total or partial removal of solid tumours (debulking), or for removal of residual disease after chemotherapy or radiotherapy.
- Radiotherapy: has an important role in specific circumstances, e.g. brain tumours.
- Chemotherapy: has a prominent role. A number of highly effective antineoplastic agents have been developed in the last four decades. Their use is based on a number of principles (see Hints & Tips). Most children are enrolled into clinical trials on diagnosis.

Chemotherapy may be used as:

- Primary therapy for disseminated malignancy, e.g. the leukaemias.
- To shrink bulky primary or metastatic disease before local treatment.
- Adjunctive treatment for micrometastases.

Bone marrow toxicity is the limiting factor for many therapeutic regimens. This can be circumvented by using bone marrow transplantation to 'rescue' patients after administering potentially lethal, but potentially curative, doses of chemotherapy or radiation.

Supportive care

Treatment produces many predictable and often severe side effects in many systems. Supportive care is a vital part of treatment (Fig. 20.4). Indwelling central venous catheters allow pain-free blood sampling and injections.

Supportive care in the treatment of cancer	
Infection	Risk of opportunistic infection from immunosuppression
Anaemia and thrombocytopenia	Blood and platelet transfusions
Nausea and vomiting	Antiemetics and steroids
Pain control	Use of appropriate analgesia
Long-term vascular access	Surgically implanted venous access

Fig. 20.4 Supportive care in the treatment of cancer.

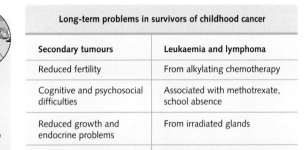

Psychosocial support is very important. Diagnosis of a potentially fatal illness provokes enormous anxiety, guilt, fear and sadness. Children and their siblings need an explanation of the illness tailored to their age. The severe stress might give rise to relationship problems between the parents and behavioural difficulties in siblings. Help with practical difficulties such as transport and finances might be required. Help from the community nursing team is very important.

Long-term problems in survivors of childhood cancer	
Secondary tumours	Leukaemia and lymphoma
Reduced fertility	From alkylating chemotherapy
Cognitive and psychosocial difficulties	Associated with methotrexate, school absence
Reduced growth and endocrine problems	From irradiated glands
Auditory Cardiac	From platinum-containing drugs From doxorubicin

Fig. 20.5 Long-term problems in survivors of childhood cancer.

For some children, a time comes when further treatment represents postponement of inevitable death rather than prolongation of life. A definite decision to concentrate on palliative care is then appropriate. For survivors, long-term follow-up is required to detect and manage long-term sequelae (Fig. 20.5).

Chemotherapy in childhood cancer:
- Chemotherapy is most likely to effect a cure when the malignant cell burden is small.
- Adverse effects are produced on rapidly dividing normal cells, e.g. those of the bone marrow, gastrointestinal tract, and hair follicles.
- Most children with leukaemia are enrolled into clinical trials.

THE LEUKAEMIAS

Leukaemia is a disease characterized by proliferation of immature white cells and is the most common malignancy of childhood. Acute leukaemias account for the majority (97%) of cases. Note that chronic myeloid leukaemia is rare and that chronic lymphocytic leukaemia is confined to adults. The malignant cells are termed 'blasts'.

The leukaemias are classified according to the white blood cell line involved:

- Acute lymphocytic (lymphoblastic) leukaemia (ALL): cells of lymphoid lineage.
- Acute myeloid leukaemia: cells of granulocytic or monocytic lineage.

It is of note that prognosis continues to improve with reductions in treatment related mortality and matching of therapies to different prognostic groups.

Clinical features

In most children with acute leukaemia, there is an insidious onset of symptoms and signs arising from infiltration of the bone marrow or other organs with leukaemic blast cells. Most will have one or more of the following:

- Pallor and malaise: anaemia.
- Haemorrhagic diathesis: purpura, easy bruising, epistaxis due to thrombocytopenia.
- Hepatosplenomegaly, lymphadenopathy: reticuloendothelial cell infiltration.
- Bone pain: due to expansion of marrow cavity.
- Infection: due to neutropenia.

Investigations

Peripheral blood investigations reveal:

- Anaemia: normocytic, normochromic.
- Thrombocytopenia.
- Neutropenia: total WBC might be low, normal or high.
- Blast cells.

Bone marrow examination reveals replacement of normal elements by leukaemic cells.

A diagnosis of leukaemia should always be confirmed by bone marrow aspiration.

Acute lymphocytic leukaemia (ALL)

This accounts for 80% of childhood leukaemia and has a peak incidence between age 3 and 6 years. It is slightly more common in boys than girls. Lymphoblasts in these children do not successfully complete the rearrangement of immunoglobulin and T cell receptor genes necessary for full maturation. Coupled with genetic alterations, which permit them to survive and proliferate, the lymphoblasts remain 'frozen' at an early stage of development.

ALL can be classified according to cell-surface antigens (immunophenotype) into:

- Non-T, non-B cell (common) ALL: 80% are mostly early B cell clone.
- T cell ALL: 15%.
- B cell ALL: 1%.

Prognostic groups in acute lymphocytic leukaemia		
Factors	Good >70% cure (all factors required)	Poor <60% cure (any factor sufficient)
Age	2–9 years	<1 year
WBC	$<50 \times 10^9$ g/L	$>50 \times 10^9$ g/L
Lineage	Non-T, non-B cell	T cell or B cell

Fig. 20.6 Prognostic groups in acute lymphocytic leukaemia.

Clinical features

Prognosis and clinical presentation varies with subtype. T cell ALL tends to occur in older children and teenagers, with a high peripheral white cell count and mediastinal mass. The prognosis is related to tumour load and can be defined according to certain clinical and laboratory features (Fig. 20.6).

Management

Overall, at least 65% of patients with ALL can now expect to be cured. Children with null cell (common) ALL have the best prognosis:

- 75% will go into remission.
- 75% survive beyond 5 years.

A typical treatment regimen can be divided into six phases:

1. Induction: an intensive regimen of between three and five drugs with the aim of reducing tumour load.
2. Early CNS-directed therapy.
3. Consolidation: continued systemic therapy after remission.
4. CNS prophylaxis without irradiation.
5. Intensification of therapy depending on risk of relapse.
6. Maintenance: chemotherapy continues for 2 years from diagnosis.

Initial preparation involves:

- Blood transfusion.
- Treatment of infection.
- Allopurinol to protect the kidneys against the effects of rapid cell lysis.

Relapses can occur in bone marrow, CNS or testes. The prognosis in these cases is poor and high-dose chemotherapy with total body irradiation and bone marrow transplantation might be necessary for survival. In ALL, bone marrow transplant is used only for high-risk groups because the benefits are counterbalanced by the risks of transplant-related mortality.

Acute myeloid leukaemia

This is classified into seven subtypes; 80% are associated with chromosomal abnormalities and the treatment is more intensive than ALL and carries a worse prognosis. Treatment approach is similar to that of ALL. Bone marrow transplant is used in high-risk groups only because of the mortality associated with the procedure and because studies in good- and intermediate-risk groups have shown no overall benefit.

LYMPHOMAS

These can be classified into:

- Non-Hodgkin's lymphoma (NHL): more common in young children.
- Hodgkin's disease: more common in adolescents and young adults.

Non-Hodgkin's lymphoma (NHL)

NHLs are a heterogeneous group of lymphomas with different characteristics and cells of origin. NHL causes 7% of all childhood cancer and 100 cases per year are seen in the UK. They can develop in immunocompromised children with HIV infection, severe combined immunodeficiency or other severe inherited immunodeficiencies.

Clinical features

NHLs tend to be aggressive and rapidly growing, and might present with:

- Peripheral lymph node enlargement: usually B cell origin.
- Intrathoracic mass: usually T cell origin.
- Mediastinal mass or pleural effusion.
- Abdominal mass: usually advanced B cell disease.
- Gut or lymph node masses.

Subtypes of ALL and NHL might represent a continuation of the same disease.

Treatment

Chemotherapy is the mainstay of treatment but extensive surgical debulking might be required for abdominal tumours. Localized disease has a 90% survival at 5 years. Complications in the acute setting are superior vena cava syndrome and tumour lysis syndrome.

Hodgkin's disease

This is characterized histologically by the Reed–Sternberg cell. It is relatively uncommon in prepubertal children and usually presents in adolescence or young adulthood, with a slight preponderance in females.

Clinical features

The usual presentation is with painless cervical or supraclavicular lymphadenopathy. Systemic symptoms are uncommon. Metastatic disease occurs in the lungs, liver and bone marrow.

Diagnosis

Diagnosis is confirmed by histological examination of a lymph node biopsy. Classification based on histopathology identifies four subtypes of different prognosis:

1. Lymphocyte predominance: best prognosis.
2. Mixed cellularity.
3. Nodular sclerosing: most common in children and adolescents.
4. Lymphocyte depletion: least common, worst prognosis.

Treatment

The disease is staged, to determine treatment, using imaging of chest, mediastinum and abdomen. (Staging laparotomy is no longer performed in the UK.) Treatment is combination chemotherapy for all except patients with localized disease, who can be treated with radiotherapy. The overall prognosis is good and 80% of patients are cured overall.

BRAIN TUMOURS

Brain tumours are the second most common form of childhood cancer and the most common solid tumour of childhood. Most are located infratentorially and present with signs and symptoms of raised intracranial pressure and cerebellar dysfunction. Metastasis is rare and diagnosis is often difficult and delayed.

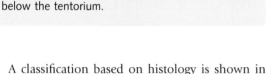

Brain tumours are the most common solid tumour of children. Two-thirds arise below the tentorium.

A classification based on histology is shown in Fig. 20.7. An example of a posterior fossa tumour with hydrocephalus is shown in Fig. 20.8.

Classification of brain tumours in childhood

Astrocytic tumours
  High-grade astrocytomas
  • Supratentorial
  Low-grade astrocytomas
  • Cerebellar
  Brainstem gliomas
Neuroepithelial tumours
  Primitive neuroectodermal tumours (PNET)
  (includes cerebellar medulloblastoma)

Fig. 20.7 Classification of brain tumours in childhood.

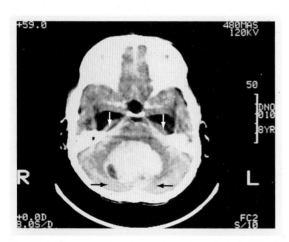

Fig. 20.8 CT of an enhancing posterior fossa tumour (black arrows) with hydrocephalus demonstrated by dilated temporal horns (white arrows).

Astrocytomas (40%)

Cerebellar astrocytomas are usually low-grade, slow-growing, cystic gliomas occurring between the ages of 6 and 9 years. Presentation might be with:

- Headache and vomiting: caused by obstructive hydrocephalus; papilloedema might be present.
- Cerebellar signs: ataxia, nystagmus and uncoordination.
- Diplopia, squint: sixth nerve palsy.

Supratentorial astrocytomas and gliomas are less common and present with focal neurological signs and seizures.

Brainstem gliomas (6%) present with cranial nerve palsies, ataxia and pyramidal tract signs.

Diagnosis is usually based on clinical findings and MR imaging as biopsy is hazardous. Prognosis is poor, with median survival less than 1 year after diagnosis despite radiotherapy.

Primitive neuroectodermal tumours (medulloblastomas) (20%)

These are the most common malignant brain tumours of childhood, with a peak incidence between the ages of 2 and 6 years, and a preponderance in boys. They usually arise in the midline and invade the fourth ventricle and cerebellar hemispheres. Unlike other CNS tumours they seed through the CNS and up to 20% have spinal metastases at diagnosis.

Presentation is usually with headache, vomiting and ataxia.

Treatment is surgical removal and whole CNS irradiation (5-year survival rates are 50%). Adjuvant chemotherapy may be added for children with higher than average risk of recurrence.

Craniopharyngioma (4%)

These arise from the squamous remnant of Rathke's pouch and are locally invasive. They present with:

- Visual field loss: due to compression of the optic chiasm.
- Pituitary dysfunction: growth failure, diabetes insipidus.

Most are calcified and are visible on skull radiographs. Treatment is surgical excision and/or radiotherapy. Prognosis is good but sequelae include visual impairment and endocrine deficiency.

NEUROBLASTOMA

Neuroblastoma is a malignancy of neural crest cells that normally give rise to the paraspinal sympathetic ganglia and the adrenal medulla. It is the second most common solid tumour of childhood, occurring predominantly in infants and preschool children with a median age at diagnosis of 2 years. It is unusual in that it can regress spontaneously in very young children (stage IV-S).

Clinical features

The clinical features depend on the location and may include:

- Abdominal mass: a firm, non-tender abdominal mass is the most common mode of presentation.
- Systemic signs: pallor, weight loss, bone pain from disseminated disease.
- Hepatomegaly or lymph node enlargement.
- Unilateral proptosis: periorbital swelling and ecchymosis from metastasis to the eye.
- Opsoclonus-myoclonus: 'dancing-eye' syndrome caused by an immune response.
- Watery diarrhoea due to secretion of vasoactive intestinal peptide.
- Extra-abdominal tumours are often well on presentation.
- Mediastinal mass on CXR.

Diagnosis

Diagnosis is usually made from the characteristic clinical and radiological features:

- Raised urinary catecholamines (vanillylmandelic acid, homovanillic acid) are useful in diagnosis and monitoring response to therapy.
- Confirmatory biopsy is usually possible and scanning using MIBG (meta-iodobenzyl guanidine), a radiolabelled tumour-specific agent, is useful to measure disease extent.

Treatment

Treatment of neuroblastoma includes:

- Surgical resection.
- Chemotherapy.
- Irradiation.

Prognosis is worse for older children and those with metastatic disease. Overexpression of the *N-myc* oncogene in tumour material is associated with a poor prognosis.

WILMS' TUMOUR (NEPHROBLASTOMA)

Wilms' tumour arises from embryonal renal cells of the metanephros. It is predominantly a tumour of the first 5 years of life with a median age of presentation of 3 years of age. Sporadic and familial forms occur. Most tumours are unilateral.

Clinical features

The most common clinical presentation is an asymptomatic abdominal mass that does not cross the midline. Other features may include:

- Abdominal pain: due to haemorrhage into the tumour.
- Haematuria.
- Hypertension: in 25% of cases. This can be caused by compression of the renal artery or renin production by tumour cells.

A Wilms' tumour susceptibility gene has been recognized from the rare association of Wilms' tumour, sporadic aniridia and deletions of part of chromosome 11. Associated abnormalities found in some children include:

- Hemihypertrophy.
- Genitourinary tract abnormalities.
- Mental retardation.
- Aniridia.

Wilms' tumour:
- Arises from embryonic renal cells.
- Usually presents as an abdominal mass in a child under 5 years old.
- Is bilateral in 5% of cases.
- Is associated with aniridia (absent iris).

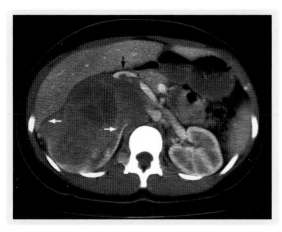

Fig. 20.9 CT scan of nephroblastoma. Wilms' tumour mass arising out of right kidney (white arrows) displacing the inferior vena cava (black arrow).

Diagnosis

Diagnosis is normally made from the characteristic appearance on CT (Fig. 20.9), which shows an *intrinsic* renal mass with mixed solid and cystic densities, and from biopsy. A search for distant metastases, which are most common in lungs and liver, should be made.

Treatment

Treatment involves surgical resection of the primary tumour, chemotherapy tailored to the stage and histology, and radiotherapy for those with advanced disease. Overall, the prognosis is good, with an 80% chance of cure if there is no metastasis, although this falls to 30% if metastases are present.

SOFT TISSUE SARCOMAS

These arise from primitive mesenchyme. The most important is rhabdomyosarcoma, but even rarer forms include fibrosarcomas and liposarcomas.

BONE TUMOURS

Primary malignant bone tumours account for 4% of childhood cancer. They are uncommon before puberty and are most common in adolescents with a preponderence in boys. The two main types are:

- Osteogenic sarcoma: older children, most common.
- Ewing's sarcoma: younger children, less common.

Osteogenic sarcoma

This is a malignant tumour of the bone-producing mesenchyme and is twice as common in males as females.

Clinical features

The usual presenting feature is local pain and swelling. Persistent bone pain precedes the detection of a mass. Half of all cases occur around the knee joint in the metaphysis of the distal femur or proximal tibia. Systemic symptoms are rare. Metastases are mainly to the lungs and are often asymptomatic.

Diagnosis

Bone X-ray shows destruction and a characteristic 'sunburst' appearance as the tumour breaks through the cortex and spicules of new bone are formed.

Treatment

Treatment involves surgery of primary and metastatic deposits. En bloc resection might allow amputation to be avoided. Aggressive neoadjuvant chemotherapy is important to treat micrometastatic disease. Survival has improved and is greater than 50%.

Ewing's sarcoma

This is less common than osteogenic sarcoma and is very rare in Afro-Caribbean children. It is an undifferentiated sarcoma of uncertain tissue of origin that arises primarily in bone, but occasionally in soft tissues.

It most commonly affects the long bones, especially the mid- to proximal femur, but can also affect flat bones such as the pelvis.

Clinical features and diagnosis

Pain and localized swelling are the usual presenting complaints. X-ray demonstrates a destructive lesion with periosteal elevation or a soft tissue mass (so called 'onion skin' appearance). Metastases occur to the lungs and other bones.

Treatment

Radiotherapy to the primary tumour is combined with chemotherapy for the prevention or treatment of metastases.

> Bone tumours:
> - Are most common in adolescence.
> - Are more common in boys.
> - Most commonly affect the long bones.

Retinoblastoma

This is a cause of an absent red reflex in the neonate. It is associated with deletion of a tumour suppressor gene on chromosome 13 and is bilateral in 40%.

LANGERHANS CELL HISTIOCYTOSIS

Formerly called histiocytosis X, this term encompasses a group of relatively rare diseases characterized by the clonal proliferation of Langerhans cells (components of the bone-marrow-derived mononuclear phagocytic system). It is not now considered a true malignancy but the potentially aggressive course and response to chemotherapy brings it within this sphere of clinical practice.

Further reading

Will A. Recent advances in the management of leukaemia. *Current Paediatrics* 2003; **13**:201–216.

Endocrine and metabolic disorders

DISORDERS OF CARBOHYDRATE METABOLISM

Diabetes mellitus

This is a heterogeneous group of disorders, characterized by hyperglycaemia and caused by reduced or absent insulin secretion or action. Type 1 diabetes (formerly called insulin-dependent diabetes) is the most common form of childhood diabetes, although other varieties might be encountered. Type 2 diabetes is characterized by insulin resistance and its increasing incidence has been associated with childhood obesity; however, the discussion below refers to type 1.

Aetiology

There is good evidence that type 1 diabetes results from T-cell-mediated autoimmune destruction of β cells in the pancreatic islets of Langerhans, perhaps triggered by environmental factors (e.g. viruses) in people with a genetic predisposition (Fig. 21.1). The incidence of the disorder is increasing in the UK.

Pathophysiology

The pathophysiological pathways are described in Fig. 21.2. Key features include:

- Insulin deficiency becomes clinically significant when 90% of the β cells are destroyed.
- Osmotic diuresis ensues when blood glucose concentration exceeds renal threshold.
- Ketoacidosis develops when insulin deficiency is severe.

Clinical features

Although type 1 diabetes can present at any age, the most common age of onset is between 7 and 15 years of age. Increasingly, type 1 diabetes is diagnosed at an early stage, when the principal features are:

- Polyuria: increased frequency of urination (possibly enuresis).
- Polydipsia: increased thirst.
- Weight loss.

Always check for glycosuria in a child with a history of polyuria and polydipsia. Never ascribe frequency of micturition to urinary tract infection without checking for glycosuria and culturing urine.

Diabetic ketoacidosis supervenes at a late stage over a short period and is characterized by abdominal pain, vomiting, features of severe dehydration and ketoacidosis (see Hints & Tips). Younger children develop more severe complications of ketoacidosis.

Fig. 21.1 Aetiology of insulin-dependent diabetes mellitus.

Aetiology of insulin-dependent diabetes mellitus

Genetic factors
Inherited susceptibility is demonstrated by increased incidence of IDDM in first-degree relatives: 2-5% in siblings and offspring. Concordance for identical twins is 30%. There is an 8-10 times risk for IDDM in people who are HLA-DR3, HLA-DR4, or both

Auto-immune factors
Auto-immune basis is supported by:
• Anti-islet cell antibodies
• Lymphocytic infiltration of pancreas
• Association with other auto-immune endocrine diseases, e.g. thyroiditis, Addison disease

Environmental factors
Triggers may include viruses and dietary proteins

Traps for the unwary regarding diabetic ketoacidosis include mistaking the abdominal pain for acute appendicitis and mistaking the hyperventilation for pneumonia.

Diagnosis

Diagnosis is confirmed in a symptomatic child by documenting hyperglycaemia—a random plasma glucose level >11 mmol/L in the absence of other acute illnesses. If there is doubt, as might occur very early in the disease process, a fasting plasma glucose >8 mmol/L or a raised glycosylated haemoglobin level will clarify the situation. Oral glucose tolerance tests are rarely needed in children.

Management

The discovery of insulin in 1922 transformed type 1 diabetes mellitus from a fatal disease into a treatable one. Initial management depends on the child's clinical condition. Long-term management of this life long condition rests on:

• Insulin replacement.
• Diet.
• Exercise.
• Monitoring.
• Education and psychological support.
• Management of complications: hypoglycaemia and diabetic ketoacidosis.

These are considered in turn.

Insulin replacement
The important features of insulin replacement are:

• Average requirement is 0.5–1.0 unit/kg/day. During the 'honeymoon' or remission phase, which can last for weeks or months after presentation, temporary residual islet cell function causes a reduction in insulin requirements.
• Insulin regimes (Fig. 21.3): (1) One, two or three injections daily—usually combination of short/rapid acting insulin with an intermediate acting insulin. It often comes premixed in specific ratios. (2) Multiple daily injections—this involves short/rapid acting insulin injections before meals and one or more separate injections of intermediate/long acting insulin. (3) Continuous subcutaneous insulin infusion using a pump.
• In the first regime, the total daily dose is divided in a 1:2 proportion between short-acting (regular, soluble) insulin and medium-acting (isophane) insulin. Two-thirds is usually given before breakfast and one-third before the evening meal, so two injections per day are administered.
• Multiple daily injection regimes usually use ultra rapid acting insulins as they are more convenient (usually taken just before a meal, or even after the meal—the dose can be titrated according to blood sugar response) and results in improved glucose control.
• Injections are given subcutaneously and can be given in upper arms, outer thighs or abdomen. The site must be rotated to avoid local complications such as fat atrophy.
• During puberty, insulin requirements increase. Multiple injections may result in better glycaemic control.

Fig. 21.2 Pathophysiology of insulin-dependent diabetes mellitus.

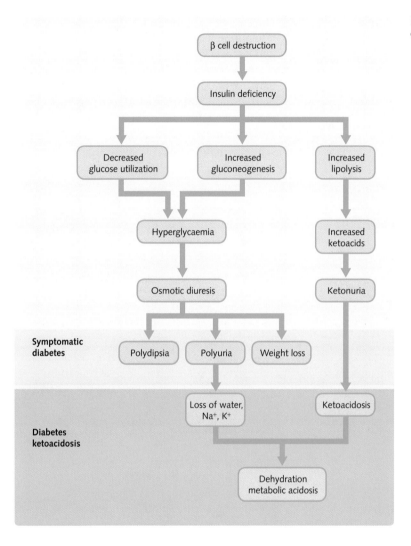

Types of insulin			
Type of insulin	**Onset of action**	**Duration of action**	**Examples**
Rapid acting	15 min	1–5 h	NovoRapid (insulin aspart)
Short acting	30–60 min	Up to 8 h	Actrapid, Humulin (soluble insulin)
Intermediate acting	1–2 h	16–35 h (peak: 4–12 h)	Isophane insulin
Long acting	Steady state in 3–4 days	Constant	Levemir (insulin detemir), Lantus (insulin glargine)
Biphasic insulin	Variable	Variable	Mixtard, NovoMix, etc.

Fig. 21.3 Types of insulin.

Diet and exercise

Food intake needs to match the time course of insulin absorption and be adjusted for unusual heavy exercise. Dietary management therefore encompasses:

- High fibre, complex carbohydrates: this provides sustained release of glucose and avoids rapid swings in blood glucose generated by refined carbohydrates (e.g. sweets or ice creams).
- Food intake is divided between the three main meals and intervening snacks.
- Food intake is increased before or after heavy exercise to avoid hypoglycaemia.

Dietary advice is an important part of the management of diabetes. Involvement of a dietitian is crucial. Once a diagnosis of diabetes is made, children are seen by the diabetic nurse and the dietitian before discharge and arrangement for follow up made. It is important to ensure that this is done before the child goes home.

Monitoring

Monitoring of blood glucose concentrations is necessary to evaluate the management and control. This is performed using finger-prick samples, which are convenient and easy to take. Readings are recorded in a diary so changes to insulin regimens can be appropriately made. 24-hour profiles are more useful than single daily records. Urine testing is more indirect, does not detect unacceptably low levels of glucose, and is often less popular, especially with teenagers. However, urine testing for ketones is important if ketoacidosis is suspected.

The measurement of glycosylated haemoglobin (HbA1c) reflects glycaemic control over the past 6–8 weeks and allows long-term glucose control to be optimized. NICE guidelines recommend a target HbA1c level less than 7.5 %, though in practice this may result in more hypoglycaemic episodes.

Education and psychological support

Children and their families require an educational programme that covers:

- A basic understanding of diabetes in lay language.
- The influence of diet and exercise on blood glucose levels.
- Practical aspects of insulin injection and blood glucose monitoring.
- Recognition and treatment of hypoglycaemia.
- Adjustments for intercurrent illness, significance of ketonuria.
- The importance of good control.

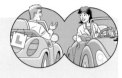

A multidisciplinary approach is essential, involving the physician, dietitian, diabetic nurse and community nurses. Children and parents should be introduced to the various members of the team before discharge if possible since they can offer valuable support regarding the practical aspects of diabetic management.

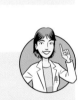

The diagnosis of type 1 diabetes provokes strong emotional responses in the child and family, including anger, guilt, resentment and fear. Adjustment to these normal responses is facilitated by open discussion. Voluntary groups (e.g. the British Diabetic Association) are important sources of support.

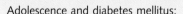
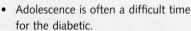

Adolescence and diabetes mellitus:
- Adolescence is often a difficult time for the diabetic.
- There might be conflict at home and with healthcare professionals.
- Problems occur with self-image, self-esteem and desire for independence.
- Denial or indifference can lead to poor compliance.
- 'Feeling well' is equated with good control and long-term risks are often ignored.
- Helpful strategies include: a united team approach, clear guidelines plus short-term goals and peer group pressure.

Management of complications

These can be divided into immediate complications, which include hypoglycaemia and diabetic ketoacidosis, and late complications.

Hypoglycaemia   The concentration of glucose in the blood can fall when there is a mismatch between insulin dose, time of administration, carbohydrate intake and exercise. Many young children are not aware of hypoglycaemic episodes and repeated hypoglycaemic episodes increase this lack of awareness.

Symptoms usually occur at blood glucose levels below 4 mmol/L. Initial symptoms reflect the compensatory sympathetic discharge and include feeling faint, dizzy or 'wobbly', sweating, tremulousness and hunger. More severe symptoms reflect glucose deprivation to the central nervous system and include lethargy, bizarre behaviour and—ultimately—coma or seizures. Unlike adults and older children, in young children the behavioural and neuroglycopenic symptoms predominate over autonomic symptoms.

Treatment of a 'hypo' is easily achieved at an early stage by administration of a sugary drink, glucose tablet or glucose polymer gel, which is well absorbed via the buccal mucosa, but this should be followed by a more complex form of carbohydate. In severe hypoglycaemia, if consciousness is impaired or there is lack of cooperation, IV glucose or 1 mg of IM glucagon is administered. Eating a sugary snack just before exercising reduces the risk of exercise-induced hypoglycaemia.

Diabetic ketoacidosis   This can occur at presentation or complicate established diabetes (e.g. if there is poor compliance or intercurrent illness). It is considered in Chapter 26.

Late complications of diabetes

Intensive insulin control with four injections daily reduces the incidence of long term vascular complications of diabetes such as:

- Retinopathy.
- Nephropathy.
- Neuropathy.

Intensive control is associated with more hypoglycaemic episodes, hence may not be suitable in young children. This is usually acceptable only in older children.

Hypoglycaemia

This is a common problem in the newborn (see Chapter 25) but is still seen occasionally in infants and children. It is important to diagnose because it is easy to treat and has serious consequences if unrecognized.

The various causes are best understood in relation to the normal factors determining glucose homeostasis. The major causes are listed in Fig. 21.4.

Clinical features

Early symptoms reflect the compensatory sympathetic response and include dizziness, faintness and hunger. Signs include tachycardia, sweating and pallor. Late features are those of neuroglycopenia: altered behaviour and consciousness, headache and seizures.

Diagnosis

The precise definition of hypoglycaemia is problematic but a useful working definition is a blood glucose less than 2.6 mmol/L. This corresponds to

Causes of hypoglycaemia beyond the neonatal period
Metabolic
Ketotic hypoglycaemia
Liver disease
Inborn errors of metabolism, e.g. glycogen storage disorders
Hormonal
Deficiency
• Adrenocortical insufficiency, e.g. Addison disease, congenital adrenal hyperplasia
• Panhypopituitarism
• Growth hormone deficiency
Hyperinsulinism
• Islet cell adenoma
• Exogenous insulin-treated IDDM

Fig. 21.4 Causes of hypoglycaemia beyond the neonatal period.

changes in the EEG. Measurements made using a glucose-sensitive strip should always be verified by a laboratory measurement. Serum and urine should be taken during the attack for further diagnostic testing e.g. for metabolic disorders.

Management

If the child is alert then giving a sugary drink is the first step; an unconscious child should be given 5 mL/kg IV 10% dextrose. Higher concentrations have been associated with rebound hypoglycaemia and should be avoided. Blood glucose should be monitored closely and a maintenance infusion of glucose can be given if the hypoglycaemia persists. Glucagon can be used in cases where glycogen stores are depleted, e.g. insulin overdose.

Ketotic hypoglycaemia

The most common cause of hypoglycaemia in children 1–4 years of age, this ill-defined entity is the result of diminished tolerance of normal fasting. The typical child is short and thin and becomes hypoglycaemic after a short period of starvation, for example, in the early morning. Insulin levels are low and there is ketonuria. Treatment is with frequent snacks and extra glucose drinks during intercurrent illness. Spontaneous resolution occurs by the ages of 6–8 years.

Regarding hypoglycaemia, at the time of blood glucose measurement, samples should be sent for measurement of:
- Plasma insulin, growth hormone and cortisol.
- β-hydroxybutyrate.
- Urine should be tested for ketones.

THYROID DISORDERS

Thyroid hormone is critical for normal growth and neurological development in infants and children. Conditions causing hypothyroidism and hyperthyroidism occur, and the gland can also be the site of benign and malignant tumours. Worldwide, the most important condition affecting the thyroid gland is iodide deficiency, estimated to affect at least 800 million people.

Hypothyroidism

This might be present at birth (congenital hypothyroidism) or develop at any time during childhood or adolescence (acquired hypothyroidism).

Congenital hypothyroidism

This has an incidence of 1 in 4000 live births. The causes include:

- Developmental defects: thyroid agenesis or failure of migration.
- Dyshormonogenesis: inborn error of thyroid hormone synthesis (accounts for 15%, a goitre usually occurs).
- Transient congenital hypothyroidism: (e.g. ingestion of maternal goitrogens).
- Congenital pituitary lesions (rare).
- Maternal iodide deficiency: the most common cause worldwide.

Clinical features

Infants may appear clinically normal at birth. The clinical features that develop include:

- Prolonged neonatal jaundice.
- Feeding problems.
- Constipation.
- Coarse facies, large fontanelle, large tongue, hypotonia and goitre.

Diagnosis and treatment

Testing for hypothyroidism is a part of the neonatal screening in the UK and most infants are diagnosed this way. Most laboratories test for raised levels of thyroid stimulating hormone (TSH), although some measure both TSH and thyroxine (T_4). Early diagnosis and treatment with oral thyroxine results in nearly normal neurological function and intelligence. Acquired hypothyroidism is treated with thyroxine. Monitoring of treatment is by regular assessment of TSH and T_4.

Hyperthyroidism

Neonatal hyperthyroidism can occur in the infants of mothers with Graves' disease from the transplacental transfer of thyroid-stimulating immunoglobulins (see Chapter 26).

Juvenile hyperthyroidism

This is most commonly caused by Graves' disease, an autoimmune condition in which one type of antibody (human thyroid stimulating immuno-globulins) mimics TSH by binding and activating the TSH receptor. It usually presents during adolescence and is much more common in girls than boys.

The clinical features are similar to those seen in adults and can also include deteriorating school performance; puberty might be delayed or accelerated.

On laboratory testing, serum levels of thyroxine (T_4) and triiodothyronine (T_3) are elevated and TSH levels are depressed. Antimicrosomal antibodies are often present.

Medical therapy with carbimazole is the first line of treatment. β-blockers can be added for relief of severe symptoms but should be discontinued when thyroid function is controlled. Subtotal thyroidectomy or radioiodine treatments are options for relapse after medical treatment. Radioiodine has not been shown to be harmful in children.

- Slow linear growth is the hallmark of hypothyroidism in childhood.
- Children with Down syndrome have an increased incidence of hypothyroidism and hyperthyroidism.

ADRENAL DISORDERS

Disorders of the adrenal cortex can result in deficiency or excess of adrenocortical hormones. The latter causes Cushing syndrome, the most common cause of which is chronic administration of corticosteroids. Disorders of the medulla (e.g. phaeochromocytoma) are exceedingly rare.

Cortisol, the major glucocorticoid, is stimulated by pituitary adrenocorticotrophic hormone (ACTH) under a negative feedback loop. Aldosterone is the principal mineralocorticoid and is controlled by the renin–angiotensin system. The major sex steroids produced by the adrenal glands are androgens.

Adrenocortical insufficiency

Diminished production of adrenocortical hormones may arise from:

- Congenital adrenal hyperplasia (CAH): an inherited inborn error of metabolism in biosynthesis of adrenal corticosteroids.
- Primary adrenal cortical insufficiency: Addison's disease.
- Secondary adrenal insufficiency: ACTH deficiency due to pituitary disease or long-term corticosteroid therapy.

Congenital adrenal hyperplasia (CAH)

This is a group of disorders caused by a defect in the pathway that synthesizes cortisol from cholesterol. Approximately 90% of cases are caused by a deficiency in 21-hydroxylase and 5–7% are due to 11-hydroxylase deficiency; other defects are seen but are rare. Prevalence is approximately 1 in 10000 and newborn screening is available in some centres. The condition is autosomal recessive and the gene is found on chromosome 6.

Clinical features
Clinical features are due to androgen excess and cortisol deficiency:

- Female virilization.
- Salt-wasting crises due to mineralcorticoid deficiency (this is less common with 11-hydroxylase deficiency). This leads to volume depletion, electrolyte imbalances and shock.
- Cortisol deficiency—hypoglycaemia, hypotension, shock.

It is difficult to diagnose male infants with this disorder because they have few clinical manifestations at birth. For this reason, screening programmes are currently being evaluated.

Diagnosis
Diagnosis rests on the demonstration of markedly elevated levels of 17α-hydroxyprogesterone in the serum. In the 'salt-losing' form, the characteristic electrolyte disturbance of hyponatraemia, hypochloridaemia and hyperkalaemia provides a clue to the diagnosis.

Management
Initial management of a 'salt-losing' crisis involves volume replacement with normal saline and systemic steroids. Parents are also taught to recognize early signs of illness and children should carry a steroid card to alert health professionals.

Long-term treatment involves:

- Cortisol replacement with hydrocortisone: to suppress ACTH and androgen overproduction. Growth is used as a monitor of therapy.
- Mineralocorticoid replacement: fludrocortisone if there is salt wasting.
- Surgical correction of female genital abnormalities.

Congenital adrenal hyperplasia is a potentially lethal but treatable cause of vomiting and dehydration in young infants.

Primary adrenal insufficiency

Addison's disease is rare in children but can be caused by:

- Autoimmune disease.
- Haemorrhage and infarction (Waterhouse–Friderichsen syndrome).
- Tuberculosis (rare).

Physical findings include postural hypotension and increased pigmentation. Intercurrent illness or trauma can trigger an adrenal crisis (characterized by vomiting, dehydration and shock).

Secondary adrenal insufficiency

This is most commonly caused by prolonged glucocorticoid use in diseases not involving the adrenal gland, e.g. severe chronic asthma. The risk is increased by increased duration of treatment but courses less than 10 days have a low risk. Reduction of steroid doses should be slow after a prolonged course and tailored to the underlying disease. This also rarely occurs with high-dose inhaled steroids.

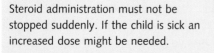

Steroid administration must not be stopped suddenly. If the child is sick an increased dose might be needed.

Causes of Cushing syndrome	
Primary	Adrenal tumour
Secondary	ACTH secretion from: Pituitary tumour Ectopic ACTH production
Iatrogenic	Long-term glucocorticoid administration

Fig. 21.5 Causes of Cushing syndrome.

Cushing syndrome

This is a cluster of symptoms and signs caused by glucocorticoid excess, due either to endogenous overproduction of cortisol or exogenous treatment with pharmacological doses of corticosteroids. The causes are listed in Fig. 21.5.

Clinical features

The clinical features include:

- Short stature.
- Truncal obesity, 'buffalo' hump.
- Rounded 'moon' facies.
- Signs of virilization, striae.
- Hypertension.

Diagnosis

Elevated serum cortisol levels are found with absence of the normal diurnal rhythm (high midnight levels). A prolonged dexamethasone suppression test might be required to distinguish Cushing disease (ACTH-driven bilateral adrenal hyperplasia: suppressible by dexamethasone) from Cushing syndrome (adrenal tumour: cortisol levels not suppressed by dexamethasone). CT or MRI of the adrenal and pituitary glands might identify an adrenal tumour or pituitary adenoma. Treatment depends on the cause and might involve surgical resection and radiotherapy.

DISORDERS OF THE PITUITARY GLAND

The pituitary gland has two distinct portions: the anterior and posterior lobes. These have different embryonic origins and separate hormonal functions. Pituitary disorders in childhood are rare.

Anterior pituitary disorders

A deficiency of the anterior pituitary hormones is more common than an excess of these and might involve individual hormones or all (panhypopituitarism). Hypopituitarism in children can be caused by:

- Cranial defects, e.g. septo-optic dysplasia and agenesis of corpus callosum.
- Tumours, e.g craniopharyngioma.
- Idiopathic hormone abnormalities.
- Trauma/surgery and radiation.

Growth retardation is a common feature, together with thyroid, adrenal and gonadal dysfunction depending on the pattern of deficiency. Isolated idiopathic growth hormone (GH) deficiency accounts for most cases of GH deficiency.

Posterior pituitary disorders

The posterior lobe (neurohypophysis) secretes arginine, vasopressin (also called antidiuretic hormone, ADH) and oxytocin.

Diabetes insipidus

This results from deficiency of ADH. It might occur as an isolated idiopathic defect or in association with anterior pituitary deficiency (e.g. due to tumours, infections or trauma).

It presents with polydipsia and polyuria. Several conditions mimic diabetes insipidus, including hypercalcaemia, chronic renal disease and psychogenic water drinking. Diagnosis is by a water deprivation test.

Syndrome of inappropriate secretion of ADH (SIADH)

Diagnosis consists of:

- Hypo-osmolality with hyponatraemia.
- Normal or increased volume status.
- Normal renal, thyroid and adrenal function.
- Elevated urine sodium and osmolality.

Symptoms occur due to effects of water intoxication: these include vomiting, behavioural changes and seizures.

SIADH is a common stress response and might be caused by several underlying conditions including:

- CNS disease: meningitis, brain tumours or head trauma.
- Lung disease: pneumonia.

Treatment is by treating the underlying cause and fluid restriction.

DISORDERS OF THE GONADS

These cause abnormalities of sexual differentiation (which usually present in the newborn) and disorders of puberty, which might be precocious or delayed.

Disorders of sexual differentiation

Abnormal sexual differentiation results in a newborn with ambiguous genitalia. Congenital adrenal hyperplasia leading to a virilized female is the most common cause. The causes can be classified as shown in Fig. 21.6.

Complete diagnostic evaluation should be undertaken as soon as possible. A definite sex cannot and should not be assigned immediately. It is worth remembering that 'sex' is determined at many different levels (Fig. 21.7). Naming and announcement

Causes of abnormal sexual differentiation
46XY males with testes and incomplete masculinization due to:
• Defects in testosterone synthesis
• Defects in androgen action, e.g. 5α-reductase deficiency
• Androgen resistance (testicular feminization syndrome)
46XX females with ovaries who are masculinized due to:
• Congenital adrenal hyperplasia
• Maternal androgen exposure

Fig. 21.6 Causes of abnormal sexual differentiation.

Sex determination
An individual's sex is determined at many different levels:
• Chromosomal
• Gonadal (testis, ovary)
• Anatomical (internal and external genitalia)
• Hormonal
• Psychological
• Sex of rearing

Fig. 21.7 Sex determination.

Features of puberty	
Male genitalia	First sign is testicular growth Followed by penis enlargement Growth spurt reached 2 years later than females
Female genitalia	Initially breast development Pubic and axillary hair development follows Menses occur late

Fig. 21.8 Features of puberty.

Causes of precocious puberty

Gonadotrophin-dependent
  Idiopathic, familial
  CNS lesions, e.g. postirradiation, surgery, tumours,
  hydrocephalus
Gonadotrophin-independent
  McCune–Albright syndrome (polyostotic fibrous
  dysplasia of bone)
  Tumours of adrenals or gonads

Fig. 21.9 Causes of precocious puberty.

Fig. 21.10 Causes of delayed puberty.

Causes of delayed puberty

Central causes—gonadotrophins low
  Constitutional delayed puberty
  Hypothalamo-pituitary disorders, e.g. panhypopituitarism, intracranial tumours,
  isolated gonadotrophin deficiency
  Severe systemic disease, e.g. cystic fibrosis, severe asthma, starvation
Gonadal failure—gonadotrophins high
  Chromosomal abnormalities, e.g. Klinefelter syndrome (47, XXY), Turner syndrome (45, XO)

of the child's sex should be delayed until the diagnostic work-up is complete. Investigations will include:

- Chromosomal analysis.
- Hormone levels: testosterone, luteinizing hormone, follicle stimulating hormone, 17-hydroxyprogesterone.
- Pelvic ultrasonography.

Management is multidisciplinary, involving:

- Endocrinology.
- Psychology.
- Paediatric urology and gynaecology.

Disorders of puberty

During normal puberty, secondary sex characteristics are acquired and reproductive capacity is attained. Features of normal puberty in males and females are listed in Fig. 21.8. Puberty can be precocious or delayed.

Precocious puberty

This refers to the development of secondary sexual characteristics before the age of 8 years in girls or 9 years in boys. There is an associated growth spurt. It should be differentiated from:

- Premature thelarche: isolated breast development in a very young girl. A non-progressive, benign condition.
- Premature adrenarche: isolated early appearance of pubic hair in either sex. A benign, self-limiting condition due to early maturation of adrenal androgen secretion, although an adrenal tumour might need to be excluded.

The causes of precocious puberty are shown in Fig. 21.9. In females, it is usually due to early onset of normal puberty. In boys, it is usually pathological and must be investigated.

Treatment depends on cause. Gonadotrophin-releasing hormone analogues (GnRHa) can be used to prevent puberty from progressing.

Delayed puberty

This can be defined as the absence of secondary sex characteristics at 14 years of age in girls or 15 years of age in boys. The problem is more common in boys and the majority of adolescents affected are normal. The causes are listed in Fig. 21.10.

Assessment should include pubertal staging and examination to exclude systemic disease. If indicated, helpful investigations are:

- Chromosomal analysis.
- Measurement of gonadotrophin levels.

Treatment is often not required for constitutional delay, but hormone therapy (e.g. oxandrolone or low-dose testosterone) can be used to accelerate growth and induce secondary sexual characteristics in boys. Oestrogen therapy can be used in girls but care must be taken to prevent premature closure of the epiphyses.

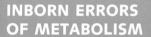

- Precocious puberty is more common in girls.
- Delayed puberty is more common in boys.

INBORN ERRORS OF METABOLISM

This term is used to describe any of the inherited disorders that result in a defect in normal biochemical pathways. Several hundred of these conditions have been described. Individually they are rare, although certain ethnic groups are at increased risk for specific diseases.

Inborn errors of metabolism are usually autosomal recessive, although some are X-linked. The main categories are listed in Fig. 21.11.

The clinical effects might be caused by accumulation of excess precursors, toxic metabolites or metabolic energy insufficiency. Clinical manifestations are non-specific and often mistaken for sepsis. Metabolic stress often precipitates symptoms, e.g. weaning, intercurrent infections and commonly during the neonatal period.

Features in the neonate that should raise the suspicion of a metabolic error include:

- Parental consanguinity.
- Previous sudden infant death.
- Previous multiple miscarriages.
- Encephalopathic episodes.
- Severe disease in whom a diagnosis has not been forthcoming.

Investigations might reveal severe metabolic acidosis, hypoglycaemia or hyperammonaemia. In older children, they should be considered as a cause of:

- Progressive learning difficulties.
- Developmental delay.
- Seizures.
- Failure to thrive.
- Coarse facies.
- Hepatosplenomegaly.

Investigations that should be undertaken for an initial screen include:

- Urea and electrolytes, liver function tests, lactate and ammonia levels.
- Acid–base status and anion gap.
- Cerebrospinal fluid (CSF) lactate.
- Blood levels of glucose and amino acids.
- Urine amino acids and organic acids: ketonuria is abnormal as neonates do not readily produce ketones in the urine.

Treatment is to stop feeds and administer dextrose to stop metabolic load and further catabolism. Correction of metabolic disturbances and ventilatory and renal support may be necessary.

Although in many conditions the prognosis is very poor, the diagnosis should be made so that prenatal diagnosis can be performed in future pregnancies.

Examples of individual inborn errors of metabolism are considered briefly in turn.

Phenylketonuria (PKU)

This autosomal recessive trait has an incidence of 1 in 10 000 live births with a carrier rate of 1 : 50. In

Categories of inborn errors of metabolism	
Category	Examples
Amino acid metabolism	Phenylketonuria
Organic acid metabolism	Maple syrup urine disease
Urea cycle disorders	Ornithine transcarbamylase deficiency
Carbohydrate metabolism	Galactosaemia Glycogen storage diseases
Mucopolysaccharidosis	Hurler syndrome

Fig. 21.11 Categories of inborn errors of metabolism.

most cases, the defect lies in the enzyme phenylalanine hydroxylase, which normally converts phenylalanine to tyrosine. Hyperphenylalaninaemia occurs, with a build-up of toxic byproducts, such as phenylacetic acid, which are excreted in the urine (hence phenylketonuria).

As PKU is relatively common and is treatable, newborn screening is carried out by the Guthrie test. This is carried out at several days of age because it is necessary for the infant to have been fed milk, which contains phenylalanine.

Infants with PKU are clinically normal at birth. Symptoms and signs appear later in infancy and childhood if the disorder is undetected and untreated. These include:

- Neurological manifestations: moderate to severe mental retardation, hypertonicity, tremors, behaviour disorders and seizures.
- Growth retardation.
- Hypopigmentation: fair skin, light hair (due to the block in tyrosine formation that is required for melanin production).

Treatment consists of dietary manipulation. The phenylalanine content of the diet is reduced. This should start early in infancy and is continued until at least 6 years of age. Some authorities recommend lifelong dietary restriction but the diet is unpalatable.

Females with PKU must be on dietary restriction if planning a pregnancy, because maternal hyperphenylalaninaemia is associated with spontaneous abortion, microcephaly and congenital heart disease.

Galactosaemia

This causes neonatal liver disfunction, coagulopathy and cataracts. It has an association with *E. coli* sepsis. It is diagnosed by the presence of reducing substances in the urine and decreased or absent galactose-1-phosphate uridyltransferase in red cells. A high suspicion of this disorder should be considered in all cases of severe neonatal jaundice. Treatment is by a lactose free diet and it is an absolute contraindication to breastfeeding.

Glycogen storage diseases

This group of conditions is caused by defects in the enzymes involved in glycogen synthesis or breakdown. There is an abnormal accumulation of glycogen in tissues. The pattern of organ involvement depends on the enzyme defect and may include liver, heart, brain, skeletal muscle or other organs. There are at least six varieties, some of which have eponyms, e.g. type 1A (von Gierke's disease; glucose-6-phosphatase deficiency). Affected children have growth failure, hypoglycaemia and hepatomegaly. Treatment is by frequent feeds throughout day and night.

Mucopolysaccharidoses (MPS)

This group of disorders is caused by defects in enzymes involved in the metabolism and storage of mucopolysaccharides. They are progressive multisystem disorders that can affect the central nervous system, eyes, heart and skeletal system. Characteristic features are:

- Developmental delay in the first year.
- Coarse facies: develop in most cases although children are normal at birth.

There are numerous types, many of which have eponymous designations, e.g. MPS I (Hurler syndrome, which is autosomal recessive). Affected children develop coarse facial features, corneal opacities, hepatosplenomegaly, kyphosis and mental retardation.

Diagnosis is made by identifying the enzyme defect and identifying the excretion in the urine of the major storage substances, the glycosaminoglycans. Treatment is by bone marrow transplant if performed early.

References

Devendra D, Liu E, Eisenbarth GS. Type I diabetes: recent developments. *British Medical Journal* 2004; **328**:750–754.

National Institute of Clinical Excellence. Diagnosis and management of type 1 diabetes in children, young people and adults. 2004.

Wraith JE, Cleary MA, Chakrapani A. Detection of inborn errors of metabolism in the newborn. *Archives of Diseases in Childhood. Fetal Neonatology Edition.* 2001.

Disorders of emotion and behaviour

Objectives

At the end of this chapter, you should be able to

- Understand the aetiology of common childhood behavioural problems.
- Understand the clinical presentations of autistic spectrum disorders.
- Understand the common causes and management options for bedwetting.
- Recognize the clinical features of ADHD.
- Outline common behavioural problems in adolescence.

Major psychoses rarely present during childhood although disturbed emotions and behavioural problems are very prevalent. The conditions encountered are, not surprisingly, age-related and range from the toddler who will not sleep to deliberate self-harm in an adolescent.

A child's personality, behaviour patterns and emotional responses are determined by an interplay between nature (genetic endowment) and nurture (predominantly provided by parents). The relative importance of genes and environment remains the subject of debate and current research.

An infant's first relationship is usually with the mother and separation anxiety typically becomes evident at about 6 months to 1 year. By the second year, emotional attachments are extended to the father and other family members, and by the age of 4–5 years separation from parents can be tolerated for several hours as occurs with school attendance.

With entry into school, the importance of others—such as teachers and fellow school children—in shaping the child's psychosocial development increases.

Early, strong, emotional bonding underpins normal emotional development.

Nature

Some children have a temperament that in itself can make it difficult for the parents to maintain a positive, loving relationship. Features might include:

- Predominantly negative mood.
- Intense emotional reactions.
- Poor and slow adjustment to new situations.

Developmental delay (e.g. slow language development) can also cause problems.

Nurture

Families are the most powerful environmental influence on a child's emotional and behavioural development. Adequate parents will endeavour to:

- Provide love and affection.
- Provide food and shelter and protect children from physical harm.
- Exert authority to establish reasonable limits on behaviour.

Risk factors with an adverse influence are shown in Fig. 22.1.

PROBLEMS OF EARLY CHILDHOOD

Behavioural problems can relate to sleeping or eating, and tantrums are common. The rare disorder of autism might present at this time.

Factors associated with disturbed emotional
and behavioural development

Parental factors
Maternal depression
Marital discord
Divorce or bereavement
Intrusive overprotection or emotional rejection
Inconsistent discipline
Socio-economic factors
Poverty, poor housing

Fig. 22.1 Factors associated with disturbed emotional and behavioural development.

Sleep-related problems

Babies

An average baby sleeps for 15 hours a day in the first 2–3 months of life, sleeping for about 4 hours and waking for 3 hours at a time. At about 4 months, night-time breastfeeds are often discontinued and the baby might sleep through for 8 hours. Some babies are 'quiet wakeners', some are not, and appear to sleep less.

Toddlers

Problems include:

- Difficulty in settling to sleep at night.
- Waking at night.
- Nightmares and night terrors.

Difficulty in getting to sleep at night

A child might not settle at night for many reasons including:

- Separation anxiety.
- Fear of darkness and silence.
- Erratic bedtime routine.
- Use of the bedroom as punishment.

Helpful strategies include creating a predictable structure around bedtime and leaving the child alone to settle for lengthening periods. Sedatives are used only as a last resort to relieve parental exhaustion (it should be pointed out that it is parents, not children, who have sleep problems).

Nightmares and night terrors

Nightmares are bad dreams that can be recalled by the child. They are common and normal unless very frequent or stereotyped in content. Reassurance is usually sufficient.

Night terrors are a form of parasomnia in which there is rapid emergence from the initial period of deep, slow-wave sleep, into a state of high arousal and confusion. The child usually cries out and is found sitting up with open eyes but disorientated and unresponsive. The child settles, with no subsequent recall of the episode. Waking the child briefly before the night terror is expected to occur might break the pattern.

Food refusal

Meal times can easily become a battleground. Parents often find that their toddler refuses to eat the meals provided or is a fussy eater. The child is invariably well nourished or small with a normal rate of weight gain. Advice can be given to avoid:

- Excessive food and drink between main meals.
- Irregular meal times.
- Unsuitable food or unreasonably large portions.
- Punitive methods, e.g. forcing a child to eat cold food.

Small amounts of food with gradual introduction of new foods in a relaxed, non-bargaining atmosphere is the best approach. No preschool child will voluntarily starve him- or herself, although some mothers find this difficult to believe.

Tantrums

Toddlers normally go through a period in which they are disinclined to comply with their parents' demands; this phase is sometimes referred to as 'the terrible twos'. Temper tantrums can occur in response to frustration. Parents might become demoralized in their attempts to assert control.

Management

Management strategies for 'toddler taming' include:

- Praising compliance and reward good behaviour.
- Avoiding threats that cannot be carried out.
- Setting reasonable limits.
- Giving clear commands.

A tantrum itself can be dealt with by ignoring it (this can be difficult, especially in a public place) or by giving the child 'time-out' (removing him or her from social interaction for a short period, e.g. in a separate room).

Autistic spectrum disorder

This rare, pervasive condition presents in early childhood with a triad of difficulties that is usually evident before the age of 3 years. It is part of a spectrum of disorders characterized by profound impairment of social interactions.

The prevalence is 0.7–21 cases out of 10 000 children with an excess of males (M : F ratio 4 : 1). Autism is an organic neurodevelopmental disorder, with a strong genetic component in its causation in most cases. On occasion, an identifiable cause or coexisting condition is present. No association with immunization has been found. Autistic features are found in patients with:

- Fragile X syndrome.
- Tuberous sclerosis.
- Untreated phenylketonuria.

The four main features include:

- Impaired social interaction: poor interactions with others and avoiding eye contact.
- Impaired communication: delayed speech and language development with poor comprehension.
- Restricted pattern of behaviour and interests: stereotypical patterns and lack of imaginative play and behaviour.
- Onset before 3 years of age.

In addition to these features, about two-thirds of affected children have a severe learning disability and a quarter of autistic individuals develop epileptic seizures during adolescence.

Autism is one end of a spectrum of disorders. Children can have autistic features and be socially and functionally impaired without fulfilling criteria for a diagnosis of autism. Children with Asperger's syndrome, for example, have near normal IQ and speech but impaired social and communication skills and obsessional interests. This syndrome tends to be recognized in later childhood.

> Autism is characterized by:
> - Delayed and abnormal language.
> - Difficulty relating to others—poor social reciprocity.
> - Restricted, stereotyped interests and activities.

Management

There are no drug treatments for autism but medical treatment for epilepsy might be necessary. However, specific indications do exist for symptomatic treatment of problems such as extreme anxiety or disruptive behaviour. Special education programmes are required to meet the complex needs of the individual child. A variety of behavioural treatment programmes has been tried and it is vital that parents receive strong professional support. Only 15% of affected individuals are independent in adult life with another 15–20% functioning well with support.

Improved outcomes are seen if communicative speech is present by 5 years of age.

PROBLEMS OF MIDDLE CHILDHOOD

Continence disorders

Enuresis

Enuresis is the involuntary discharge of urine at an age after continence has been reached by most children (see Hints & Tips). Enuresis is usefully subcategorized as shown in Fig. 22.2.

Fig. 22.2 Classification of enuresis.

Classification of enuresis
Primary or secondary?
Children with primary enuresis have never been continent for a period of at least 3 months
Secondary enuresis is incontinence after a prolonged period of bladder control
Nocturnal or diurnal?
Nocturnal enuresis occurs only at night (85% enuretic children)
Diurnal enuresis occurs during the day (5% enuretic children)
10% have a mixed type

Urinary continence (dryness) is achieved by most girls by age 5 years and boys by age 6 years.

Nocturnal enuresis

Nocturnal enuresis, or 'bedwetting', is the involuntary voiding of urine during sleep beyond the age at which dryness at night has been achieved in a majority of children. Children under 5 years of age who regularly wet the bed can be regarded as normal. About 1 in 6 five-year-olds regularly wets the bed; this drops to 1 in 20 at age 10 years.

Nocturnal enuresis is usefully classified into:

- Primary, in which dryness has never been achieved.
- Secondary, in which it has.

The aetiology of primary nocturnal enuresis is multifactorial with genetic, emotional and cultural factors contributing. Organic causes of either are uncommon but include:

- Urinary tract infection.
- Polyuria due to diabetes mellitus or chronic renal failure.
- Neuropathic bladder.
- Genital abnormalities.
- Faecal retention causing bladder neck dysfunction.

History and examination

The history should establish the frequency (50% or more wet nights over 2 weeks is severe) and time of night that wetting occurs. The presence of any daytime urgency or wetting should be established as this suggests an underlying cause. A family history might be present and an assessment should be made of any emotional stresses either at school or at home.

Physical examination must include:

- A review of growth and measurement of blood pressure to identify unrecognized renal failure.
- Careful abdominal palpation to exclude an enlarged bladder.
- Inspection of the genitalia.

The spine and overlying skin should be inspected for any deformity, hairy patch or sinus and the neurology of the lower limbs examined thoroughly. Investigation should include:

- Urinalysis: tests for proteinuria and glycosuria.
- Microscopy and culture of a clean catch midstream urine.

Management

Important general measures include the establishment of a supportive and trusting relationship with the child and parents. A simple explanation of how the bladder works as a muscular balloon and the problem of being unaware of a full bladder during sleep should be given. Parental intolerance should be discouraged (by a reminder of how common enuresis is) and 'functional payoffs' (e.g. sleeping in parents' bed) should be identified and stopped. A diary of wetting should be kept for at least 4 weeks and frequent, regular supervision by the doctor should be arranged.

Further management is age-dependent:

- Under 5 years: the situation should improve with reassurance.
- Over 5 years: in addition to the above methods, star charts and appropriate praise might be of value.
- Over 7 years: in addition to the above methods, alarms can be used. A choice of body-worn or pad and buzzer type alarm should be offered. The alarm rings when urination begins, causing the child to wake up and 'hold-on' to the sensation of a full bladder. A high degree of compliance and motivation is required and 60–70% of children will attain dryness after a few months.

Tricyclic antidepressants are rarely used in the treatment of enuresis. Desmopressin (a synthetic analogue of antidiuretic hormone) is available in tablet form and provides effective short-term relief. A percentage of patients who attain dryness on desmopressin remain dry when it is stopped. Oxybutinin is also used for this purpose.

Encopresis (faecal soiling)

Encopresis is involuntary faecal soiling at an age beyond which continence should have been achieved (normally about 4 years). Children with encopresis fall into two main groups:

- Retentive: those with a rectum loaded with faeces. There is overflow incontinence (the majority).

- Non-retentive: children without constipation and a loaded rectum who have a neurogenic sphincter disturbance or psychiatric illness.

A number of factors predispose to chronic stool retention. These include:

- Environmental problems: lack of toilet facilities, harsh toilet training.
- Idiopathic: some children's rectums only empty occasionally, perhaps due to poor coordination with anal sphincter relaxation.
- Transient constipation: an episode of constipation due to dehydration or an anal fissure might lead to chronic retention.
- Organic constipation: associated with Hirschsprung's disease, drugs or hypothyroidism.

Once established, a large bolus of faeces in the rectum might be impossible for the child to expel. The loaded rectum becomes dilated and might habituate to distension, so the child is unaware of the need to empty it. Psychological factors can be both a cause and a result of encopresis. Soiling disturbs the child and can have a profound impact in school, social life and in the family.

Onset of soiling in middle childhood, without a previous history of constipation, suggests a primary psychiatric cause. It might occur in the setting of a chaotic family with high levels of emotional deprivation, neglect and disturbed behaviour.

Diagnosis
Assessment must include a full bowel history, assessment of the family's psychological functioning and careful examination of the neurological system and abdomen. Rectal examination and abdominal palpation will determine whether there is faecal retention.

Management
The key objective in management of encopresis due to faecal retention is to empty the rectum as soon as possible. This might require an enema but can often be achieved by a combination of stool softener (e.g. lactulose) and laxative (e.g. senna). Regular defecation should then be encouraged by:

- Regular laxatives.
- Star charts.
- Sitting on the toilet after meals.
- Dietary changes: increased fibre.

The distended rectum will take several weeks to shrink to normal size. It is unusual for the problem to persist into adolescence. Agents such as picosulphate or movicol can be used in different cases.

Attention-deficit hyperactivity disorder (ADHD)
The three hallmarks of ADHD are:

- Inattention beyond the child's normal for age.
- Hyperactivity.
- Impulsiveness.

Incidence and aetiology
In the USA, this diagnosis is applied if either inattention or hyperactivity and impulsiveness persist in two or more situations. In the UK, the diagnosis of ADHD is made only if all three features:

- Are present for at least 6 months.
- Persist in more than one situation (home and school).
- Impair function.

Hyperkinetic syndrome is a more severe subtype of ADHD with a prevalence of 1 in 200 (ADHD affects 2–4% of school children). Hyperkinetic syndrome is four times more common in boys than girls and is characterised by significant hyperactivity.

Twin studies suggest a genetic contribution to aetiology. Perinatal problems and delays in early development appear to be more common in hyperkinetic syndrome. Disturbed relationships, such as might occur with an emotionally rejecting parent or institutional upbringing, seem to exacerbate it.

Hyperkinetic syndrome is a severe subtype of ADHD. It is more common in boys than girls.

Clinical features
Features of ADHD:

- Inattention: manifests as an easily distracted child who changes activity frequently and does not persist with tasks.

- Hyperactivity: an excess of movement with persistent fidgeting and restlessness that can be distinguished from normal high-spirited, energetic behaviour by the interference with normal social functioning.
- Impulsiveness: acting without reflection: affected children act impetuously and erratically.

Although these features might be present in the pre-school years, they often come to clinical attention with the increased demands of the classroom. Physical examination should include a search for:

- Developmental delay, clumsiness.
- Deficits in hearing or vision and specific learning difficulties.
- Dysmorphic features.

Most children do not have a sudden onset or an identifiable brain disorder and do not need special investigations such as electroencephalography or brain imaging. Between 18 and 35% will have an additional psychiatric disorder.

Management

A behaviour-modifying and educational approach is the mainstay of treatment but drug treatment should be considered if these strategies fail. It is important to explain the nature of the disorder to the parents and school staff. Parent support groups might provide reassurance and help.

Behavioural therapy

About 50% of children respond to behavioural therapy comprising:

- A structured environment.
- Positive reinforcement.
- Cognitive approaches emphasizing relaxation and self-control.

Extra help in the classroom and modification of the curriculum might be required.

Drug therapy

Studies have shown that the addition of drugs to behavioural therapy is effective. These are central stimulant drugs such as methylphenidate (Ritalin). Side effects include slowing of growth and hypertension. A drug holiday should be given once per year. Atomoxetine and dexamfetamine are also used, though less frequently.

Alternative therapies

Numerous alternative therapies have been advocated. Diets can have a role in a minority of children and the parents' observations that a particular food aggravates hyperactivity should be heeded. A trial of an exclusion diet might be warranted. (Few children react to additives alone and a diet just excluding foods with synthetic dyes or preservatives is unlikely to be helpful.)

Hyperactivity itself does not usually persist as a predominant feature into adulthood. However, affected children tend to do poorly at school and low self-esteem together with antisocial traits might turn them into disadvantaged adults.

Symptoms diminish over time but approximately half will continue to have symptoms in adolescence and adulthood.

Recurrent pain syndromes

Recurrent pain without an organic cause is not uncommon in children. The usual sites are the abdomen, head or limbs.

A strict dichotomy between organic and psychological causation for recurrent pain is unhelpful and explains only a minority of cases. In most cases the pain is best explained as dysfunctional, a result of mild individual differences in physiology that render the child vulnerable to pain in response to stress.

- Apley's law: the further the pain is from the umbilicus, the more likely it is to be organic.
- The more localized limb pain is, the less likely it is to be 'growing pains'.
- Measure the blood pressure and examine the fundi in a child with recurrent headaches.

Clinical features and diagnosis

The history should establish:

- Onset, frequency and duration of the pain and associated symptoms.
- Family functioning.
- Stressors, e.g. bullying at school.

Organic causes of recurrent pain	
Site	**Cause**
Abdominal pain	Genitourinary problems: UTI, obstructive uropathy Gastrointestinal disorders: inflammatory bowel disease, peptic ulcer
Headache	Refractive disorders Migraine Hypertension Raised intracranial pressure
Limb pain	Neoplastic disease, e.g. leukaemia, bone tumour Orthopaedic: Osgood–Schlatter disease

Fig. 22.3 Organic causes of recurrent pain.

Physical examination is directed towards excluding an organic cause (Fig. 22.3). Investigations have a low yield if physical examination is normal and should be kept to a minimum. Full blood count, erythrocyte sedimentation rate and urinalysis might be indicated.

Management

For dysfunctional pain, normal activity should be encouraged. Symptomatic relief should be offered (e.g. mild analgesics) and the patient should be encouraged to keep a symptom diary.

School refusal

Repeated absence from school might be due to illness or truancy but in a few cases it is due to school refusal, i.e. an unwillingness to attend because of anxiety. School refusal might be associated with:

- Separation anxiety (under 11 years).
- Adverse life events (bereavement, moving).
- Stressors (bullying).

School refusers tend to be good academically but oppositional at home.

True school phobia is seen in older, anxious children, who typically have problems beginning school in the autumn and returning to school after weekends and holidays. Unlike school refusal, they are poor academically and have a lack of desire rather than anxiety about school.

Management

Management requires an early, graded return to school with support for the parents and treatment of any underlying emotional disorder. Two-thirds of school refusers will return to school regularly.

ADOLESCENT PROBLEMS

This is a period during which a number of important disorders might present, including emotional disorders such as anxiety and depression, conduct disorders and disorders of eating.

Eating disorders

Anorexia nervosa

This eating disorder is characterized by:

- Refusal to maintain an expected bodyweight for height with weight less than 85% of expected bodyweight.
- Intense fear of gaining weight or being fat.
- Disturbed body image: feeling fat when actually emaciated.
- Denial of the danger of serious weight loss or low body weight.
- Amenorrhoea for at least three cycles (in postmenarchal girls).

The prevalence rate is 1% with a peak age of onset of 14 years (and girls outnumbering boys by 20 to 1). The aetiology is unknown. The patient often displays obsessive, overachieving, perfectionist and controlling personality traits.

Clinical features and diagnosis
Physical examination may reveal:

- Emaciation and muscle wasting.
- Fine lanugo hair over trunk and limbs.

- Bradycardia and poor peripheral perfusion.
- Slowly relaxing tendon reflexes.

Laboratory investigations may reveal:

- Reduced plasma proteins, vitamin B_{12} and ferritin.
- Endocrine abnormalities: elevated cortisol, reduced T_4, luteinizing hormone and follicle stimulating hormone.

In boys, cranial computed tomography should be undertaken to exclude a brain tumour.

Management and prognosis

The immediate goal is to make a therapeutic alliance with the patient to restore normal bodyweight by re-feeding. This can be attempted initially as an out-patient, aiming at a gain of 500 g per week. Failure to meet this target necessitates hospital admission for re-feeding under nursing supervision. This can be difficult because affected young people might hide food and lie about their weight. Tube feeding might be required if there is continued weight loss in hospital.

Once weight gain is achieved, psychotherapeutic approaches are adopted. This aims to provide counselling on handling conflict, relationships and personal autonomy.

Prognosis is variable with an eventual 5% mortality rate from malnutrition, infection or suicide. Fifty per cent make a good recovery, 30% show partial improvement and 20% have a chronic relapsing course. Good prognostic factors are:

- Young age at onset.
- Supportive family.
- Less denial and improved self-esteem.

Emotional disorders

Depression

Depression as a clinical syndrome is more than just a transitory low mood or misery in response to adverse life circumstances. It is characterized by:

- Persistent feelings of sadness or unhappiness.
- Ideas of guilt, despair and lack of self-worth.
- Social withdrawal.
- Lack of motivation and energy.
- Disturbances of sleep, appetite and weight.

It is increasingly recognized in prepubertal children but is predominantly a problem of adolescence. Aetiology is multifactorial but there is a clear genetic

contribution. Dysfunctional families or adverse life events might contribute.

Management

Treatment includes selective serotonin re-uptake inhibitor (SSRI) antidepressants and family therapy.

- Suicide is the third most common cause of death in adolescents and young adults.
- Most intentional overdoses are not taken with suicidal intent but an important minority are, so psychiatric evaluation is important in all cases.

Conduct disorder

This is a syndrome characterized by the persistent (6–12 months) failure to control behaviour within socially defined rules. This involves three overlapping domains of behaviour:

- Defiance of authority.
- Aggressiveness.
- Antisocial behaviour: violating other people's property, rights or person.

This affects approximately 4% of all children and is more prevalent in boys. The aetiology is multifactorial, with genetic and environmental contributions. In many children, it is preceded by the so-called oppositional defiant disorder, i.e. children who demonstrate a persistent pattern of angry, negative, vindictive and defiant behaviour.

Management and prognosis

Family behavioural therapy with social support is helpful. A significant number (40%) of children with conduct disorder become delinquent young adults with ongoing behaviour problems and disrupted relationships. Those with onset before adolescence are most at risk.

Chronic fatigue syndrome

This refers to generalized fatigue persisting after routine tests and investigations have failed to identify an obvious underlying cause. It is classically exacerbated by mental and physical exertion and usually associated with non-specific pain in muscles and joints. Headaches, sleep difficulties, depressed mood, sore throat, tender lymph nodes and abdominal pain can also occur. A full history and examination is important to characterise symptoms and basic screening tests are important to exclude other diagnosis e.g. anaemia and hypothyroidism. Definite diagnosis allows a multidisciplinary approach to management.

Management and prognosis

- Activity management strategy.
- Psychological and educational support.
- Symptom relief.

Psychosis

Chronic disorders such as schizophrenia and bipolar affective disorder might present in adolescence. The prevalence of drug abuse in this age group renders drug-induced psychosis an important problem.

Further reading

Evans JHC. Evidence based management of nocturnal enuresis. *British Medical Journal* 2001; **323**: 1167–1169.

Volkmar FR, Pauls D. Autism. *Lancet* 2003; **362**: 133–141.

Social and preventive paediatrics

Objectives

At the end of this chapter, you should be able to

- Understand the importance of prevention in child health.
- Outline the current UK immunization schedule.
- Know the contraindications to routine immunization in children.
- Understand the importance of neonatal screening.
- Recognize the different types of child abuse.
- Outline the causes and prevention of sudden infant death syndrome.
- Understand some of the legal issues pertaining to paediatrics.

This includes all aspects of promoting health and preventing illness such as child health surveillance, immunization, health education and accident prevention. In addition, community paediatric services are closely involved with the problems of child abuse, adoption and foster care, and children with special needs. Important legislation concerning children and health in the UK exists, in particular the Children Act and the Education Act.

PREVENTION IN CHILD HEALTH

There remains a high level of morbidity from preventable conditions including:

- Infectious diseases.
- Congenital disorders.
- Accidents.
- Malnutrition.
- Smoking in teenagers.

Strategies for prevention include:

- Immunization.
- Screening.
- Child health surveillance.
- Health promotion and education.

Immunization

Immunization has probably conferred more benefit on the world's children than any other medical advance or intervention. It has allowed the prevention of many major diseases such as diphtheria and polio, which killed or crippled millions of children, and the complete eradication of smallpox. In recent times, the highly successful introduction of immunization against *Haemophilus influenzae* type B (Hib) has dramatically reduced the incidence of invasive infections such as Hib meningitis and epiglottitis.

Immunization is effective against major bacterial diseases, such as diphtheria and tuberculosis (TB), and viral diseases, such as measles, mumps, rubella and hepatitis. Bacille Calmette–Guérin (BCG) vaccination against TB is effective in some parts of the world. However, a vaccine has yet to be developed against the important parasitic disease, malaria.

Immunity: active and passive

Immunity can be induced either actively (long term) or provided by passive transfer (short term) against a variety of bacterial and viral agents.

Active immunity is induced by using:

- A live, attenuated form of the pathogen, e.g. oral poliomyelitis vaccine (OPV), measles, mumps, rubella vaccine (MMR), BCG vaccine for TB.
- An inactivated organism, e.g. inactivated poliomyelitis vaccine (IPV), pertussis.
- A component of the organism, e.g. Hib, pneumococcal vaccine, hepatitis B and meningitis C.
- An inactivated toxin (toxoid), e.g. tetanus vaccine, diphtheria vaccine.

In many individuals, live, attenuated viral vaccines promote a full, long-lasting antibody response after one dose. Several doses of an inactivated version or toxoid are usually required.

Passive immunity is conferred by the injection of human immunoglobulin. There are two main types:

- Human normal immunoglobulin (HNIG).
- Specific immunoglobulins for tetanus, hepatitis B, rabies and varicella zoster (VZIG).

Routes of administration are:

- By mouth: oral polio vaccine.
- Intradermal: BCG.
- Subcutaneous or intramuscular injection: all other vaccines.

In infants, the upper outer quadrant of the buttock or the anterolateral aspect of the thigh are the recommended sites for the injection of vaccines.

Immunization schedule

In the UK, the schedule for primary immunization has been changed recently to include pneumococcal vaccine. This schedule provides earlier and more effective protection against haemophilus, pneumococcal and pertussis infections, which are more dangerous to the very young. Added benefits have included fewer side effects and better completion of the full course.

The new schedule is shown in Fig. 23.1.

The timing of childhood immunization is critical: too early and the immune response might be inadequate, too late and the child could acquire the disease before being protected.

Indications and contraindications to immunization

Every child should be protected against infectious diseases and a denial of immunization should not be allowed without serious consideration of the consequences.

Special risk groups can be identified for whom the risk of complications from infectious disease is high and who should be immunized as a priority. These include children with:

- Chronic lung and congenital heart disease.
- Down syndrome.
- HIV infection.
- Low birth weight.
- No spleen or hyposplenism.

General contraindications

These include:

- Acute illness with fever >38°C: postpone until recovery has occurred.

UK immunization schedule		
Age	Vaccine	Comments
2 months	DTaP/IPV/Hib; PCV (pneumococcal vaccine)	2 injections (DTaP/Hib/IPV is a 5 in 1 vaccine)
3 months	DTaP/IPV/Hib; Men C	2 injections
4 months	DTaP/Hib/IPV; Men C; PCV	3 injections
12 months	Hib / Men C	1 injection
13 months	MMR; PCV	2 injections
3 years 4 months to 5 years	dTaP/IPV or DTaP/IPV and MMR	2 injections
13–18 years	Td/IPV	1 injection

Fig. 23.1 UK immunization schedule.

- A definite history of a severe local or general reaction to a preceding dose.

Live vaccines: special risk groups Live vaccines pose a risk for certain individuals whose immunity is impaired. These include children:

- Being treated with chemotherapy or radiotherapy for malignant disease.
- On immunosuppressive treatment after organ or bone marrow transplant.
- On high-dose systemic steroids.
- With impaired cell-mediated immunity, e.g. severe combined immunodeficiency syndrome or Di George syndrome.

Children positive for antibodies to HIV, with or without symptoms, should be given all vaccines except BCG (there have been reports of dissemination of BCG in HIV-positive individuals), yellow fever and oral typhoid.

- Immunization should be postponed if the child has an acute febrile illness.
- Premature babies can be immunized following the recommended schedule according to chronological age, i.e. immunization should not be postponed.
- Live vaccines are contraindicated in immunocompromised children.

Specific contraindications

Particular vaccines are contraindicated in certain circumstances:

- Measles vaccination is contraindicated if there is allergy to neomycin. MMR is safe for those with egg allergies. If there is concern, immunization should be given under hospital supervision.
- Pertussis: it has never been conclusively demonstrated that this vaccine ever causes permanent brain damage. The current acellular pertussis vaccine is safer than the previous cellular vaccine. There are no specific contraindications (in particular, a family or personal history of epilepsy is not a contraindication). Immunization is best delayed in patients with progressive neurological disease until the condition is stabilized.

'False' contraindications

The following are *not* contraindications to immunization:

- Family history of adverse reaction to immunization.
- Prematurity.
- Stable neurological conditions, e.g. cerebral palsy.
- Asthma, eczema, hay fever.
- Under a certain weight.
- Over the age recommended in standard schedule.
- Minor afebrile illness.
- Child's mother being pregnant.

Adverse reactions associated with specific vaccines are shown in Fig. 23.2.

Screening

An effective and worthwhile screening programme should satisfy certain criteria:

Adverse reactions associated with specific vaccines		
Vaccine	Minor reaction	Major reaction
Diphtheria/tetanus	Local	Neurological (very rare)
Pertussis	Fever, crying	Convulsions (1:300 000) Encephalopathy (very rare)
Polio	—	Vaccine-associated polio (1 in 2 million)
MMR	Fever, rash, arthropathy	Encephalopathy (very rare) Thrombocytopenia
BCG	Local abscess	Adenitis

Fig. 23.2 Adverse reactions associated with specific vaccines.

- The condition screened for should be an important health problem.
- There should be a sensitive and specifc test.
- Treatment should improve the condition.
- It should be cost-effective.
- The screening method should be acceptable to child and parents.

Screening can be targeted at a 'high-risk' population or carried out opportunistically when a patient presents for some other reason at the relevant age.

Child health promotion

A programme of health surveillance is undertaken to identify important conditions that have a better outcome if diagnosed and treated early (e.g. congenital dislocation of the hip and deafness). This programme includes:

- Neonatal examination.
- 6-week check.
- 6–9 month check.
- 18–24 month check.
- 36–42 month check.

Neonatal examination

Full physical examination looking for congenital anomalies such as congenital dislocation of the hips, undescended testes and absence of the red reflex. Hearing is tested by otoacoustic emission (and/or brainstem auditory evoked potentials in some centres) in all babies in the first few days.

Guthrie test: Usually between days 5 and 8, a heel prick blood sample is taken to screen for phenylketonuria cystic fibrosis and hypothyroidism. Screening for MCADD (medium chain acyl CoA dehydrogenase deficiency) is done in certain centres.

6-week check

Physical examination with emphasis on:

- Surveillance for congenital anomalies, e.g. cardiac, undescended testes and dislocated hips.
- Growth: weight, length and head circumference.
- Development: alert, makes eye contact, smiles in response.
- Vision and hearing (explore parental concerns).

Assessment should also be made of the family's adjustment to the new infant, quality of parent–child interactions and signs of maternal depression.

6–9 months

- Squint assessment.
- Distraction test for hearing.
- Assess growth and development.
- Anticipatory guidance on feeding, safety and injury prevention, sleep habits.

18–24 months

This is done by the health visitor but in some areas it is no longer performed.

- Assess development: confirm walking with normal gait and age-appropriate vocalization and language.
- Growth: height and weight.
- Anticipatory guidance on toilet training, temperament and behaviour.

36–42 months

This is a physical examination that aims to detect health problems before school.

- Growth: height and weight.
- Hearing and vision tests.
- Developmental tests.

CHILD ABUSE

Although it is probable that children have been abused throughout history, it is only in the last few decades that the extent to which children can be abused by their parents or carers has been recognized. In the UK, one child in 2000 suffers severe physical abuse and as many as 100 children are killed each year. Several types of abuse are recognized and these often occur together (Fig. 23.3).

Diagnosis

Certain families and children are at particular risk. Adults who abuse are often young, immature, isolated, poor and subject to social or marital stress. Alcoholism, drug abuse and personality or psychiatric disorders (e.g. postnatal depression) might be

Physical (non-accidental injury)
Sexual
Emotional
Neglect
Munchausen by proxy (fictitious illness)

Fig. 23.3 Types of abuse.

Features of non-accidental bruises

Any bruises in a (non-mobile) baby
Bruises on face, back, buttocks as opposed to forehead
and shins in toddler
Bruises in pattern of finger-tips, hand-print, belt
(follow shape and size of object used)
Bruises of different ages

Fig. 23.5 Features of non-accidental bruises.

Features of non-accidental injury

History
Delay in seeking medical help
Injury inconsistent with history or changing story
Cause of trauma inappropriate for age and activity
Previous unexplained injury
Parents unconcerned or concern about minor unrelated problem
Examination
Signs of neglect
Withdrawn personality
Frenulum lacerations
Genital injury
Old injuries

Fig. 23.4 Features of non-accidental injury.

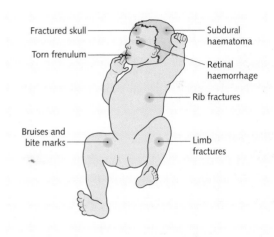

Fig. 23.6 Battered or shaken baby syndrome.

contributory. Young children under the age of 3 years and babies born prematurely are at particular risk.

Child abuse might present directly to the GP or hospital doctor; or a health visitor, social services, police, school, a relative or even a neighbour might raise a suspicion of abuse. Diagnosis is difficult and, of course, false accusations cause great anguish. Each type is considered in turn.

Types of abuse

Physical abuse or non-accidental injury (NAI)
Certain features in the history of a physical injury should raise the suspicion that it might be non-accidental (Fig. 23.4). Actual injuries can include bruises (Fig. 23.5), bite marks, burns or scalds, and head injuries or fractures. Accidental fractures of long bones are rare in babies but common in mobile children aged 3–4 years. Metaphyseal fractures and posterior rib fractures should raise the suspicion of NAI. Direct blows to the mouth or forcing a bottle into the mouth can tear the frenulum. Violent shaking of a baby might tear the vessels that cross the subdural space leading to subdural haemorrhage (Fig. 23.6). This is associated with irritability, poor

feeding and signs of raised intracranial pressure (increasing head circumference, a tense fontanelle and retinal haemorrhages).

Neglect and emotional abuse
Neglect can manifest as failure to thrive, developmental delay and poor hygiene. Emotional abuse includes rejection and withdrawal of love, and persistent malicious criticism or threats. The child typically improves when taken to a different environment, e.g. hospital.

Fabricated or induced illness
This was previously called 'Munchausen syndrome by proxy'. The carer, usually the mother, fabricates illness in the child by inventing symptoms or faking signs (e.g. by putting blood or sugar in the urine, or contaminating microbiological specimens). This can result in a wide range of clinical symptomatology and significant harm might also come from investigating such symptoms. Harm to the child can also result from treatments used. As diagnosis can

be difficult, consulation with other members of the child health team and other specialists might be useful.

Sexual abuse

Child sexual abuse (CSA) can involve either sex at any age, but is more common in girls. It has been defined as the involvement of dependent, immature children or adolescents in sexual activities that they do not fully understand and are unable to give informed consent to. It should be remembered that medical examination is rarely diagnostic. Physical findings such as tears or abrasions around genitalia, bruising around the genitalia or genital infection are present in less than 30% of abused children. Vulval soreness is very common in young girls and is rarely due to abuse; 80% of sexual abuse is perpetrated by someone the child knows.

Management

Extra care should be taken to record the history and physical findings in detail and with great accuracy. Physical findings should be measured, drawn and—if appropriate—photographed (with parental consent). As always, all notes should be dated, timed and signed, as this is particularly important in relation to any subsequent legal proceedings. If child abuse is suspected in the UK, the Social Services Child and Family department must be informed.

Treatment of any physical injury might be required and, if abuse is suspected, a decision made as to whether the child needs immediate protection. This might mean admission to hospital or placement in a foster home; if parental consent is not given, legal enforcement might be necessary. Senior staff should be involved from the beginning because experience is required in handling what is always a very difficult situation.

Investigations are often indicated. In the presence of suspicious bruising it is advisable to do a full blood count and coagulation screen to exclude thrombocytopenia and other bleeding diatheses, which often present with multiple and excessive bruising. A skeletal survey by X-ray should be carried out in any infant with suspected physical abuse. Forensic samples must be taken in suspected sexual abuse, and this might have to be done under anaesthetic. Emergency protection orders are available to secure admission for abused children if the parents are not cooperative (Fig. 23.7).

Orders in emergency child protection	
Emergency protection order	Applicants from social services or NSPCC Lasts up to 8 days Can be renewed once at 7 days Can be challenged at 72 h
Police protection order	If a police officer believes a child might come to harm, the officer can remove the child to police protection or prevent removal from a safe place for up to 72 h without a court order

Fig. 23.7 Orders in emergency child protection.

In most cases, further management will involve evaluation of the family by social workers and the convening of a Child Protection Conference. The conference should include the paediatrician, GP, health visitor, social workers, police and nursing staff. Parents usually attend all or part of the conference. A decision will be made on whether to place the child's name on the Child Protection Register, whether court proceedings are required and whether the child can be returned safely to the family. A child protection care plan will be produced and will define the level of supervision and medical follow-up.

SUDDEN INFANT DEATH SYNDROME (SIDS)

This is defined as the sudden death of an infant under 1 year of age, which remains unexplained after the performance of a complete post-mortem examination and examination of the scene of death. In the UK, SIDS occurs in 0.4 in 1000 live births; there are thought to be numerous aetiologies.

Risk factors are numerous but include:

- Sleeping prone.
- Maternal smoking.
- Overheating at home.
- Bed sharing.
- Preterm birth.

All paediatric units should have a protocol on dealing with SIDS and the most senior paediatrician must fully examine the child, take appropriate laboratory specimens and inform the coroner.

The family needs support and counselling and there are numerous agencies that provide ongoing help and support.

CHILDREN AND THE LAW

The principal legislation concerning children and health in the UK is contained in:

- The Children Act (England and Wales 1989, Scotland 1995).
- The Education Act (1993).
- The UN Convention on the Rights of the Child (1989).

The Children Act

This integrates the law relating to private individuals with the responsibilities of public authorities towards children. It aims to strike a balance between family independence and child protection. The essential components include:

- Parental responsibilities are defined. Responsibilities replace rights. Parents have the prime responsibility for their children and this is retained in all circumstances except adoption.
- The welfare of the child is paramount. The wishes and feelings of the child must be respected and courts should ensure that any orders made positively benefit the child or children concerned.
- Professionals are encouraged to work in partnership with parents.
- Defines responsibilities for 'children in need'. Local authorities are required to provide supportive services to assist parents in bringing up their children. A register must be kept of children with disabilities and special services provided for those whose health or development may be impaired.
- The court must consider the child's race, religion, culture and language.
- A child should remain with his or her family whenever possible.
- Describes court orders in relation to custody and access, and child protection. The latter includes: Emergency Protection Order, Child Assessment Order, Care and Supervision Order, Police Protection Order

Foster care

The purpose of foster care is to provide a safe, temporary placement for a child who is at physical, emotional or social risk. Common reasons for foster placement include:

- Child abuse.
- Death or absence of parents.
- Babies awaiting adoption.

Foster care does not provide legal rights and these remain with the natural parents, local authority or courts.

Adoption

The annual number of adoptions in the UK has fallen from 21 000 in 1975 to fewer than 6000 by 1995; baby adoptions fell from 4500 to 300. This fall is partly attributable to wider use of contraception and abortion and also to the greater social acceptance of single parenthood.

Most children available for adoption are in local authority care, either with foster parents or in a children's home. Unfortunately, the children available for adoption—many of whom are older, disabled or have suffered abuse or neglect—are not always the kind that adopting couples are looking for.

Adoption is a legal procedure encompassing several important features:

- It is arranged by registered agencies.
- Adopters must be aged over 21 years.
- An adoption cannot be reversed except in exceptional circumstances.
- An adopted child loses all legal ties with his or her birth parents (i.e. has no claim to maintenance or inheritance) and becomes a full member of the new family, taking on the nationality of the adoptive parents.
- The original parents have no right of access, although contact for older children is often maintained.
- The natural parents must give informed consent, unless they cannot be found or are judged unlikely to ever be able to look after the child adequately.
- The child lives with the adoptive parents for 3 months before the order is finalized.
- At age 18, an adopted child is entitled to his or her original birth certificate.

Consent to medical care

A person older than 16 years can legally give his or her own consent. Below the age of 16, the consent of a parent or guardian (person with parental responsibility for the child) is required unless:

- Emergency treatment is required.
- The child consents and the doctor considers that the child is of sufficient understanding to make an informed decision and the child will not consent to a parent being asked (the Gillick principle).

If a child is deemed competent, the parents cannot override consent.

If the parent(s) of a child younger than 16 years refuse a life-saving treatment, a court can give consent.

Confidentiality

A person aged 16 years and over has full rights to confidentiality. However, the duty of confidentiality owed to a patient under 16 years old is as great as that owed to any other person. Information can be disclosed to parents if it is in the interests of the child.

THE CHILD WITH A DISABILITY

Many children have complex and long-lasting neurodevelopmental disabilities that require early identification and support in the community. It is useful to define some of the terms used:

- Impairment: any loss or abnormality of physiological or anatomical structure.

- Disability: any restriction or loss of ability in performing an activity (in a way considered normal for a particular age) that is caused by an impairment.
- Handicap: a disadvantage for an individual arising from a disability that prevents the achievement of desired goals.

For example, an intraventricular haemorrhage with periventricular leucomalacia (impairment of motor tracts) might cause a hemiparesis (the disability), resulting in difficulty playing the piano (handicap). The use of the term 'handicap' with its connotation of dependency has fallen out of favour.

Disabilities can give rise to 'special needs', which in the terms of the Education Act (1993) are educational needs not normally met by the normal provisions for a child of that age.

Presentation of children with disabilities

The kinds of conditions under consideration include, for example:

- Speech and language problems.
- Behavioural problems.
- Down syndrome.
- Cerebral palsy.
- Spina bifida.
- Hearing or visual impairment.
- Learning disability.

Examples of how different problems tend to present at different ages are shown in Fig. 23.8.

Fig. 23.8 Presentation of disabilities by age.

Presentation of disabilities by age	
Age	**Disability**
Neonatal period	Chromosomal abnormality or syndrome, e.g. Down syndrome Hypoxic–ischaemic encephalopathy
Infancy	Cerebral palsy Severe visual or hearing impairment
Preschool	Speech and language delay Abnormal gait Global delay Loss of skills from neurodegenerative disorder
School age	Learning difficulties—specific or general Clumsiness

Telling parents about a disability

Diagnosis of a disability might be sudden and unexpected, or the culmination of protracted concern and investigation. In any event, the news is likely to provoke reactions of grief accompanied by anger, guilt, despair or denial. The initial interview requires sensitive handling

Breaking news to parents about a disability:

- They should be told as soon as possible.
- They should be told together, not separately.
- Tell them in a quiet place with a colleague, e.g. a nurse.
- Adopt an honest and direct approach.
- Arrange a period of privacy for the parents after the initial interview.
- Arrange a second meeting to allow questions after the news has been assimilated.

Assessment

It is necessary to assess what a child is able to do and what the main difficulties are in several areas:

- Hearing, language and communication.
- Vision and coordination.
- Physical health and mobility.
- Behaviour and emotions.
- Social interactions and self-care, including continence.
- Learning disabilities.

Medical problems commonly encountered in children with disabilities are shown in Fig. 23.9.

Management: the multidisciplinary team

Management of a severe or complex disability requires a multidisciplinary clinical team, working in concert with the social services, local education authorities and voluntary agencies. The balance changes with age:

- Preschool children: community-led child development team, voluntary agencies.

Medical problems in children with neurodisability	
System	**Problem**
Nervous system	Vision and hearing impairment Epilepsy Behavioural disorders
Skeleton	Postural deformities, e.g. scoliosis
Gastrointestinal tract	Feeding difficulties Gastro-oesophageal reflux Constipation or faecal incontinence
Respiratory system	Recurrent aspiration pneumonia
Genitourinary tract	Renal failure Urinary incontinence

Fig. 23.9 Medical problems in children with neurodisability.

- School-age children: education authorities, community health services.
- School-leavers/young adults: Social Services, community disability teams.

Members of the child development team will usually include:

- Paediatricians.
- Physiotherapists.
- Occupational therapists.
- Speech and language therapists.
- Psychologists.
- Social workers.
- Nurses and health visitors.

Statementing

Education authorities have a duty to identify children with special needs and provide appropriate resources. A detailed assessment is undertaken with reports from the educational psychologist, members of the multidisciplinary team and the parents. The resulting 'statement' sets out the child's educational and non-educational needs and the provision of services required to meet those needs. Regular reviews of the statement are also undertaken.

HUMAN RIGHTS ACT 1998

All UK law is interpreted in accordance with the European Convention of Human Rights and individuals can take action if these rights are breached:

- Article 2: Right to life.
- Article 3: Prohibition of torture.
- Article 6: Right to a fair trial.
- Article 8: Right to respect for private and family life.

Further reading

Department of Health. *Immunisation Against Infectious Disease.* London, HMSO, 1996.

Department of Health. *Working Together to Safeguard Children.* London, The Stationary Office, 1999.

Royal College of Paediatricians and Child Health. *Fabricated and Induced Illness By Carers.* London, Royal College of Paediatricians and Child Health, 2002.

Wynne J. The childrens act 1999 and child protection: What paediatricians need to know. *Current Paediatrics* 2001; **11**:113–119.

Genetic disorders

Objectives

At the end of this chapter, you should be able to

- Know the common patterns of inheritance of genetic disorders.
- Know more about common genetic disorders.
- Know the principles of genetic counselling.

The human genome comprises 46 chromosomes, which include 22 pairs of autosomes and 1 pair of sex chromosomes. With the recent mapping of the human genome, our understanding of genetics will increase greatly over the next few years. Many genetic disorders are common during childhood and infancy; those that are associated with a poor prognosis and a short lifespan are not seen during adulthood. As our understanding of genetics has advanced, many new diagnostic technologies have become clinically relevant and therapies for genetic diseases are emerging.

Clinical manifestations are highly variable but it is worth remembering that many dysmorphic syndromes have a genetic basis.

Dysmorphism and syndromes:

- Dysmorphism is an abnormality in form or structural development, often manifested in the facial appearance and often due to an underlying genetic disorder.
- A syndrome is a recognizable pattern of structural and functional abnormalities or malformations known or presumed to be the result of a single cause. Dysmorphism is often a feature.
- Syndromes might be of unknown cause, due to teratogens (e.g. fetal alcohol syndrome), chromosomal anomalies (e.g. Turner syndrome) or single gene disorders (e.g. Marfan syndrome).

BASIC GENETICS

Some useful definitions are shown in Fig. 24.1. The key symbols used in drawing a family tree are shown in Fig. 24.2.

SINGLE GENE DISORDERS

Disorders of single nuclear genes are recognizable because of their Mendelian pattern of inheritance, which can be:

- Autosomal dominant.
- Autosomal recessive.
- X-linked.

Examples of important single gene disorders are shown in Fig. 24.3.

AUTOSOMAL DOMINANT DISORDERS

An affected person has just one copy of the abnormal gene. The disease is manifested in the heterozygote. Each offspring has a 50% chance of inheriting the abnormal gene. Thus, each child of an affected individual has a 50% chance of being affected. A typical pedigree of an autosomal dominant (AD) disorder is shown in Fig. 24.4. The features of an AD pedigree are:

Basic genetics—some definitions	
Term	**Definition**
Karyotype	A display of the set of chromosomes extracted from a eukaryotic somatic cell arrested at metaphase
Genome	The totality of the DNA contained within the diploid chromosome set of a eukaryotic species and within extra-nuclear structures such as the mitochondrial genome
Gene	A sequence of DNA occupying its own place (locus) on a chromosome and containing the information necessary for biosynthesis of a gene product such as a protein or ribosomal RNA molecule
Allele	Any one of the variations of a gene or polymorphic DNA marker found in the members of a species. Numerous alleles may exist, but any individual usually possesses at most two alleles of the gene or polymorphic marker
Genotype	The pair of alleles of a variable gene possessed by an individual, or the pairs of alleles of any number of variable genes possessed by an individual
Phenotype	The entire physical, biochemical, and physiological makeup of an individual as determined by genotype and environment

Fig. 24.1 Basic genetics: some definitions.

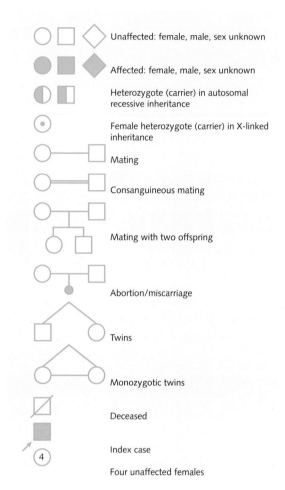

Fig. 24.2 Pedigree symbols.

- Several generations with affected individuals.
- Equal numbers of males and females are affected.
- Male-to-male transmission occurs.

Several complicating factors can occur. These include:

- Variable expression: the pattern and severity of disease varies in affected individuals within the same family.
- Non-penetrance: some individuals with the disease allele have no clinical signs or symptoms.
- Sporadic cases: a new mutation in the ovum or spermatocyte of a parent will give rise to a 'sporadic' case with no family history of the disease. The recurrence risk for new offspring from those parents is then very low.

New mutations are common in some AD disorders. For example, over 80% of individuals with achondroplasia have unaffected parents.

Achondroplasia

This autosomal dominant disorder is characterized by short limbs, large head and abnormalities in neu-

Single gene disorders: examples
Autosomal dominant (total number approximately 3000)
Myotonic dystrophy
Marfan syndrome
Neurofibromatosis type 1
Tuberous sclerosis
Achondroplasia
Autosomal recessive (total number approximately 1500)
Cystic fibrosis
Thalassaemia
Sickle cell disease
Congenital adrenal hyperplasia
Inborn errors of metabolism (majority), e.g. phenylketonuria
X-linked recessive (total number approximately 300)
Haemophilia A and B
Duchenne muscular dystrophy
Fragile X syndrome
Glucose-6-phosphate dehydrogenase (G6PD) deficiency
Colour blindness (red–green)

Fig. 24.3 Single gene disorders: examples.

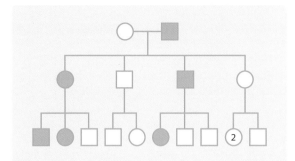

Fig. 24.4 Typical pedigree with autosomal dominant inheritance.

Major clinical features of achondroplasia	
Limbs	Shortened limbs: proximal>distal Bow legs
Neurological	Hydrocephalus Motor developmental delay Normal intelligence
Spine	Short stature Thoracolumbar kyphosis Lumbar lordosis
Ear	Recurrent otitis media

Fig. 24.5 Major clinical features of achondroplasia.

Fig. 24.6 Pedigree of an autosomal recessive disorder.

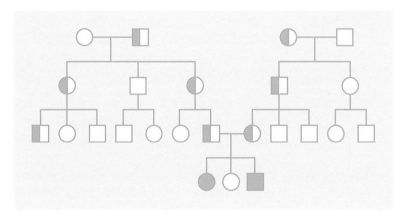

rology. The gene is found on the short arm of chromosome 4 and is a fibroblast growth receptor gene (FGFR3 gene). It affects 1 in 2500 births; typical clinical features are shown in Fig. 24.5.

AUTOSOMAL RECESSIVE DISORDERS

An affected individual has two copies of the abnormal gene inherited from each parent and is said to be homozygous for the disease alleles. The parents are heterozygous carriers if they have only one copy of the abnormal gene. Many recessive disorders are caused by mutations in the genes coding for enzymes. As half of the normal enzyme activity is usually sufficient, a person with only one mutant allele will not normally be affected.

A typical pedigree of an autosomal recessive disorder is shown in Fig. 24.6.

- Autosomal dominant disorders are often caused by mutations in a gene encoding a structural protein.
- Autosomal recessive disorders are often caused by mutations in a gene encoding a functional protein, such as an enzyme.

The risk of each child being affected when both parents are carriers is 25%. Males and females are equally likely to be affected. There is usually no positive family history other than affected individuals within the sibship.

Parental consanguinity increases the risk of a recessive disease occurring in the offspring. Everyone probably carries at least one recessive disease gene allele. A couple who are first cousins, for example, are more likely to have inherited the same abnormal recessive disease gene allele from their common ancestor.

Certain recessive disorders show a founder effect. Affected individuals have inherited a founder mutation that occurred on an ancestral chromosome many generations ago. Carrier rates may be high within inbred populations (e.g. Tay–Sachs disease in Ashkenazi Jews).

Important autosomal recessive diseases are described elsewhere, including cystic fibrosis (Chapter 14), thalassaemia, sickle-cell disease (Chapter 19), congenital adrenal hyperplasia (Chapter 21) and inborn errors of metabolism (Chapter 21).

X-LINKED DISORDERS

Several hundred disease genes are found on the X chromosome and give rise to the characteristic pattern of X-linked inheritance. Most X-linked disorders are recessive. In the carrier female there is a disease allele on one X chromosome but the normal allele on her other X chromosome provides protection from the disease. The male is hemizygous for the gene because he has only a single X chromosome. The abnormal allele is not balanced by a normal allele and he manifests the disease.

A typical pedigree for X-linked recessive inheritance is shown in Fig. 24.7.

The characteristic features are:

- Males only are affected.
- Females are carriers and are usually healthy.
- Females might show mild signs of the disease depending on the pattern of X-chromosome inactivation (note that the Lyon hypothesis suggests that only one of the two X chromosomes in any cell is transcriptionally active).
- Each son of a female carrier has a 50% chance of being affected and each daughter of a female carrier has a 50% chance of being a carrier.
- Daughters of affected males are all carriers.
- Sons of affected males are never affected because a father passes his Y chromosome to his son (i.e. there is no male-to-male transmission).

New mutations are common, so there might be no family history. Several important X-linked recessive diseases, including haemophilia (Chapter 19) and Duchenne muscular dystrophy (Chapter 17), are discussed elsewhere. Additional examples are fragile X syndrome and ornithine transcarbamylase deficiency.

Fragile X syndrome

This is an example of a trinucleotide repeat disorder. After Down syndrome, this is the most common cause of severe learning impairment (mental retardation) with an incidence of 1 in 1000 men and 1 in 2000 women. The disorder is due to expansion of a triplet repeat (CGG) in the FRAXA gene FMR1.

The clinical features of fragile X syndrome are listed in Fig. 24.8.

A number of unusual features are accounted for in part by the triplet repeat amplification:

- The number of repeats determines status: normal individuals have fewer than 50 triplet

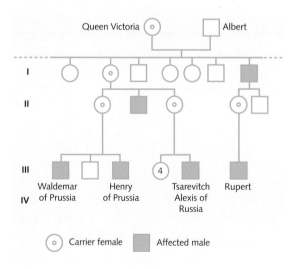

Carrier female ⦿ | Affected male ▪

Fig. 24.7 Typical pedigree for X-linked recessive inheritance. Haemophilia in a royal family.

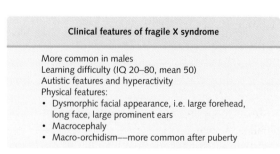

Clinical features of fragile X syndrome
More common in males
Learning difficulty (IQ 20–80, mean 50)
Autistic features and hyperactivity
Physical features:
• Dysmorphic facial appearance, i.e. large forehead, long face, large prominent ears
• Macrocephaly
• Macro-orchidism—more common after puberty

Fig. 24.8 Clinical features of fragile X syndrome.

repeats, carriers with a 'pre-mutation' have 50–200 triplet repeats and affected men or women have over 200 triplet repeats.

- The number of repeats becomes amplified when the gene is inherited from a mother but not usually when inherited from a father.
- One-third of obligate female carriers have mild learning difficulties.
- 'Normal transmitting males' occur, who pass the disorder on to their grandchildren through their daughters.

Cytogenetic analysis or direct DNA analysis confirms the diagnosis.

Ornithine transcarbamylase deficiency

This is an X-linked recessive disorder caused by mutations in the gene for the urea-cycle enzyme that causes hyperammonaemia. Males are most severely affected and usually present with an overwhelming and sometimes fatal illness a few days after birth when protein-containing feeds are given.

Up to 30% of female carriers manifest symptoms, depending on the pattern of lyonization in hepatic cells (the enzyme is expressed in the liver). They might present with learning difficulties or headache and vomiting after high-protein meals.

MULTIFACTORIAL DISORDERS

These conditions are believed to be caused by a combination of genetic susceptibility, due to the interaction of several genes (polygenic), and environmental (non-genetic) factors. Multifactorial inheritance accounts for several common birth defects as well as a number of other important diseases with onset in childhood or adult life (Fig. 24.9).

A feature of the familial clustering of multifactorial diseases is that the recurrence risk is low, often in the range 3–5% (most significant for first-degree relatives and decreases rapidly with more distant relatedness). Factors that increase the risk to relatives include:

- Severely affected proband (e.g. greater in bilateral cleft lip and palate than unilateral cleft lip).
- Multiple affected family members.

Conditions with multifactorial inheritance

Congenital malformations
Neural tube defects
Orofacial clefts (lip and palate)
Pyloric stenosis
Talipes
Common diseases
Asthma
Insulin-dependent diabetes mellitus (IDDM)
Epilepsy
Hypertension
Atherosclerosis
Psychiatric disorders, e.g. autism

Fig. 24.9 Conditions with multifactorial inheritance.

- The affected proband is of the less often affected sex (if there is a difference in the M : F ratio of affected individuals).

In many multifactorial disorders, the environmental factors remain obscure.

CHROMOSOMAL DISORDERS

An alteration in the amount or nature of the chromosomal material is seen in 5 in 1000 live births and is usually associated with multiple congenital anomalies and learning difficulties. A high proportion (40%) of all spontaneous abortions are caused by chromosome abnormalities.

Most chromosome defects arise de novo. They are classified as abnormalities of number or structure, and might involve either the autosomes or the sex chromosomes. Examples of important chromosomal disorders are shown in Fig. 24.10.

The indications for chromosome analysis are shown in Fig. 24.11. Chromosome studies are carried out on dividing cells. Most commonly, T cells from peripheral blood are used after stimulation of mitosis with phytohaemagglutinin.

Chromosomal abnormalities

Three autosomal trisomies are found in live born infants; others are not compatible with life and are found only in spontaneously aborted fetuses. These are:

- Down syndrome: trisomy 21 (1 : 700 live births).

Fig. 24.10 Chromosomal disorders.

Chromosomal disorders			
Type	Class	Name	Defect
Numerical	Autosomal	Down syndrome Edwards syndrome Patau syndrome	Trisomy 21 Trisomy 18 Trisomy 13
	Sex chromosomes	Klinefelter syndrome Turner syndrome	47, XXY 45, XO
Structural	Deletions	Prader–Willi syndrome Cri-du-chat syndrome Wilms tumour with aniridia	15q deletion 5p deletion 11p deletion

Indications for chromosome analysis

- Phenotype consistent with known chromosomal disorder
- Multiple congenital abnormalities
- Dysmorphic features
- Recurrent pregnancy losses
- Spontaneously aborted or stillborn fetuses
- Bone marrow in leukaemia, solid tumours

Fig. 24.11 Indications for chromosome analysis.

Risk of Down syndrome (for live births) by maternal age at delivery

Maternal age (years)	Risk
All ages	1:700
30	1:900
35	1:380
40	1:110
44	1:37

Fig. 24.12 Risk of Down syndrome (for live births) by maternal age at delivery.

- Edward syndrome: trisomy 18 (1:8000 live births).
- Patau syndrome: trisomy 13 (1:15 000 live births).

Trisomy refers to the fact that three, rather than the normal two copies of a specific chromosome are present in the cells of an individual. Trisomies occur because of a meiotic error called non-dysjunction in the gamete of mother or father.

Down syndrome

Trisomy 21 is the most common autosomal trisomy compatible with life. The extra chromosomal material can result from non-dysjunction, translocation or mosaicism.

Non-dysjunction

Ninety-five per cent of children with Down syndrome have trisomy 21 due to non-dysjunction. The pair of chromosomes 21 fails to separate at meiosis, so one gamete has two copies of chromosome 21. Fertilization of this gamete gives rise to a zygote with trisomy 21.

Ninety per cent of non-dysjunctions are maternally derived and the risk rises with maternal age, increasing steeply in mothers over 35 years (Fig. 24.12).

However, because a higher proportion of pregnancies occur in younger women, most children with trisomy 21 are born to women under 35 years of age. The recurrence risk for parents of children with trisomy 21 increases to 1–2% (unless the age-related risk is higher).

Translocation

Four per cent of Down syndrome children have 46 chromosomes with a translocation of the third chromosome 21 to another chromosome (most commonly 14). Three-quarters of cases are *de novo* and, in one-quarter, one of the parents has a balanced translocation involving one chromosome 21. If the mother is the translocation carrier, the recurrence risk might be as high as 15%; if the father is the carrier, the risk is 2.5%.

Mosaicism

In 1% of cases the non-dysjunction occurs during mitosis after formation of the zygote so that some cells are normal and some show trisomy 21. The phenotype might be milder in mosaicism.

Clinical features

Down syndrome is often suspected at birth because of the characteristic facial appearance but the diagnosis can be difficult on clinical features alone. A senior paediatrician should confirm clinical suspicion. Chromosome analysis takes several days though faster results can be obtained by using FISH (Fluorescent in situ hybridization). The phenotypic features are listed in Fig. 24.13.

Management and prognosis

Parents need information about the implications of the diagnosis and the assistance available from professionals and self-help groups. Feelings of disappointment, anger and guilt are common. Genetic counselling for recurrence risks will be required. Life expectancy in Down syndrome has increased and issues relating to employment and living situations in adulthood will need to be addressed.

Treatment of trisomy 21 again involves a multidisciplinary approach. In addition to the healthcare agencies there are many voluntary organizations offering help and support to such families. The Down's syndrome association is one such organization.

Sex chromosome disorders

Turner syndrome

In this condition, there are 44 autosomes and only one normal X chromosome. It affects 1 in 2500 live born females. Various underlying chromosomal defects are seen:

- In 55% of girls, the karyotype is 45, XO.
- In 25%, there is a deletion of the short arm of one X chromosome, or a so-called isochromosome with duplication of one arm and loss of the other.
- In 15%, there is mosaicism due to postzygotic mitotic non-dysjunction. (45, XO/46, XY).

The incidence does not increase with maternal age and the recurrence risk is the same as the general population risk.

Clinical features of Down syndrome	
Dysmorphic facial features	Round face Epicanthic folds, flat nasal bridge Protruding tongue Small ears Brushfield spots on iris
Other dysmorphic features	Single palmar creases Flat occiput Incurved little fingers Gap between first and second toes (sandal toe gap) Small stature
Structural defects	Cardiac defects in 50% Duodenal atresia
Neurological features	Hypotonia Developmental delay Mean IQ = 50
Late medical complications	Increased risk of leukaemia Respiratory infections Hypothyroidism Alzheimer's disease Atlantoaxial instability

Fig. 24.13 Clinical features of Down syndrome.

Clinical features of Turner syndrome
Dysmorphic features Lymphoedema of hands and feet (at birth) Neck webbing Widely spaced nipples Wide carrying angle (cubitus valgus) Short stature **Structural and functional abnormalities** Gonadal dysgenesis Congenital heart disease, particularly coarctation of the aorta Renal anomalies

Fig. 24.14 Clinical features of Turner syndrome.

The hallmarks of Turner syndrome are short stature and primary amenorrhoea. Intelligence is normal but there might be specific learning difficulties.

Clinical features and diagnosis

The clinical features are shown in Fig. 24.14. Diagnosis may be made:

- Prenatally by ultrasound scan.
- At birth by presence of puffy hands and feet (lymphoedema).
- During childhood because of short stature.
- In adolescence because of primary amenorrhoea and lack of pubertal development.

Diagnosis is confirmed by a peripheral blood karyotype.

Management

Therapy with growth hormone improves final height. Ovarian hormones are not produced due to the gonadal dysgenesis (streak ovaries). Oestrogen therapy is given at the appropriate age (11 years) to produce maturation of secondary sexual characteristics including breast development. Towards the end of puberty, progestogen is added to maintain uterine health and allow monthly withdrawal bleeds (periods). Although pregnancy can occur naturally, most patients are infertile. Pregnancy can be achieved with *in vitro* fertilization.

Structural chromosomal abnormalities

These arise from chromosome breakage and include deletions, duplications, inversions and unbalanced translocations. Deletions are the most common. Most arise de novo but they can also arise from inheritance of an unbalanced translocation. Examples of conditions associated with chromosomal deletions include:

- Cri-du-chat syndrome: caused by deletion of short arm of chromosome 5 (5p-). Affected children have profound mental retardation and a cat-like cry.
- Prader–Willi syndrome: caused by deletions of the paternal copy of 15q11-13
- Angelman syndrome: caused by deletions of the maternal copy of 15q11-13

MITOCHONDRIAL INHERITANCE

Mitochondrial disorders are inherited maternally. Examples include:

- Mitochondrial encephalopathy, lactic acidosis, stroke-like episodes (MELAS).
- Mitochondrially inherited diabetes mellitus.

Imprinting:
- Some genes are 'imprinted'. The copy derived from one parent (either male or female) is active and the other is not.
- Deletions of chromosomal regions that are 'imprinted' have different effects according to the parent of origin of the deleted chromosome.
- The most well-known example is deletion of 15q11-13. Paternal chromosome deletion causes Prader–Willi syndrome (obesity, learning difficulties). Maternal chromosome deletion causes Angelman syndrome (happy puppet syndrome: ataxia, learning difficulties, 'happy' disposition).

The mitochondria contain genetic material as a 16.5-kilobase circular chromosome. They have no introns and a mixture of normal and abnormal mitochondria (heteroplasmy) can exist within tissues. It is worth noting the similarities between mitochondrial and prokaryotic genetics.

POLYMERASE CHAIN REACTION

This is a technique of obtaining a large amount of DNA copied from a small initial sample. It has applications in detection of specific DNA sequences or differences in genes. Its main clinical use is in detection of mutations and rapid diagnosis of bacterial or viral infection. It has a very high sensitivity and is being increasingly used in clinical practice.

Information base in genetic counselling:
- Magnitude of risk.
- Severity of disorder.
- Availability of treatment.
- Parental cultural and ethical values.
Options in antenatal genetic counselling:
- Not to have offspring.
- To ignore the risk.
- Antenatal diagnosis and termination of pregnancy.
- Pre-implantation diagnosis.
- Artificial insemination by donor or ovum donation.

GENETIC COUNSELLING

This is usually carried out as a specialist service by trained medical staff and specialist nurses. The main aim is to provide information about hereditary disorders so that parents will have greater autonomy and choice in reproductive decisions

The basic elements of counselling include:

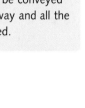

- Establishing a diagnosis: this might involve physical examination of proband and family members and special investigations including DNA, cytogenetic and biochemical analysis.
- Estimation of risk: the risk for future offspring is determined by the mode of inheritance of the disease.
- Communication: information must be conveyed in an unbiased and non-directive way and all the possible options should be discussed.

Fetal and neonatal life are best regarded as a continuum and the term 'perinatal' medicine is sometimes used to encompass the care of the pregnant mother and fetus, as well as the newborn infant. Many factors from before conception to delivery influence the health of the newborn infant.

Introduction: perinatal statistics and definitions

Terms used in perinatal statistics are defined in Fig. 25.1.

Nearly half of all neonatal deaths occur in the first 24 hours. The perinatal mortality rate in developed countries has fallen steadily over the last 20 years and seems to be approaching an irreducible lower limit set by deaths from lethal malformations. However, disadvantaged people continue to have the highest rates of perinatal deaths and congenital malformations.

MATERNAL AND FETAL HEALTH

Mother and fetus are a single physiological unit and any serious maternal disease or condition can affect the fetus. Action to optimize the chances of a healthy baby can begin even before conception. The chance of a good outcome can be enhanced by:

- Avoiding smoking, excess alcohol and medication.

- Avoiding infections: rubella immunization before pregnancy, avoiding exposure to toxoplasmosis (via cat's litter) and avoiding exposure to listeriosis (unpasteurized dairy products).
- Folic acid supplements reduce the risk of neural tube defects.
- Optimizing treatment of maternal conditions such as hypertension and diabetes mellitus.
- Genetic counselling for couples at risk of inherited diseases.

FETAL ASSESSMENT AND ANTENATAL DIAGNOSIS

Methods for assessing the growth, maturation and well-being of the fetus are available. They include:

- Ultrasound: for assessing age and growth.
- Doppler blood flow studies.

Antenatal diagnosis is now available for many disorders using the methods shown in Fig. 25.2.

Antenatal diagnosis can allow the option of termination to be offered in certain disorders, therapy to be given or neonatal management to be planned in advance. Medical treatment can be given to the fetus via the mother or directly (e.g. fetal blood transfusion for anaemia in severe rhesus isoimmunization).

Definitions for perinatal statistics	
Term	**Definition**
Still birth	A fetus born after 24 weeks of gestation who shows no signs of life after delivery
Low birthweight	A baby weighing 2500 g or less at birth
Preterm	A baby born at any time before 37 weeks' gestation
Term	A baby born between 37 and 42 completed weeks' gestation
Post-term	A baby born after 42 weeks' gestation
Neonatal period	First month of life
Perinatal mortality rate	Still births and deaths within the first 6 days per 1000 live and still births (i.e. total births)
Neonatal mortality rate	Deaths of liveborn infants during the first 28 days of age per 1000 live births

Fig. 25.1 Definitions for perinatal statistics.

MATERNAL CONDITIONS AFFECTING THE FETUS

The fetus can be affected by:

- Maternal diseases: diabetes mellitus, thyrotoxicosis and auto-immune disorders (e.g. systemic lupus erythematosus, myasthenia gravis and thrombocytopenia).
- Maternal drugs, e.g. medications, alcohol and narcotics.
- Maternal infections: congenital infections.

Thus, many conditions affecting the first and second trimesters lead to organ dysfunction or structural abnormality.

Maternal diseases

Diabetes mellitus

The outlook for the infant of a mother with insulin-dependent diabetes mellitus has improved greatly and is enhanced by good diabetic control during the pregnancy. Potential fetal problems include:

- Congenital malformations: there is a three-fold increase (especially cardiac malformations).
- Macrosomia: the fetal insulin response to hyperglycaemia promotes excessive growth, which predisposes to difficulties during delivery.

Potential neonatal problems include:

- Hypoglycaemia: transient early hypoglycaemia occurs due to fetal hyperinsulinism; early feeding can usually prevent this.
- Respiratory distress syndrome (RDS).
- Polycythaemia (haematocrit >0.65).

Maternal drugs affecting the fetus

Drugs taken by the mother might cause congenital malformations (Fig. 25.3), adverse effects by their pharmacological action on the fetus or placenta, or transient problems at birth.

Maternal drugs and the fetus:
- Teratogenic drugs taken during organogenesis can cause spontaneous abortions or congenital malformations.
- Drugs given during labour can have adverse effects, e.g. analgesics and anaesthesia (suppression of spontaneous breathing at birth), sedatives (sedation, hypotension).
- IV fluids: excess hypotonic fluids can cause hyponatraemia.

Maternal infections and the fetus

A number of infections acquired by the mother could affect the fetus or newborn (Fig. 25.4). Transmission can occur in utero, during labour or post-partum (Fig. 25.5).

Rubella

For rubella, see Chapter 10.

Varicella zoster

More than 85% of women of childbearing age have evidence of past infection with chickenpox, so a minority of pregnant women are at risk.

Infection in the first trimester does not usually cause fetal damage but about 5% develop the so-called 'congenital varicella syndrome' characterized by:

- Cicatricial skin lesions (scars).
- Malformed digits.
- Cataracts.
- CNS damage, chorioretinitis.

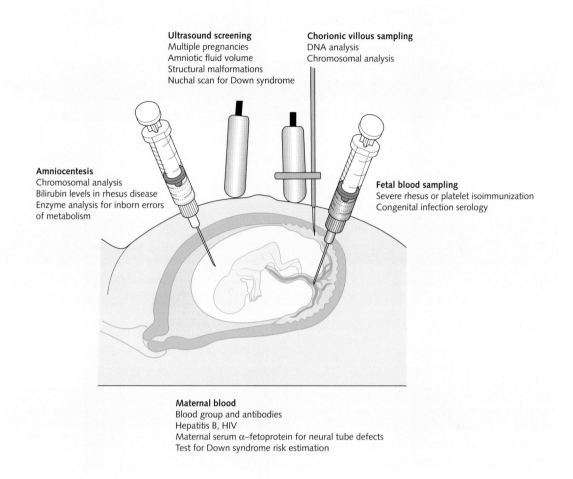

Ultrasound screening
Multiple pregnancies
Amniotic fluid volume
Structural malformations
Nuchal scan for Down syndrome

Chorionic villous sampling
DNA analysis
Chromosomal analysis

Amniocentesis
Chromosomal analysis
Bilirubin levels in rhesus disease
Enzyme analysis for inborn errors
of metabolism

Fetal blood sampling
Severe rhesus or platelet isoimmunization
Congenital infection serology

Maternal blood
Blood group and antibodies
Hepatitis B, HIV
Maternal serum α–fetoprotein for neural tube defects
Test for Down syndrome risk estimation

Fig. 25.2 Antenatal diagnosis: various methods and the disorders they are used to diagnose.

The principal problem is infection acquired late in pregnancy, particularly within 5 days before and 2 days after delivery. The fetus receives a high viral load but little in the way of maternal antibodies. Severe infection can ensue with a mortality of up to 5%.

Exposed susceptible women can be treated with varicella zoster immune globulin (VZIG) and aciclovir. Infants exposed in the high-risk period should also be treated with VZIG. Intravenous aciclovir should be used if lesions develop in the newborn infant.

Cytomegalovirus
For cytomegalovirus, see Chapter 10.

Human immunodeficiency virus (HIV)
Vertical transmission from mother to infant can occur in utero, during birth or postnatally by breast-feeding. The exact risk of infection by each of these routes is uncertain but overall vertical transmission rates is now less than 1% (see Chapter 10).

Use of zidovudine given to the mother during pregnancy and delivery, and to the neonate for the first 6 weeks of life, reduces the transmission risk.

- Diagnosis of HIV during infancy is rendered difficult by the passage of maternal antibody, which can persist for up to 18 months.
- Breastfeeding can increase the risk of vertical transmission by 15%.

Maternal medication that may harm the fetus	
Drug	**Adverse effects**
Cytotoxic agents	Congenital malformations
Phenytoin	Fetal hydantoin syndrome (growth retardation, microcephaly, hypoplastic nails)
Sodium valproate	Neural tube defects
Carbamazepine	Growth retardation, craniofacial abnormalities
Warfarin	Interferes with cartilage formation, risk of cerebral haemorrhage, and microcephaly
Progestogens (androgenic)	Masculinization of fetus
Diethylstilboestrol	Adenocarcinoma of vagina
Thalidomide	Limb shortening (phocomelia)
Drug abuse	
Alcohol	Fetal alcohol syndrome (characteristic facies, septal defects, mental retardation)
Opiates (heroin/methadone)	Growth retardation, prematurity, drug withdrawal in neonate (tremors, hyperirritability, seizures)
Cocaine	Spontaneous abortion, prematurity, cerebral infarction

Fig. 25.3 Maternal medication that can harm the fetus.

Toxoplasmosis

Infection with the protozoan parasite *Toxoplasma gondis* occurs from the ingestion of raw or undercooked meat, or from oocytes excreted in the faeces of infected cats. Most infections are asymptomatic. Serological epidemiological studies show that in some countries (e.g. France and Austria), 80% of women of childbearing age are immune, whereas in the UK only 20% have antibodies.

About 40% of women who acquire an acute infection during pregnancy transmit the infection to the fetus. The risk of severe damage is highest following infection in the first trimester. About 10% of infected infants have clinical manifestations at birth, which can include:

- Hydrocephalus.
- Intracranial calcification.
- Chorioretinitis.
- Neurological damage.

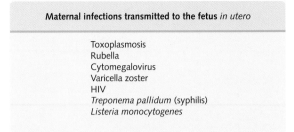

Maternal infections transmitted to the fetus *in utero*
Toxoplasmosis
Rubella
Cytomegalovirus
Varicella zoster
HIV
Treponema pallidum (syphilis)
Listeria monocytogenes

Fig. 25.4 Maternal infections transmitted to the fetus in utero.

Infections acquired during delivery
Group B haemolytic streptococci
E. coli
HIV
Hepatitis B
Herpes simplex
Gonococci
Chlamydia trachomatis
Echoviruses

Fig. 25.5 Infections acquired during delivery.

Infants with asymptomatic infection may still develop chorioretinitis in later life.

In some countries, serological screening for infection is carried out during pregnancy. If positive (and fetal infection is confirmed by cordocentesis), termination or treatment with spiramycin can be offered, although the efficacy of the latter remains uncertain. An infected newborn infant is treated with alternating courses of pyrimethamine with sulphadiazine and spiramycin until the age of 1 year.

NORMAL NEONATAL ANATOMY AND PHYSIOLOGY

There are characteristic features of newborn anatomy and physiology that are important and these are considered in turn.

Size and growth

The average term infant in the UK weighs about 3500 g. Boys weigh approximately 250 g more than girls. Infants of 2500 g or less are classified as 'low birthweight'. This important category is considered separately.

During the first 3–5 days, up to 10% of birth-weight is lost. This is regained by 7–10 days. In the first month, average weight gain per week is 200 g.

Skin

The newborn skin is immature, with a thin epithelial layer and incompletely developed sweat and sebaceous glands. Combined with the high surface area to body mass ratio, this renders the baby prone to heat and water losses.

Numerous benign skin lesions occur (see Chapter 12). The skin is covered with a greasy protective layer, the vernix caseosa.

Head

The average occipitofrontal head circumference is 35 cm. Significant moulding of the head might occur during birth. Two soft spots or fontanelles are present. The anterior fontanelle closes between 9 and 18 months of age and the posterior closes by 6–8 weeks.

Respiratory system

Changes occur at birth that allow the newborn to convert from dependence on the placenta to breathing air for the exchange of respiratory gases:

- *In utero*, the airways and lungs are filled with fluid that contains surfactant in the later stages of pregnancy.
- The lung fluid is removed by the squeezing of the thorax during vaginal delivery and by reduced secretion and increased absorption mediated by fetal catecholamines during labour and after birth.
- Surfactant lines the air–fluid interface of the alveoli and reduces the surface tension thereby facilitating lung expansion. This is associated with a fall in pulmonary vascular resistance.

Newborn infants breathe mainly with the diaphragm. The rate is variable and normally ranges between 30–50 breaths/min. Brief (up to several seconds) self-limiting apnoeic spells might occur during sleep. Small babies are obligate nose-breathers.

Cardiovascular system

Major changes in the lungs and circulation allow adaptation to extrauterine life.

In the fetal circulation, the right-sided (pulmonary) pressure exceeds the left-sided (systemic) pressure. Blood flows from right to left through the foramen ovale and ductus arteriosus (Fig. 25.6). At birth, these relationships reverse:

- Left-sided (systemic) pressure rises with clamping of umbilical vessels.
- Right-sided (pulmonary) pressure falls as the lungs expand and the rising PO_2 triggers a prostaglandin-mediated vasodilatation.
- The foramen ovale and ductus arteriosus close functionally shortly after birth. The ductus closes due to muscular contraction in response to rising oxygen tension.

Gastrointestinal system

Most infants over 35 weeks' gestation have developed the coordination necessary to 'latch on' and feed from breast or bottle. At term, the secretory and absorbing surfaces are well developed, as are digestive enzymes, with the exception of pancreatic amylase.

Meconium is usually passed within 6 hours and delay beyond 24 hours is considered abnormal.

With normal feeding, 'changing stools' replace meconium on day 3 or 4, and thereafter the yellowish stools of the milk-fed infant develop.

Immaturity of the liver enzymes responsible for conjugation of bilirubin is responsible for the 'physiological jaundice', which can occur from the second day of life.

Genitourinary system

Urine production is occurring during the second half of gestation and accounts for much of the amniotic fluid. The infant might micturate during delivery (unnoticed) and should void within the first 24 hours of life. Renal concentrating ability is diminished in neonates.

Haematopoietic and immune system

The newborn's red cells contain fetal haemoglobin (HbF) and has a higher affinity for oxygen than adult haemoglobin. The haemoglobin concentration of cord blood ranges from 15 to 20 g/dL (mean 17 g/dL). A large volume of blood is present in the placenta and late clamping causes this blood to

Fig. 25.6 Fetal circulation.

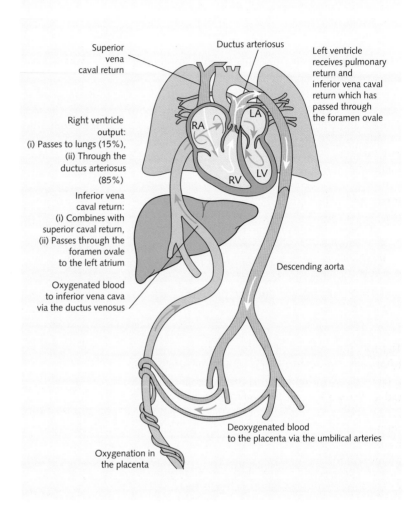

Superior vena caval return

Ductus arteriosus

Left ventricle receives pulmonary return and inferior vena caval return which has passed through the foramen ovale

Right ventricle output:
(i) Passes to lungs (15%),
(ii) Through the ductus arteriosus (85%)

Inferior vena caval return:
(i) Combines with superior caval return,
(ii) Passes through the foramen ovale to the left atrium

Descending aorta

Oxygenated blood to inferior vena cava via the ductus venosus

RA   LA

RV   LV

Deoxygenated blood to the placenta via the umbilical arteries

Oxygenation in the placenta

enter the baby. This can lead to polycythaemia. In the preterm baby it is advantageous.

The neonatal immune system also is incomplete compared to older children and adults:

- Impaired neutrophil reserves.
- Diminished phagocytosis and intracellular killing capacity.
- Decreased complement components.
- Low IgG_2, leading to infections with encapsulated organisms.

The presence of maternal antibody in babies born greater than 30 weeks gestational age provides some protection against infection.

Central nervous system

The central nervous system (CNS) is relatively immature at birth. Myelination is incomplete and continues during the first 2 years of life.

A limited behavioural response repertoire is sufficient for survival, comprising a sleep and wake cycle, sucking and swallowing, and crying:

- Newborn infants sleep for a total of 16–20 hours each day.
- The touch of a nipple on the baby's face initiates the sequence of rooting, latching on and the complex coordination of lip, tongue, palate and pharynx required for sucking and swallowing.

- Crying (without tears) is the main means of communication. Usually this is in response to hunger, thirst or pain, but some newborns cry without obvious reason and are difficult to pacify.

BIRTH

The short journey down the birth canal from the intrauterine environment to the external world is potentially hazardous. Various risk factors can be identified during labour; the most important of which is prematurity. The problems of the preterm infant are dealt with separately. Here we consider the:

- Normal care and resuscitation of the term newborn.
- Problems of birth asphyxia and birth injuries.

Assessment and care at a normal birth

The infant is usually delivered after a short period of oxygen deprivation and begins to breathe within a few seconds. The Apgar score is a useful quantitative assessment of the infant's condition (Fig. 25.7) and is commonly determined at 1 and 5 minutes after birth. The Apgar score is influenced by several factors including intrapartum asphyxia, maternal sedation or analgesia, the gestational age and any cardiac, pulmonary or neurological disease in the infant. Most babies will establish respirations spontaneously after delivery or if apnoeic respond to airway opening manoeuvres. However a few will need more extensive resuscitation (see Fig. 25.9).

Birth asphyxia

This refers to a condition in which the fetus is acutely deprived of oxygen and is commonly due to utero-placental insufficiency. The incidence has fallen to 1.5–6 per 1000 live births but in 75% of newborns neurological damage is antenatal, 20% is antenatal and intrapartum and only 5% is intrapartum alone.

Asphyxia (which literally means 'absent pulse' and was a term for 'suffocation') is manifested during labour by various fetal responses (previously termed 'fetal distress'). There is fetal hypoxia, hypercapnia, and acidosis, which may be detected by:

- Abnormalities in fetal heart rate: there may be fetal bradycardia (rate under 120 beats/min), fetal tachycardia (rate over 160 beats/min) or an abnormal pattern of deceleration during or after uterine contractions.
- Acidosis: sampling of fetal blood from scalp or cord will demonstrate significant acidosis (pH <7.20).
- Meconium staining of the liquor: the asphyxiated infant passes meconium.

These signs are an indication for prompt delivery of the fetus. The effects of asphyxia are seen in Fig. 25.8.

The postnatal symptoms and signs of asphyxia vary with the degree of asphyxia, which can be classified as mild, moderate or severe. Neonatal encephalopathy is the term used to describe the neurological manifestations.

Apgar score evaluation of the newborn			
Criteria	Score		
	0	1	2
Heart rate	Absent	<100 beats/min	>100 beats/min
Respiratory effort	Absent/weak	Irregular/gasping	Regular
Muscle tone	Limp	Some flexion	Active movements
Reflex response to stimulation	None	Weak	Cries
Colour	Blue or pale	Extremities blue	Pink

Fig. 25.7 Apgar score evaluation of the newborn.

Neonatal encephalopathy (hypoxic–ischaemic encephalopathy)

The manifestations of the effects of asphyxia on the brain vary with its severity:

- Mild: initial lethargy followed by a period of hyperalertness with irritability, staring of the eyes and impaired feeding for 1–2 days. There are no focal signs. Prognosis is good.
- Moderate: as above with generalized seizures occurring 12–24 hours after the episode of asphyxia and resolving within a few days. Depressed conscious level. Variable prognosis.
- Severe: coma and intractable seizures worsening over 1–3 days as delayed or 'secondary' injury develops. Multiorgan failure is often present. Death is common and survival is associated with poor long-term outcome.

As neuronal injury continues after resuscitation, good supportive care is required. Management involves:

- Respiratory support.
- Anticonvulsants for seizures.
- Fluid restriction.
- Circulatory support with inotropes if necessary.

Complications of perinatal asphyxia (severe)	
Organ	Complication
Brain	Hypoxic–ischaemic encephalopathy
Heart	Hypoxic cardiomyopathy, hypotension
Lungs	Persistent pulmonary hypotension
Guts	Ileus and necrotizing enterocolitis
Kidneys	Acute tubular necrosis
Blood	Disseminated intravascular coagulation

Fig. 25.8 Complications of perinatal asphyxia (severe).

Fig. 25.9 Neonatal resuscitation.

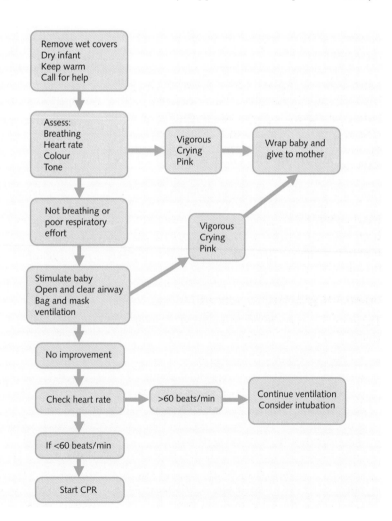

- Application of mild hypothermia after perinatal asphyxia may improve the functional outcome.

MRI and EEG can assist in predicting the outcome. Cystic lesions or cerebral atrophy may appear in the ensuing weeks.

BIRTH INJURY

Physical injury during labour and delivery is now relatively uncommon, partly because the availability of caesarean section obviates the need for heroic attempts at vaginal delivery. Predisposing factors include:

- Breech presentation.
- Cephalopelvic disproportion.
- Assisted delivery: manual or instrumental (forceps or ventouse extraction). Injuries can occur to soft tissues, nerves or bones.

DISEASES OF THE NEWBORN

Much neonatal care is directed towards the problems of low-birthweight infants, especially those born prematurely, many of whom require intensive care. It is therefore useful to consider the disorders of low-birthweight and term infants separately, although there is, of course, significant overlap.

Size and gestational age

Newborn infants might be small because they have been born preterm or because they are small in relation to their gestational age (small for dates). Some useful definitions are shown in Fig. 25.10.

Small for gestational age infants

These infants have intrauterine growth retardation (IUGR), which can be caused by:

- An intrinsic fetal problem: poor growth is symmetrical, with head circumference proportionally reduced, e.g. chromosomal disorders, small normal fetus and congenital infections.
- Placental insufficiency: poor growth is asymmetrical, with brain growth relatively spared (an adaptive response), e.g. maternal pre-eclampsia, hypertension, renal disease, sickle-cell disease and multiple pregnancy.

Definitions for size and gestational age	
Term	**Definition**
Preterm	Gestation <37 completed weeks
Post-term	Gestation >42 completed weeks
Low birthweight	<2500 g
Very low birthweight	<1500 g
Extremely low birthweight	<1000 g
Small for gestational age	Birthweight <10th centile for gestational age
Large for gestational age	Birthweight >90th centile for gestational age

Fig. 25.10 Definitions for size and gestational age.

The fetus with IUGR is at risk from hypoxia and death and is closely monitored using cardiotocography and Doppler ultrasound to profile blood flow velocity in the uterine and umbilical arteries.

Postnatal problems encountered by the fetus with IUGR include:

- Hypothermia.
- Hypoglycaemia from low fat and glycogen stores.
- Hypocalcaemia.
- Polycythaemia (haematocrit >0.65).

Large for gestational age infants

The most common cause of macrosomia is maternal diabetes mellitus. Potential associated problems include birth asphyxia from a difficult delivery and birth trauma, especially from shoulder dystocia.

The preterm infant

About 3 in every 100 babies are born prematurely (before 37 weeks' gestation) and are classified as 'preterm'. Most weigh less than 2500 g and are therefore 'low-birthweight' babies. These infants provide much of the work in neonatal units and account for 60% of neonatal deaths.

The major problems encountered by preterm infants are determined by the immaturity of their organ systems, particularly the lungs (Fig. 25.11). The limits of viability are currently in the region of 23–24 weeks' gestation.

Major problems in preterm infants	
Temperature	Hypothermia
Respiratory	Respiratory distress syndrome Pneumothorax Chronic lung disease Pneumonia Pulmonary hypertension
Cardiac	Patent ductus arteriosus Hypotension
Gastrointestinal	Feed intolerance Vomiting and gastro-oesophageal reflux Jaundice Necrotizing enterocolitis
Infection	Group B streptococci Staphylococcus epidermidis Gram-negative cocci Fungi, e.g. Candida species
Nervous	Intraventricular haemorrhage Retinopathy of prematurity Developmental delay
Bone	Osteopenia of prematurity
Fluids and electrolytes	High transepidermal water loss Hypoglycaemia
Haematology	Anaemia

Fig. 25.11 Major problems in preterm infants.

Characteristics of the preterm infant

A typical infant of 28 weeks' gestation would have the following features:

- Large head in relation to the chest, which is small and narrow.
- Shiny, smooth skin.
- Skull soft, ears floppy and lacking cartilage.
- Eyes closed.
- Extended posture, jerky, frog-like movements.
- Weak cry.

The physiology of the major organ systems and bodily functions are immature as shown by:

- Temperature control: heat production is low (no brown fat, limited muscle activity). Heat loss is high (high surface area to volume, lack of fat insulation).
- Blood and circulation: hypotension, easy bruising and bleeding.
- Respiratory system: narrow nasal airways, soft thoracic cage, poor cough reflex, unstable respiratory drive with irregular breathing and apnoea. Alveolar collapse due to surfactant deficiency.
- Gastrointestinal tract: uncoordinated suck or swallow (before 32–34 weeks). Regurgitation common. Increased severity and incidence of 'physiological' jaundice.
- Renal function: tendency to lose sodium but unable to excrete fluid load. Oedema and hyponatraemia might occur.
- Immune system: active and passive immunity are both limited.

General care of the preterm infant

Some basic principles apply to the care of all preterm infants. These are considered separately from the specific problems that arise in different systems. Attention must be paid to:

- Prevention and predelivery care.
- Resuscitation at birth.
- Maintaining body temperature.
- Avoiding infection.
- Nutrition and fluids.
- Physiological monitoring.

Prevention and predelivery care

Preterm labour can be avoided in the presence of risk factors by bed rest and β-mimetic drugs, e.g. ritodrine. Once labour has started it can be delayed by using the same group of drugs. This might give time for the administration of a corticosteroid to reduce the risk of respiratory distress syndrome (hyaline membrane disease).

Parents should be given the opportunity to speak to a paediatrician prior to the delivery of a premature infant and, if possible, visit the neonatal unit. At this time, they should be made aware of the possible complications of preterm delivery and the chances of survival and disability. It is also important to tell them what happens soon after delivery and briefly about the resuscitation. They should also be prepared for a long stay in the neonatal intensive care.

Resuscitation at birth

Delivery should ideally take place in a location with full paediatric backup, including a neonatal special care unit. At birth the baby should be handled gently, dried and placed under a source of radiant heat.

Many preterm infants of 32 weeks' gestation or less will not achieve adequate spontaneous ventilation and intermittent positive pressure ventilation or nasal continuous positive airways pressure is advisable. Surfactant administration in <29 weeks should be considered at this stage.

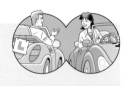

Parents would often want to know the chances of survival of an extremely premature infant. Studies show that babies born earlier than 23 weeks have less than 10% chances of survival and those who do survive will have disabilities, often severe. At 25 weeks this is about 50% and about 20% of babies born at 25 weeks survive without severe disability. At 28 weeks most babies survive and do not have major disability although minor learning difficulties can occur.

Body temperature

Preterm infants rapidly lose heat through evaporation, radiation and convection (see Hints & Tips), and have limited heat-production mechanisms. Strategies for maintaining body temperature have to take into account the need for observation and access. They include:

- Ambient temperature: incubators provide a controlled microenvironment.
- Insulation with clothing: monitoring equipment can be attached to a clothed infant so most do not need to be kept naked. A bonnet prevents excessive loss from the relatively large head.
- Radiant heat: this is useful in the resuscitation area as access is optimized, but it causes excessive fluid loss over prolonged periods.

Body temperature in the preterm infant:
- Heat loss is excessive due to high surface area to volume ratio, poor insulation and transepidermal water loss.
- Heat generation is limited by reduced muscular activity, lack of brown fat and inability to shiver.

Avoiding infection

Meticulous attention to hand-washing before and after handling is the most important safeguard against transmitting infection. Obviously, staff with skin or bowel infections should not be at work until clear. Good skin care will reduce the incidence of *Staphylococcus epidermidis* infection.

Nutrition and fluids

Infants of 35 weeks' gestation or more are usually able to take oral feeds of milk from breast or bottle without difficulty. Although preterm infants can digest and absorb enteral feeds, their sucking and swallowing reflexes might be ineffective and some or all of the feeds must be delivered through a small-bore polyethylene tube passed via the nose or mouth into the stomach. The approach to giving nutrition and fluids therefore depends on the size and maturity of the individual baby.

Enteral feeding in very low-birthweight babies should be slow to allow the gut to adapt to feeds.

The majority of small preterm infants (under 1500 g) require their fluid and calorie requirements intravenously during the first few days. Feeds should be slowly introduced and in the <1000 g babies parenteral nutrition commenced early as full enteral feeding will take longer to establish.

If enteral feeds by mouth or nasogastric tube are not tolerated, more prolonged maintenance of nutrition is achieved by total parenteral nutrition. A mixture of amino acids, dextrose, lipids and electrolytes is given intravenously via a long line, the lumen of which is placed centrally in the vena cava or right atrium.

Which milk for preterm infants? Although breast milk alone does not provide enough calories or minerals, it is better tolerated than artificial feeds and its use is encouraged in the early setting for this reason, and to protect against necrotizing enterocolitis (NEC). Once feeding is established, a preterm formula to increase calories and electrolytes can be added.

Supplements Breastfed preterm infants need supplements of phosphate and vitamin D to ensure adequate bone mineralization. A multivitamin preparation is usually given from the third week and an iron supplement from 4–6 weeks of age onwards. This is continued until 1 year of life but vitamins can be up to 5 years.

DISORDERS OF THE PRETERM INFANT

Respiratory disorders

Surfactant deficiency (hyaline membrane disease, respiratory distress syndrome)

This syndrome is caused by a deficiency of surfactant associated with immaturity of the type II alveolar cells. Surfactant is a lipoprotein that lowers surface tension in the alveoli and prevents collapse of the alveoli during expiration. At postmortem, an exudate of proteinaceous hyaline material is seen in the alveoli and terminal bronchioles (hence, the alternative term 'hyaline membrane disease' for this disorder).

Surfactant deficiency is uncommon in term infants but will occur in the majority born before 30 weeks' gestation. It tends to be worse in boys and hypoxia, acidosis or hypothermia exacerbates surfactant deficiency.

Clinical features

Respiratory distress is the major feature. This might be present from birth or could develop within the first 4 hours. The signs include:

- Tachypnoea.
- Cyanosis.
- Subcostal and intercostal recession.
- Expiratory grunting.

The disease displays a spectrum of severity from mild to severe and life threatening. A chest X-ray (CXR) will show a diffuse granular or 'ground glass' appearance of the lungs and an air bronchogram outlining the larger airways.

Management

Glucocorticoids given antenatally for 48 hours stimulate fetal surfactant production but, of course, many preterm births occur without this period of warning. Effective resuscitation, at birth, of infants at risk reduces the severity of the disease.

The mainstays of management include:

- Surfactant therapy.
- Oxygen.
- Assisted ventilation.

Exogenous surfactant therapy given after birth reduces mortality and morbidity and many babies can be rapidly weaned off ventilatory support after treatment.

An increased concentration of inspired oxygen is required and in more severe disease this needs to be supplemented with continuous positive airways pressure via the nasal airways or intermittent positive pressure ventilation via an endotracheal tube. Ventilation is guided by monitoring of the arterial blood gas tensions (PaO_2 and $PaCO_2$). High frequency oscillatory ventilation can be used as the sole mode of ventilation but often reserved for severe lung disease. Complications of RDS are shown in Fig. 25.12.

Surfactant deficiency itself resolves spontaneously in 3–7 days as endogenous surfactant is produced. Extremely preterm, very low-birthweight infants, have lungs that are both anatomically immature as well as surfactant deficient. Also, ventilation itself can cause lung injury so ventilatory support might be required for weeks or months and chronic lung disease might ensue.

Complications of respiratory distress syndrome	
Pulmonary	Pneumothorax
	Interstitial emphysema
	Secondary infection
	Chronic lung disease
Non-pulmonary	Intraventricular haemorrhage
	Patent ductus arteriosus

Fig. 25.12 Complications of respiratory distress syndrome.

- Mechanical ventilation can cause acute lung injury in preterm ventilated babies with RDS.
- Overventilation is harmful and contributes to chronic lung disease.
- A lower oxygen saturation limit should be used to minimize ROP and to reduce mechanical ventilator requirements.

Apnoeic attacks

Many small, preterm infants display 'periodic respiration' with some spells of very shallow breathing or complete cessation of breathing for up to 20 seconds. This reflects immaturity of the respiratory centre.

Apnoeic is defined as cessation of respirations for at least 20 seconds and might be associated with bradycardia and desaturations. Predisposing factors include:

- Respiratory distress syndrome (RDS).
- Hypoxia.
- Infection.
- Cranial pathology, especially haemorrhage.

The differential diagnosis includes seizures, which can mimic apnoeic attacks.

Apnoea alarms set to respond at an appropriate interval are useful for alerting staff to the need for action. Breathing will usually start again with physical stimulation. If frequent, and in the absence of an underlying cause, they can be prevented by oral caffeine. Ventilatory support might be needed if severe.

Cardiovascular problems

Patent ductus arteriosus

A patent ductus arteriosus (PDA) is a common problem in preterm infants and is often associated with RDS. Failure of closure occurs because of gestational immaturity and hypoxia. Presentation occurs after 2–3 days.

As the pulmonary vascular resistance falls, blood is shunted across the ductus from left to right. The clinical features are a widened pulse pressure with prominent peripheral pulses, tachycardia and a systolic murmur. This shunt often causes difficulty in weaning ventilated infants. Diagnosis is by echocardiography.

Treatment

Spontaneous closure is the rule but treatment is used if the baby is ventilated or cardiac failure occurs. Fluid restriction and diuretics might be sufficient initially but a prostaglandin inhibitor, such as indomethacin or ibuprofen, could be used to facilitate closure. (The local action of prostaglandin maintains an open ductus.) Surgical closure might occasionally be required.

Intracranial lesions

Preterm infants are at risk of:

- Intracranial haemorrhage: into the germinal matrix or ventricles.
- Ischaemia: of the periventricular white matter.

Risk factors for both include pneumothorax, asphyxia, hypovolaemia, hypotension and hypoxia in association with RDS. Hydrocephalus is a late complication of intracranial haemorrhage.

Gastrointestinal problems

Necrotizing enterocolitis (NEC)

This is a necrosis of the intestine involving usually the distal ileum or proximal colon. The aetiology is uncertain but established predisposing factors include:

- Preterm birth.
- Polycythaemia.
- PDA.
- Asphyxia.
- Early rapid oral feeding with formula milk: early feeding with breast milk is protective.

Clinical features include abdominal distension, vomiting, and bloody stools. Abdominal X-rays might show intramural gas, a pathognomonic finding. Bowel perforation may occur in 20–30%.

Treatment

This comprises:

- Gastric aspiration and parenteral nutrition.
- Antibiotics: penicillin, gentamicin and metronidazole.
- In severe cases, surgical resection of the necrosed segment might be required.

Long-term sequelae and prognosis

Although the majority of preterm infants survive intact without sequelae, a number of significant problems can persist, especially in the very low-birthweight group. These include:

- Retinopathy of prematurity (retrolental fibroplasia).
- Chronic lung disease of prematurity. (bronchopulmonary dysplasia).
- Neurodevelopmental problems.

Retinopathy of prematurity

This comprises a spectrum of vascular abnormalities of the retina that occur in preterm infants in response to various injurious factors especially hyperoxia (PaO_2 >12 kPa). There is abnormal vascular proliferation, which might progress to fibrosis, retinal detachment and blindness.

All infants weighing less than 1500 g or <32 weeks' gestational age should have their eyes screened 6–8 weeks after birth by indirect ophthalmoscopy until 36 weeks corrected gestational age. Most cases resolve spontaneously but laser therapy might be indicated for severe disease.

Chronic lung disease of prematurity

Chronic lung disease of prematurity or bronchopulmonary dysplasia is defined as requiring supplemental oxygen beyond 36 weeks corrected gestation or 28 days of age, whichever is later. It occurs in newborns who, for any reason require prolonged assisted ventilation with high pressures and high concentrations of oxygen. It is particularly common in very low-birthweight infants and positive pressure ventilation causing volutrauma and barotrauma in association with an inflammatory reaction (possibly secondary to infection) is believed to be the causative factor. The CXR shows widespread opacities with patchy translucent areas.

Treatment
- Initially, there might be a continued requirement for assisted ventilation or continuous positive airways pressure and supplemental O_2.
- Dexamethasone is effective in weaning from ventilatory support but increases the risk of

neurodevelopmental impairment, so is used only in severe cases.
- Strict attention to nutrition.

Complete recovery of lung function occurs over several months but severely affected babies are at high risk of respiratory infections, which carry a high mortality.

Neurodevelopmental problems

The prospects for normal survival in preterm infants are good, especially for those weighing more than 1500 g at birth. However, very low-birthweight infants and those with a gestation period of under 28 weeks are at risk of a range of neurodevelopmental problems including:

- Cerebral palsy.
- Cognitive delay.
- Visual impairment.
- Hearing loss.
- Seizures.
- Behavioural problems.
- Educational difficulties.

Of infants born at ≤25 weeks gestational age, 23% have severe neurological disability. This improves with babies born later but all should have regular monitoring of developmental progression. Low-birthweight infants also show educational disadvantages into adulthood.

DISORDERS OF THE TERM INFANT

Respiratory disorders

Respiratory distress in term infants is characterized by:

- Tachypnoea.
- Cyanosis.
- Nasal flaring and recession.
- Expiratory grunting.

The causes are considered in Chapter 9 and are listed again in Fig. 25.13.

The pulmonary causes are considered in turn.

Transient tachypnoea of the newborn

This is caused by delay in reabsorption of fetal lung fluid and is more common after birth by caesarean

Respiratory distress in full-term infants
Pulmonary
Transient tachypnoea of the newborn
Pneumonia
Pneumothorax
Meconium aspiration
Persistent fetal circulation
Milk aspiration
Diaphragmatic hernia
Non-pulmonary
Congenital heart disease
Severe anaemia
Metabolic acidosis

Fig. 25.13 Respiratory distress in term infants.

section. There is early onset of mild to moderate respiratory distress and the CXR shows prominent pulmonary vasculature and fluid in the horizontal fissure. Treatment with increased ambient oxygen might be required. The condition usually settles spontaneously but antibiotic cover is given because infection cannot be ruled out in the early stages.

Pneumonia

Early onset, congenital pneumonia is acquired prenatally, especially when the membranes have been ruptured for more than 24 hours before the onset of labour. It is most commonly caused by the group B haemolytic streptococcus. Respiratory distress is the chief sign and the condition can mimic surfactant deficiency in preterm infants. Preterm infants with respiratory distress are therefore given antibiotics.

Chlamydia should be suspected if there is concurrent purulent conjunctivitis.

Treatment
This comprises:

- Physiotherapy to prevent local accumulation of secretions.
- Respiratory support with oxygen and ventilation if severe.
- Careful fluid balance and nutrition.
- Intravenous antibiotics.

Pneumothorax

A pneumothorax can occur spontaneously but is most commonly seen as a complication of positive pressure ventilation. Tension pneumothorax results in partial collapse of the lung with a sudden deterio-ration in the infant's condition manifested by cyanosis and hypotension. Diagnosis is confirmed by transillumination with a fibre-optic cold light source, or CXR. Urgent treatment by insertion of a chest drain is indicated.

Chylothorax

This refers to the accumulation of lymphatic fluid in the pleural cavity and is usually iatrogenic, following surgery or birth trauma. Rarely, it may be due to a congenital abnormality of the lymphatic system or associated with various syndromes, e.g. trisomy 21. But most often, it is idiopathic and a cause is never found. It needs drainage using a percutaneous chest drain and often resolves subsequently. Dietary elimination of long chain fatty acids may hasten resolution.

Meconium aspiration

Passage of meconium into the amniotic fluid is triggered by fetal distress in term or post-term infants. The infant is at risk of inhaling meconium and developing meconium aspiration syndrome. This severe condition causes respiratory distress and cyanosis and has a high mortality rate. It can be ameliorated by suctioning thick meconium from the upper airway as soon as the head is delivered and by suctioning any meconium from the trachea under direct vision after delivery. However, most severe cases are probably due to antenatal aspiration in utero and cannot be prevented by suction at delivery.

Persistent fetal circulation

This condition is characterized by high pulmonary vascular resistance and is usually found in term or post-term infants. There is right-to-left shunting of blood at atrial and ductal levels with severe cyanosis. Persistent fetal circulation may be primary or secondary to birth asphyxia, meconium aspiration, or respiratory distress syndrome.

A CXR shows a normal cardiac shadow and pulmonary oligaemia and an echocardiogram might be necessary to exclude cyanotic congenital heart disease.

Treatment
This includes:

- Assisted ventilation.
- Inhaled nitric oxide for pulmonary vasodilatation.

- Extracorporeal membrane oxygenation for severe cases.

Milk aspiration

Aspiration of milk or stomach contents into the lungs may occur especially in:

- Preterm infants with RDS or neurological problems.
- Infants with chronic lung disease of prematurity.
- Infants with cleft palate.
- Infants with tracheo-oesophageal fistula.

Diaphragmatic hernia

See Chapter 9. This congenital malformation:

- Occurs in 1 in 4000 live births.
- Is usually left-sided.
- Can be diagnosed on antenatal ultrasound.
- Is repaired surgically.
- Has a high mortality due to coexisting pulmonary hypoplasia.

Gastrointestinal and hepatic disorders

Congenital anomalies of the gastrointestinal tract including cleft lip and palate, tracheo-oesophageal fistula, duodenal stenosis or atresia, and exomphalos or gastroschisis are considered in Chapter 9.

Small bowel obstruction

This presents with:

- Persistent, bile-stained vomiting.
- Delayed or absent passage of meconium.
- Abdominal distension.

Important causes are listed in Fig. 25.14.

Causes of small bowel obstruction
Duodenal atresia
Midgut volvulus and malrotation
Gastroschisis and exomphalos
Meconium ileus

Fig. 25.14 Causes of small bowel obstruction.

Diagnosis is made on clinical features and abdominal X-ray. Treatment depends on the cause and is often surgical. In the presence of meconium ileus it is important to exclude cystic fibrosis. Administering gastrograffin contrast medium might relieve meconium ileus.

Large bowel obstruction

Hirschsprung's disease or rectal atresia can cause this.

Hirschsprung's disease

Congenital aganglionic megacolon, or Hirschsprung's disease, is a genetic disorder in which there is absence of ganglion cells from the myenteric and submyenteric plexuses of a segment of the large bowel (see Chapter 15).

Clinical features
Presentation is usually in the neonatal period with failure to pass meconium in the first 24 hours followed by abdominal distension and bile-stained vomiting. Diarrhoea might occur and alternate with periods of constipation. A major complication is enterocolitis.

Diagnosis
An unprepped barium enema can suggest the diagnosis but definitive diagnosis requires demonstration of the absence of ganglion cells on a suction rectal biopsy.

Management
Treatment is surgical. A preliminary colostomy is usually performed in the neonatal period followed later by an operation to anastomose normally innervated bowel to anus.

Jaundice

Clinical jaundice appears in newborns when the serum bilirubin exceeds 80–120 μmol/L. The causes are considered in Chapter 9.

Jaundice is important because it might be indicative of underlying problems such as infection and because unconjugated bilirubin can be deposited in the brain and cause bilirubin encephalopathy (previously called 'kernicterus'). Causative conditions are most usefully considered by age of onset of the jaundice.

- Physiological jaundice is the most common cause of jaundice in the newborn. It is associated with unconjugated hyperbilirubinaemia.
- Conjugated hyperbilirubinaemia, in excess of 15% of total serum bilirubin, suggests cholestasis due to hepatobiliary disease.

Jaundice in the first 24 hours

This is always pathological. The most common cause is haemolysis, which can be due to:

- Haemolytic disease of the newborn: Rhesus or ABO incompatibility.
- Intrinsic red cell defects: spherocytosis, G6PD deficiency or pyruvate kinase deficiency.

Congenital infections can also cause early-onset jaundice.

Haemolytic disorders Isoimmune haemolysis is caused by the destruction of fetal and neonatal red blood cells by maternal IgG antibodies that cross the placenta during pregnancy. Maternal sensitization is caused by fetal–maternal transfusion during current or previous pregnancies, or from mismatched blood transfusions.

The incidence of Rhesus (Rh) haemolytic disease has fallen since the introduction of anti-D immune globulin, which is given to the Rh-negative mother immediately after birth of a Rh-positive infant. Affected infants are usually diagnosed antenatally and given fetal therapy as necessary. Severe haemolysis causes anaemia and hydrops fetalis, which is treated by intrauterine blood transfusion.

ABO incompatibility is more common than Rh haemolytic disease. The usual combination is a group O mother with a group A, or less commonly group B infant. The anti-A or anti-B haemolysins are comparatively weak. There is mild anaemia, no organomegaly, a weakly positive Coombs' test and mild jaundice peaking in the first few days.

G6PD deficiency and congenital spherocytosis can cause neonatal jaundice.

Jaundice at 2 days to 2 weeks of age

The most common cause is physiological jaundice, due to the combination of liver enzyme immaturity and an increased load of bilirubin from red cell breakdown. Prematurity, bruising or polycythaemia (haematocrit >0.65) can exacerbate it. Physiological jaundice usually peaks on the third day of life.

Infection, particularly of the urinary tract, also causes unconjugated hyperbilirubinaemia at this time.

Jaundice at more than 2 weeks of age

Persistent (prolonged, protracted) jaundice is usually an unconjugated hyperbilirubinaemia, which can be due to:

- 'Breast milk' jaundice: affects 15% of healthy breastfed infants. The cause is unknown. It usually resolves by 3–4 weeks of age.
- Infection: particularly of urinary tract.
- Congenital hypothyroidism: this should have been detected on neonatal screening.

Prolonged conjugated hyperbilirubinaemia is usually associated with dark urine and pale stools. Causes include neonatal hepatitis syndrome and biliary atresia. Early diagnosis of biliary atresia is important because delay in surgical treatment beyond 6 weeks of age compromises outcome.

Management of neonatal jaundice

Investigations are directed towards establishing the cause (see Chapter 9). Clinical estimation of the severity is unreliable and a plasma bilirubin must be measured in any significantly jaundiced infant. The main concern is to prevent bilirubin encephalopathy.

Bilirubin encephalopathy occurs when unconjugated bilirubin is deposited in the brain, especially in the basal ganglia and cerebellum. This presents initially with lethargy, rigidity, eye-rolling and seizures. The long-term sequelae include choreoathetoid cerebral palsy, sensorineural deafness and learning difficulties.

Many factors in addition to the bilirubin level influence this risk. These include:

- The infant's gestational age: risk increases for preterm infants.
- The postnatal age: risk decreases with increasing postnatal age.
- The serum albumin level: risk increases with hypoalbuminaemia.
- Coexistent asphyxia, acidosis or hypoglycaemia.

Charts exist indicating levels at which treatment should be initiated, bearing those factors in mind.

Treatment options are:

- Phototherapy.
- Exchange transfusion.

Phototherapy   Blue light (not ultraviolet) of wavelength 450 nm converts the bilirubin in the skin and superficial capillaries into harmless water-soluble metabolites, which are excreted in urine and through the bowel. The eyes are covered to prevent discomfort and additional fluids are given to counteract increased losses from skin.

Exchange transfusion   This is required if the bilirubin rises to levels considered dangerous despite phototherapy. It rapidly reduces the level of circulating bilirubin, and in isoimmune haemolytic disease also removes circulating antibodies and corrects anaemia. Techniques vary, but conventionally the exchange is done via umbilical artery and vein catheters. Aliquots of baby's blood (10–20 mL) are withdrawn, alternating with infusions of donor blood of the same volumes. Twice the infant's blood volume (i.e. 2×80 mL/kg) is exchanged over about 2 hours.

Haematological disorders

Haemolytic diseases of the newborn are considered with jaundice.

Haemorrhagic disease of the newborn

This is caused by a relative deficiency of the vitamin-K-dependent coagulation factors II, VII, IX and X. It characteristically affects the fully breastfed infant between the third and sixth day of life, because breastmilk does not contain adequate amounts of vitamin K. Mothers taking anticonvulsant drugs that interfere with vitamin K metabolism, such as phenytoin, are at increased risk.

Bleeding usually occurs from the gastrointestinal tract but can rarely be intracranial or from the umbilical stump.

A single intramuscular dose of vitamin K prevents this disease but three doses of oral vitamin K can also be given. It is important that all three doses are administered.

Infections

The newborn infant is vulnerable to infection by bacteria, viruses and fungi. In utero, infection can take place across the placenta or by ascending the birth canal.

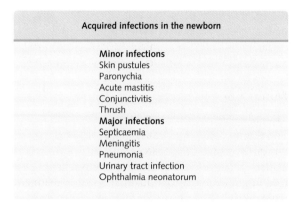

Acquired infections in the newborn

Minor infections
Skin pustules
Paronychia
Acute mastitis
Conjunctivitis
Thrush
Major infections
Septicaemia
Meningitis
Pneumonia
Urinary tract infection
Ophthalmia neonatorum

Fig. 25.15 Acquired infections in the newborn.

After birth, the skin and umbilicus are colonised by staphylococci, the gut by *Escherichia coli* and the upper respiratory tract by streptococci. Important bacterial pathogens in the neonate include:

- Group B β-haemolytic streptococci.
- *Escherichia coli*.
- *Staphylococcus epidermidis*: found in preterm babies on intensive care.

The range of acquired infections in the newborn is shown in Fig. 25.15.

Neonatal abstinence syndrome

This refers to the cluster of withdrawal symptoms that develop in babies born to substance abusing mothers. This includes both unsupervised recreational drug abuse, e.g. heroin or supervised use of methadone from a drug dependency unit.

Clinical features

This includes yawning, sweating, jitteriness and pyrexia. More severe symptoms include seizures or tremors, high pitched or inconsolable cry, projectile vomiting and watery diarrhoea.

Diagnosis

This is mainly clinical based on history and examination. This can be confirmed by a urine toxicology screen. These babies are also at high risk of other diseases like hepatitis B, hepatitis C and HIV—so the mother's serology should be checked.

Management

The symptoms are scored using various scoring systems and if high, treatment is initiated with oral morphine and gradually weaned over the next few days to weeks. It is also important to deal with the social issues and communicate with the community team, health visitor or social services as needed.

Minor infections

Skin pustules and paronychia

These are caused by staphylococcal infection and typically occur in moist areas such as the groin and axillae. Inflammation of the skin in the area of a nail fold might evolve into a pustular lesion. Treatment with oral flucloxacillin is indicated in severe cases but most resolve spontaneously.

Acute mastitis

This is an inflamed swelling under the nipple in a febrile infant. It is usually caused by *Staphylococcus aureus* infection in an engorged neonatal breast. Flucloxacillin is the antibiotic of choice.

Conjunctivitis

A 'sticky eye' in the first day or two of life is often due to chemical irritation and clears spontaneously. Conjunctivitis with a purulent discharge might be due to:

- Staphylococci, streptococci, *Escherichia coli.*
- Gonococci: ophthalmia neonatorum (see below)—usually between days 2 and 5 of life.
- *Chlamydia trachomatis*: usually between days 7 and 10 of life.

Gonococcal and chlamydial infections need systemic antibiotic treatment because the risk of scarring and blindness is high. Erythromycin or a cephalosporin is used and ophthalmological review is mandatory. It is also important to treat the parents.

Thrush (moniliasis)

Infection with *Candida albicans* can affect the mouth or nappy area. Oral thrush appears as white plaques on the tongue and inside of the mouth. Nystatin suspension 1 mL (100 000 units) after feeds for 7–10 days is usually effective. Perineal thrush responds to topical nystatin.

Major infections

Septicaemia

Neonatal sepsis carries a high mortality and morbidity and can be rapid and fulminant. As signs are non-specific (Fig. 25.16), a low threshold for inves-

---

Signs suggestive of neonatal infection

Irritability or lethargy
Persistent tachycardia
Tachypnoea or grunting
Frequent apnoeas or bradycardias and desaturations
Poor response to handling
Acute onset of pallor
Temperature instability
Feeding intolerance

Fig. 25.16 Signs suggestive of neonatal infection.

---

tigation and empirical treatment with antibiotics is needed. As this results in a high number of treated infants, to reduce unnecessary antibiotic usage antibiotics should be stopped if cultures are negative in 48 hours. Unlike adults, the incidence of false-negative blood cultures is less in neonates.

The incidence of serious acute infections in the newborn period is about 3 per 1000 live births in the UK.

Initial presentation is often non-specific with:

- Lethargy and drowsiness or excessive irritability.
- Poor feeding, vomiting.
- Temperature and cardiovascular instability.
- Pallor.
- Acidosis or glucose instability.

Specific signs relating to a site of infection may then emerge. These include:

- Tense fontanelle, seizures: meningitis.
- Respiratory distress: pneumonia.

Group B streptococcal infection

Genital tract colonization with this organism is found in 20–30% of all women and infection carries a high mortality and morbidity. It presents in two ways: early (within the first week) or late (after the first week). Early disease is associated with a worse outcome but can be reduced with preventive measures.

Diagnosis   If systemic infection is suspected, prompt investigation is essential. The following investigations are performed to confirm the diagnosis and identify a causative organism.

- 'Septic' screen: blood culture, urine culture, lumbar puncture, and cerebrospinal fluid culture. Swabs from the throat, nose, and ear.
- Rapid antigen testing on blood and cerebrospinal fluid (CSF).
- Gram stain of CSF.

Treatment Group B streptococcal (GBS) infection is usually sensitive to penicillin and aminoglycosides are added for additional synergistic effects. Cephalosporins can be also used for their high CSF penetration but they are associated with secondary coliform infections.

Meningitis

Neonatal meningitis is usually due to a different range of pathogens from that in the older infant or child. In infants, the infective organisms include:

- *Escherichia coli.*
- Group B streptococci.
- *Listeria monocytogenes.*

Meningeal infection usually follows a septicaemic stage. Clinical features include poor feeding, pallor and temperature instability. Fullness of the anterior fontanelle and fits are late signs.

Diagnosis Lumbar puncture is required to confirm the diagnosis.

Treatment and outcome High-dose intravenous antibiotics for 14–21 days are required. Penetration of drugs occur through the inflamed meninges. Mortality is 30–60% and a high incidence of neurological impairment occurs in survivors.

Pneumonia

This is most commonly due to the group B streptococcus. Respiratory distress is the chief presenting sign together with features of septicaemia.

Urinary tract infection

The most common pathogen is *Escherichia coli*, although other Gram-negative organisms are occasionally responsible. There is a relatively high incidence of underlying congenital anomalies or vesicoureteric reflux.

Symptoms and signs are usually non-specific. Urine must be cultured in all infants with poor feeding, lethargy, vomiting, failure to thrive and jaundice.

The optimal way of obtaining a specimen is a suprapubic aspirate. Any growth is diagnostic of a UTI.

IV antibiotics are used for treatment and imaging of the renal tract to look for structural abnormalities once the infant has recovered.

Further reading

Gomella TG. Neonatology: management, procedures, on-call problems. In *Diseases and Drugs,* 4th edn. Philadelphia, Appleton Lange, 1999.

Hack M et al. Outcomes in young adulthood for low birthweight infants. *New England Journal of Medicine* 2002; **346**:149–157.

MacLennan A. A template for defining a causal relation between acute intrapartum events and cerebral palsy: international consensus statement. *British Medical Journal* 1999; **319**:1054–1059.

Wood NS et al. for the EPICure study group. Neurological and developmental disability after extremely preterm birth. *New England Journal of Medicine* 2000; **343**:378–384.

Accidents and emergencies

Objectives

At the end of this chapter, you should be able to

- Know the common causes of trauma in children.
- Assess the seriously ill child.
- Learn the guidelines for basic paediatric life support.
- Know the management of common paediatric emergencies.

ACCIDENTS

Accidents in children are extremely common and are the leading cause of death between the ages of 1 and 14 years. The pattern of accidents varies with age (Fig. 26.1). Road traffic accidents account for the majority of fatal accidents (Fig. 26.2). Child abuse needs to be considered in any child presenting with injury.

Trauma

Physical trauma causing multiple serious injuries is an important cause of death. Early, appropriate management of the multiply injured child is vital to reduce mortality and long-term morbidity. Injuries to the head are the most important class of local injury.

Major trauma

Initial assessment and management is described in Fig. 26.3. Events during the first 'golden hour' determine the outcome. Once the initial steps of immediate resuscitation have been carried out, a careful secondary survey of the complete child must be undertaken to detect and treat all injuries (Fig. 26.4).

Head injury

Minor head injuries in children are very common and most children recover without ill effect. A small minority, about 1 in 800 of those admitted, develops serious complications such as intracranial haemorrhage. Causes of head injury include:

- Road traffic accidents (RTAs): the most common cause of severe and fatal head injuries.
- Falls from trees, walls, bicycles, etc.
- Child abuse: especially 'shaking' injuries in infants.

Damage to the brain might be primary or secondary (Fig. 26.5).

The history should establish:

- The mechanism of injury.
- Was consciousness lost?
- Subsequent symptoms: vomiting, drowsiness, seizures, bleeding from nose or ears.
- Anterograde amnesia >30 minutes.

Clinical features

Clinical examination should look for the following signs:

- Head: external injury including haematoma, laceration, depressed fracture. In babies, the anterior fontanelle tension provides a useful indicator of intracranial pressure, as does the head circumference. Look for blood or cerebrospinal fluid leak from the ears or nose.
- Central nervous system: assess Glasgow coma scale/AVPU scale, fundi and pupillary reflexes. Examine for focal neurological signs.
- General: full examination to exclude other injuries.

Diagnosis

Investigations include:

- Skull X-ray: now not routinely indicated, useful only if non-accidental injury is suspected.

Accidents in childhood
Toddlers are prone to: Falls Scalds Drowning Accidental ingestion Choking **School-age children are prone to:** Falls while climbing Road traffic accidents

Fig. 26.1 Accidents in childhood.

Causes of fatal accidents	
Age range	**Leading cause of death (highest at top)**
4-52 weeks	Congenital abnormalities Cot death Infection
1-4 years	Trauma Congenital abnormalities Cancer Infection
5-14 years	Trauma Cancer Congenital abnormality Infection

Fig. 26.2 Causes of fatal accidents.

Fig. 26.3 Major trauma. Initial assessment and management—A, B, C, D and E

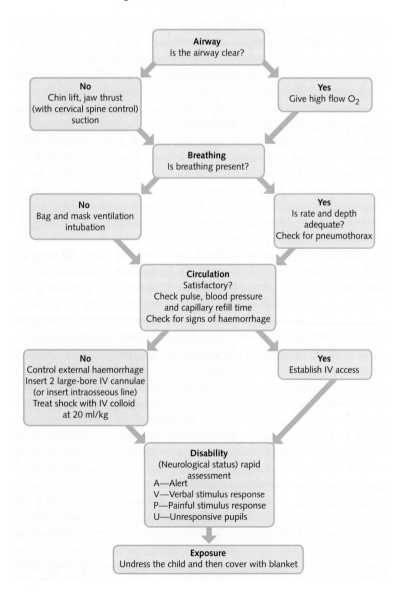

Secondary survey and treatment—multiple trauma	
Head	Examine for bruising, lacerations, CSF leak from ears or nose. Mini neurological exam
Face	Look for bruising, fractures and loose teeth
Neck	Cervical spine stabilization. Examine for bony tenderness, bruising or wounds.
Chest	Look for wounds, bruising. Feel trachea and auscultate breath and heart sounds
Abdomen	Observe movement, bruising and palpate for tenderness. PR not routinely indicated in children.
Pelvis	Inspect perineum and for bony deformity. Look for blood at urethral meatus
Spine	Done by log-rolling: look for swelling, palpate vertebrae and assess motor and sensory function
Extremities	Assess movement, deformity, bruising and tenderness. Test sensation and peripheral circulation
Radiological investigations as necessary and a full history	

Fig. 26.4 Secondary survey and treatment—multiple trauma.

Brain damage in head injury	
Primary damage	Cerebral laceration and contusion Diffuse axonal injury Dural sac tears
Secondary damage	Ischaemia from shock, hypoxia or raised intracranial pressure Hypoglycaemia CNS infection Seizures Hyperthermia

Fig. 26.5 Brain damage in head injury.

- Cranial computed tomography (CT): if fracture suspected clinically (CSF otorrhoea, rhinorrhoea, Panda eyes, etc.), decreased conscious level, seizures, excessive vomiting, amnesia, focal neurological signs or high impact injury or laceration/bruising/haematoma more than 5 cm in a child under 1 year (NICE Guidelines 2007; www.nice.org.uk).

Minor and moderate injuries
These are the majority. Admit to hospital for observation if:

- History of seizure or loss of consciousness.
- Declining level of consciousness.
- Severe headache or persistent vomiting.

- Skull fracture.
- Suspected non-accidental injury.
- Child has a bleeding tendency.
- Supervision at home is inadequate.

If the child is not admitted, the parents should be given written instructions to bring the child back if there is severe headache, recurrent vomiting or a declining level of consciousness.

If admitted, neurological observations should be made at intervals dictated by the child's clinical state and existing guidelines.

Severe injuries
These usually occur in the context of multiple major trauma requiring intensive care.

Additional measures in severe head injury are directed towards the management of complications such as raised intracranial pressure, intracranial bleeding, seizures and risk of infection.

Urgent referral to a neurosurgeon is indicated if there is any evidence of an expanding haematoma, such as:

- Declining level of consciousness.
- Focal neurological signs.
- Depressed skull fracture.
- Signs of rising intracranial pressure: bradycardia, rise in systolic blood pressure and irregular respirations.

Fig. 26.6 Assessment of the depth of burn.

Assessment of the depth of burn		
Superficial	**Partial thickness**	**Full thickness**
• Red	• Pink or mottled	• Painless
• No blisters	• Blisters	• White or charred
• Affects only epithelial layer	• Some dermal damage	• Full dermal and nerve damage

Burns and scalds

Scalds from contact with hot liquids are the most common form of thermal trauma in childhood (most of the fatalities are from house fires but those are due to gas and smoke inhalation rather than burns). Burns and scalds can be non-accidental. Toddlers are most at risk of accidental scalds.

- Electrical burns are usually full thickness.
- Most scalds are deep, partial thickness.

Assessment

The extent, depth and distribution of the injury should be estimated (Figs 26.6 and 26.7 and see Hints & Tips).

Diagnosis

Investigations should include:

- Full blood count: packed cell volume is increased with significant hypovolaemia.
- Urea and electrolytes.
- Group and save (if burns are greater than 15–20%).
- Serum albumin.

Location of the burn is important, as well as extent:
- Face—potential airway involvement, scarring.
- Hands—contractures and functional loss.
- Genitalia—difficult to nurse, risk of infection.

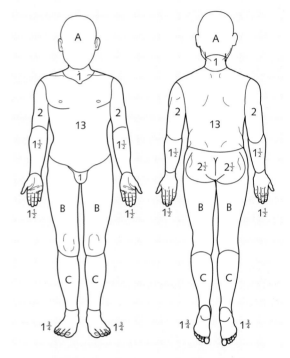

Area indicated	Surface area at			
	1 year	5 years	10 years	15 years
A	8.5	6.5	5.5	4.5
B	3.25	4.0	4.5	4.5
C	2.5	2.75	3.0	3.25

Fig. 26.7 Assessment of the extent of a burn. The percentage body surface area affected is calculated from this standard body diagram. Note that the area corresponding to head and lower limbs (A, B, C) changes with age. The small child has a relatively big head and short legs.

Management

Recommended first aid is:

- Run cold water over the affected part for 5 minutes.
- Cover the burn with a clean dressing.

Management of burns	
Analgesia	IV morphine for major burns
IV fluids	Treat shock with 20 mL/kg If >10% burn will need IV fluids: Normal fluid requirements with additional fluids at: % burn×weight (kg) ×4 per day (Half of this given within 8 h) Keep urine output >1 mL/kg/h
Wound care	Sterile towels and avoid excessive re-examination

Fig. 26.8 Management of burns.

Prognostic indicators for near drowning	
Prognostic indicators	Poor if:
Immersion time	Submerged for >8 minutes
Time to first gasp	No gasp after 40 minutes resuscitation
Rectal temperature	<33°C on arrival
Conscious level	Persisting coma
Arterial blood pH	<7.0 despite treatment
Arterial blood O2	<8.0 kPa despite treatment
Type of water	No difference on prognosis

Fig. 26.9 Prognostic indicators for near drowning.

Admit to burns centre if:

- The extent is over 5% full thickness or over 10% partial thickness.
- A difficult area is involved, e.g. face, hands and feet, perineum or genitalia.
- There is any inhalational injury, e.g. smoke inhalation.

The important aspects of management are shown in Fig. 26.8.

Near drowning

Drowning is more common in boys than girls. It is the third most common cause of childhood accidental death in the UK. In the UK, drowning incidents are more common in freshwater canals and lakes, swimming pools and domestic baths than in the sea.

The two principal problems in near drowning are:

- Hypoxia: laryngospasm results in asphyxia. Only a small amount of water initially enters the lungs.
- Hypothermia: this leads to bradycardia and asystole (extreme hypothermia can be protective).

Haemolysis or electrolyte problems caused by the ingestion or inhalation of large amounts of water are unusual.

Management

Skilled resuscitation and warming is vital. Cervical injury should be assumed. All children should be hospitalized for at least 24 hours. Patients admitted in asystole or respiratory arrest should undergo cardiopulmonary resuscitation in the normal way. Resuscitation must be continued until the core temperature has been raised to above 32°C because many arrythmias are refractory at temperatures below 30°C.

Prognostic indicators of near drowning

The prognostic indicators are shown in Fig. 26.9.

Late respiratory sequelae can occur in the 72-hour period after near drowning. These include pneumonia and pulmonary oedema.

Poisoning

Most cases of poisoning in young children follow accidental ingestion by an inquisitive, fearless toddler; in adolescents most poisoning is deliberate self-harm. Children can also be poisoned deliberately by their parents (or inadvertently by their doctors). Although many thousands of children attend hospital each year, very few die as a result of accidental ingestion.

The history should establish:

- What was ingested: identify from carton or bottle.
- Amount ingested: usually an approximation.
- Time ingested: important in relation to management.

The toxicity of the ingested substance can then be assessed (Fig. 26.10) or the Regional Poisons Information Centre contacted if there is any doubt concerning the agent's identity or toxicity.

Clinical features

Examination should include the following:

- Inspect oropharynx and any vomitus.
- Assess level of consciousness.
- Look for features specific to various poisons, e.g. small pupils (opiates or barbiturates), tachypnoea (salicylate poisoning) or cardiac arrhythmias (tricyclic antidepressants or digoxin).

Diagnosis

Relevant investigations include:

- Blood levels (at optimum time after ingestion) can be measured for salicylates, paracetamol, digoxin, iron, lithium and tricyclic antidepressants.
- Keep specimens of vomitus and urine for analysis.

Management

If the agent ingested was relatively innocuous the patient can be allowed home or observed briefly in hospital. Efforts should be made to remove the poison if there has been a large ingestion of a highly toxic substance. These include:

- Activated charcoal: give 1 g/kg, if necessary by nasogastric tube. It binds a wide range of toxic drugs, with the exception of iron and lithium. It is most efficacious if used within 1 hour of ingestion.

Specific treatment is indicated for certain drugs and toxins (see Fig. 26.10).

Deliberate self-poisoning in older children

This is a serious occurrence that can reflect a significant underlying psychiatric disorder such as depression. In most cases, there is no serious suicidal intent. Drug or alcohol intoxication is often a predisposing element. All children who deliberately poison themselves should be admitted to hospital and assessed by a child and adolescent psychiatrist.

EMERGENCIES

Children differ from adults in important ways that are relevant to emergency care (Fig. 26.11).

The seriously ill child

A seriously ill child is on one of the pathways leading to cardiopulmonary arrest (Fig. 26.12). Such arrests in children are rarely unheralded but preceded by a period of progressive circulatory, respiratory or central neurological failure. It is vital to recognize such a critically ill child and intervene to prevent the progression to cardiac arrest.

Rapid assessment

An initial ABCD assessment should be carried out to identify features of:

- Airway and breathing: airway obstruction and hypoxia.
- Circulation: shock.
- Disability: central neurological failure.

Fig. 26.10 Poison-specific adverse effects and treatments.

Poison-specific adverse effects and treatments		
Poison	Adverse effects	Specific treatment
Iron	Shock, gut haemorrhage	IV desferrioxamine
Paracetamol	Liver failure	IV N-acetylcysteine
Salicylates	Metabolic acidosis	Alkalinization of urine with bicarbonate
Ethylene glycol Tricyclic antidepressants	Widespread cellular damage Cardiac dysrhythmias	Ethanol, dialysis if severe Alkalinization of urine with bicarbonate
Ecstasy	Hyperpyrexia and rhabdomyolysis Dysrhythmias	Active cooling

Anatomical and physiological characteristics of young children	
Anatomy	Airway (see Chapter 2) Large surface area to volume ratio Small airways and elastic ribs Obligate nasal breathers until 5 months old
Physiology	Increased oxygen consumption and metabolic rate Compliant chest wall: leading to airways collapse Inefficient respiratory muscles Low stroke volume: cardiac output dependent on heart rate

Fig. 26.11 Anatomical and physiological characteristics of young children.

Respiratory assessment	
Effort of breathing	Respiratory rate Inspiratory or expiratory noises Grunting Use of accessory muscles Nasal flaring
Efficacy of air entry	Presence of breath sounds Pulse oximetry
Adequacy of oxygenation	Heart rate Skin colour Mental status

Fig. 26.13 Respiratory assessment.

Fig. 26.12 The critically ill child: pathways to cardiopulmonary arrest.

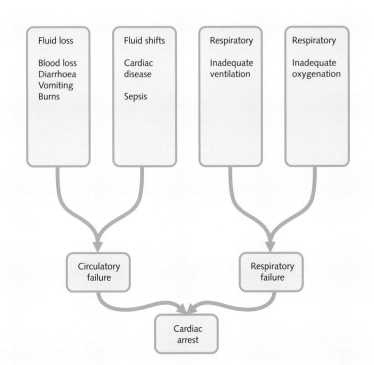

Airway and breathing

A critical state is indicated either by:

- An increase in the work of breathing (respiratory distress).
- Absent or decreased respiratory effort (exhaustion or respiratory depression).

Key signs include (Fig. 26.13):

- Efficacy of breathing.
- Effort of breathing.
- Signs of inadequate respiration.

Circulation

Signs of potential circulatory failure (shock) include:

- Tachycardia.
- Pulse volume reduction: absent peripheral pulses and weak central pulses are serious signs of advanced shock.
- Capillary refill time of over 2 seconds.
- Blood pressure: hypotension is a late and preterminal sign of circulatory failure.

The effects of circulatory failure encompass:

- Metabolic acidosis with increased respiratory rate.
- Skin: mottled, cold, pale skin peripherally.
- Mental state: agitation followed by drowsiness due to reduced cerebral perfusion.
- Urine output: oliguria due to renal hypoperfusion.

Always go back to assessing airway, breathing and circulation (ABC) if the child's condition changes.

Disability

Signs of potential central neurological failure are:

- Level of consciousness: reduced (see Hints & Tips).
- Posture: most are hypotonic; seizures reflect brain dysfunction.
- Pupils: most sinister signs are dilatation, unreactivity and inequality.

Central neurological failure has important effects on both respiration and circulation:

- Respiratory depression.
- Abnormal respiratory patterns.
- Systemic hypertension with sinus bradycardia (Cushing's response) indicates herniation of the cerebellar tonsils through the foramen magnum.

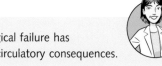

Central neurological failure has respiratory and circulatory consequences.

Cardiorespiratory arrest

A standard procedure exists for applying basic life support in the event of a cardiorespiratory arrest (Figs 26.14–26.19).

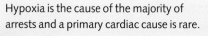

Hypoxia is the cause of the majority of arrests and a primary cardiac cause is rare.

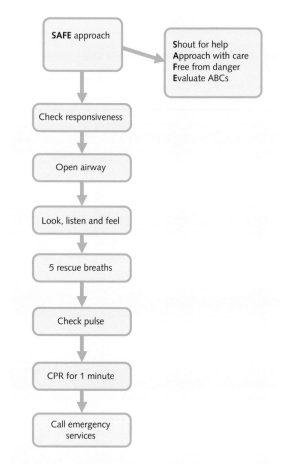

SAFE approach

Shout for help
Approach with care
Free from danger
Evaluate ABCs

Check responsiveness

Open airway

Look, listen and feel

5 rescue breaths

Check pulse

CPR for 1 minute

Call emergency services

Fig. 26.14 Basic life support.

After basic life support procedures, it might be necessary to proceed to:

- Intubation and ventilation.
- Circulatory access: venous or intraosseous.
- ECG monitoring: to identify the rhythm, asystole is most common. The protocol for drug use in asystole is shown in Fig. 26.16.

Asystole is the most common arrest rhythm in children.

Neurological emergencies

Coma

There are many causes of a reduced conscious level. Evaluation is done by the Glasgow coma scale or

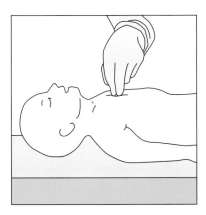

A Infant chest compression: Two finger technique

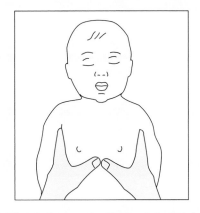

B Infant chest compression: Hand-encircling technique

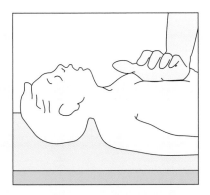

C Chest compression in small children

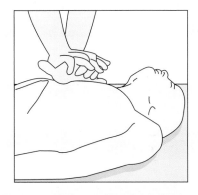

D Chest compression in older children

Fig. 26.15 Cardiac compression techniques.

AVPU (see Chapter 5). Some are self-evident but others might be identified only after careful clinical evaluation and special investigations.

Assessment

A rapid history should include information about:

- Chronic medical conditions such as epilepsy and diabetes mellitus.
- Any recent injury.
- Access to poisons including drugs.
- Normal neurological state.

Clinical examination should pay attention to:

- Airway, breathing and circulation.
- Fever or rash: especially a purpuric rash.
- Signs of injury.

- CNS: Glasgow coma score (see Fig. 5.5) or AVPU, signs of meningism (neck stiffness), focal neurological signs and posture, pupil size and reaction to light, fundi-papilloedema or haemorrhages.

Diagnosis

Investigations are determined by the clinical evaluation and may include:

- Blood analysis for glucose, electrolytes.
- Urine for toxins.
- Lumbar puncture for suspected meningitis.
- Brain imaging: cranial CT or magnetic resonance imaging.
- EEG for seizures, metabolic encephalopathy.

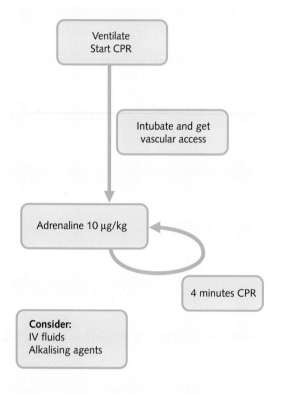

Fig. 26.16 Protocol for drug use in asystole.

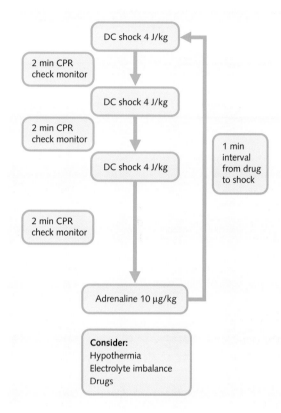

Fig. 26.17 Protocol for ventricular fibrillation.

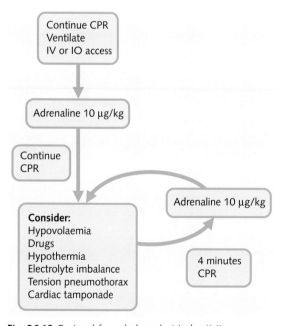

Fig. 26.18 Protocol for pulseless electrical activity.

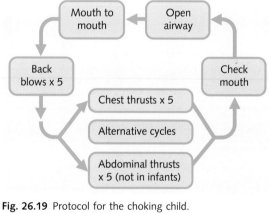

Fig. 26.19 Protocol for the choking child.

Check blood sugar in a comatose or convulsing child to identify treatable hypoglycaemia.

Hypoglycaemia is an important cause of both coma and seizures in children. Recognition and treatment is simple. If missed, brain damage can result.

Management

Initial management should be directed towards maintaining airway, breathing and circulation. Further specific treatment depends on aetiology. All children with a GCS <8 or P on the AVPU scale need airway protection with endotracheal intubation.

Secondary brain damage is minimized by maintaining oxygenation and perfusion.

Convulsions

The causes of a convulsion vary with age (Fig. 26.20). The most common cause in young children is a 'febrile convulsion' (see Chapter 17).

A continuous convulsion lasting more than 30 minutes, or repeated convulsions without recovery of consciousness between attacks, is called 'convulsive status epilepticus' (CSE).

Prolonged convulsions can result in brain damage or death from hypoxia. Cerebral blood flow and oxygen consumption increase five-fold to meet the extra metabolic demand. Oxygen delivery to the brain will be impaired if there is inadequate ventilation or hypotension.

Management

An algorithm for management of the convulsing child is shown in Fig. 26.21.

While initiating emergency management, establish the history and examine the child:

History
- Duration of convulsion.
- History of recent trauma.
- Known epileptic? If so, medication regime.
- Known diabetic?
- Preceding illness.

Examination
- Cardiorespiratory status.
- Signs of head trauma.
- Fever, petechial rash, meningism.
- Nature of convulsion: generalized or focal.

If lorazepam fails to stop the seizure, further options include, in order:

Causes of convulsions	
Age	**Causes**
All ages	Hypoglycaemia Head injury Poisoning Meningitis Epilepsy
Birth to 6 months	Hypoglycaemia Hypocalcaemia Inborn errors of metabolism Meningitis
6 months to 5 years	Febrile convulsion Meningitis
>5 years	Epilepsy (most common cause)

Fig. 26.20 Causes of convulsions.

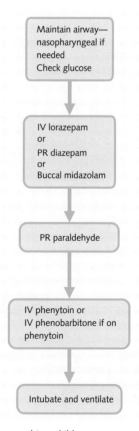

Fig. 26.21 The convulsing child.

1. Paraldehyde: rectal administration as 10% solution 1 mL/year of age. Safe and usually effective within 5 minutes.
2. Summon senior anaesthetic help.
3. IV phenytoin: give as an infusion under ECG and blood pressure monitoring.

Status epilepticus (convulsive)

Protracted convulsions (of over 30 minutes) can occur in:

- Epilepsy.
- Febrile convulsion.
- Head injury.
- Intracranial infection: meningitis or encephalitis.
- Metabolic seizures: hypoglycaemia or poisoning.

Lorazepam, paraldehyde and phenytoin are used in order, as in Fig. 26.21. If convulsions persist, the child should be paralysed, ventilated and managed on an intensive care unit where a thiopentone or benzodiazepine infusion can be safely instituted.

Cardiac emergencies

Cardiac emergencies in children occur more commonly than previously thought, although hypoxia still predominates as a cause of cardiorespiratory arrest. The causes and management of heart failure are considered elsewhere (see Chapter 2), as is the management of circulatory failure (shock) and cardiac arrest. Cardiac arrhythmias, uncommon but treatable conditions in childhood, are considered in Chapter 13.

Respiratory emergencies

The pattern of severe respiratory illness in children is determined by features of the anatomy and physiology of their respiratory system, including:

- Small airways: easily obstructed with rapid increase in airways resistance.
- Compliant thoracic cage: reduced breathing efficiency.
- Inefficient respiratory muscles: rapid development of fatigue.
- Susceptibility to infection.

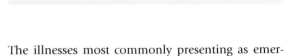

Not all respiratory distress has a respiratory cause:
- Metabolic acidosis causes deep, rapid breathing
- Heart failure is associated with tachypnoea.

The illnesses most commonly presenting as emergencies are:

- Upper airway obstruction: croup, acute epiglottitis.
- Lower airway obstruction: asthma, bronchiolitis.
- Pneumonia.

Upper airways obstruction

The cardinal sign of upper airway obstruction is stridor. This is a noise associated with breathing and due to obstruction of the extrathoracic airway. It tends to be worse on inspiration.

The important common causes of acute stridor are:

- Croup: acute laryngotracheobronchitis.
- Inhaled foreign body.
- Epiglottitis.

Features suggesting severe upper airway obstruction are shown in Fig. 26.22. Epiglottitis has become uncommon since the introduction of Hib vaccination.

Croup

This is dealt with in detail in Chapter 14. The key principles of its acute management include:

- Gentle, confident handling.
- Monitoring of O_2 saturation and heart rate.
- O_2 therapy.

Clinical features
Exhaustion
Decreased conscious level
Poor air entry on auscultation
Tachycardia
Cyanosis
Chest wall recession

Fig. 26.22 Features of severe upper airway obstruction.

- Nebulized budesonide or oral dexamethasone.
- Nebulized adrenaline (epinephrine): gives transient relief of severe obstruction and helps to buy time for the steroids to work or for intubation if needed.

The differential diagnosis of croup includes acute bacterial tracheitis.

Acute epiglottitis

This is dealt with in Chapter 14. The principles of management of acute epiglottitis include:

- Call for help—paediatric team, senior anaesthetist, ENT surgeon.
- Any distress to the child—examination, venepuncture, etc. can further compromise the airway and should be deferred until full support is available.
- Arrange examination under anaesthesia
- Once the diagnosis is confirmed, secure the airway by endotracheal intubation; take blood cultures and start intravenous antibiotics (e.g. ceftriaxone).

Usually these children can be extubated within a day or two and full recovery occurs by one week.

Lower airways obstruction

Acute asthma

An algorithm for the management of acute asthma is given in Fig. 26.23. Features of life threatening asthma are shown in Fig. 26.24.

Fig. 26.23 Management of acute severe asthma.

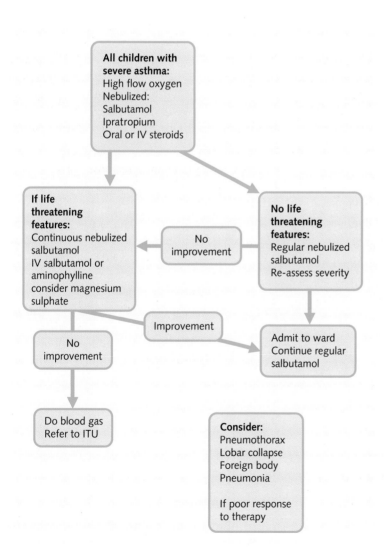

All children with severe asthma:
High flow oxygen
Nebulized:
Salbutamol
Ipratropium
Oral or IV steroids

If life threatening features:
Continuous nebulized salbutamol
IV salbutamol or aminophylline consider magnesium sulphate

No improvement

No life threatening features:
Regular nebulized salbutamol
Re-assess severity

Improvement

No improvement

Admit to ward
Continue regular salbutamol

Do blood gas
Refer to ITU

Consider:
Pneumothorax
Lobar collapse
Foreign body
Pneumonia

If poor response to therapy

Clinical features of life-threatening asthma
Decreased conscious level
Exhaustion or agitation
Poor respiratory effort
Silent chest
Oxygen saturation <85% in air

Fig. 26.24 Clinical features of life-threatening asthma.

β_2 bronchodilators, steroids and oxygen are the mainstays of treatment of acute asthma:

- Inhaled bronchodilator therapy given by spacer is as effective as nebulized bronchodilators, although in severe cases it is given by nebulizer due to ease of giving O_2.
- Short course (3–4 days) oral steroids can reduce the severity of the attack and should be given early as they take up to 6 hours to act. If the child cannot take oral steroids or is vomiting, intravenous hydrocortisone can be given.
- If the child does not respond adequately to appropriate doses of inhaled bronchodilators, then intravenous aminophylline or salbutamol is recommended early.
- Nebulized bronchodilators can be given continuously, but it is important to watch out for hypokalaemia and sinus tachycardia. If intravenous fluids are used, it should be restricted to two-thirds of normal requirement as there is often excess ADH secretion.

Antibiotics or chest X ray are rarely required unless there are clear signs of infection. Mechanical ventilation is rarely required.

Bronchiolitis

This is the commonest serious respiratory infection in infancy, characterized by tachypnoea (rate >60), irregular breathing or recurrent apnoea and hypoxia sometimes needing more than 60% O_2. The management is mainly supportive and involves:

- Monitoring O_2 saturation, respiratory rate and heart rate.
- Humidified O_2 by headbox or nasal cannulae to maintain O_2 saturation above 94%.
- Maintaining adequate fluid and nutrition intake by giving nasogastric or intravenous fluids.

Antibiotics, steroids and bronchodilators have no role.

Three phases of shock	
Phase	**Clinicopathological features**
Compensated shock	Vital organ function (brain, heart) is preserved by sympathetic response. Pallor, tachycardia, cold periphery, poor capillary return but systolic blood pressure is maintained
Decompensated shock	Inadequate perfusion leads to anaerobic metabolism, metabolic acidosis, and, on occasion, a bleeding diathesis. Blood pressure falls, acidotic breathing, very slow capillary return, altered consciousness, anuria
Irreversible shock	A retrospective diagnosis. Damage to heart and brain irreversible, with no improvement even if circulation is restored

Fig. 26.25 Three phases of shock.

Causes of shock	
Mechanism	**Causes**
Hypovolaemia	Fluid loss • Haemorrhage • Burns • Diarrhoea and vomiting • Diabetic ketoacidosis Fluid shifts • Septicaemia • Anaphylaxis • Peritonitis
Cardiogenic	Arrhythmias Heart failure

Fig. 26.26 Causes of shock.

Shock (circulatory failure)

Shock is a clinical syndrome resulting from acute failure of circulatory function leading to poor tissue perfusion. It tends to progress through three phases (Fig. 26.25):

- Compensated.
- Uncompensated.
- Irreversible.

The two common causes of shock are hypovolaemia and septicaemia (Fig. 26.26).

Clinical features

A brief history might identify the cause. The early physical signs of shock include:

- Pallor: due to vasoconstriction.
- Tachycardia with reduced pulse volume.
- Poor skin perfusion: capillary refill time >2 seconds, core/toe temperature difference of >2°C.
- Hypotension.

The late physical signs include:

- Rapid deep breathing: response to metabolic acidosis.
- Agitation, confusion: due to brain hypoperfusion.
- Oliguria: urine flow less than 2 ml/kg/h in infants and 1 ml/kg/h in children.

Management of shock: general

(See algorithm Fig. 26.27.) If there is no rapid improvement or if there is evidence of organ failure, transfer to an intensive care unit for assisted ventilation, intensive monitoring and inotropic support.

> Poor capillary refill should not be used in isolation to diagnose shock. The clinician must look at heart rate, blood pressure, base excess and clinical signs of organ perfusion, e.g. conscious level and urine output.

Specific shock syndromes

The three important specific syndromes in which shock occurs are:

- Anaphylactic shock.
- Septicaemic shock.
- Diabetic ketoacidosis.

Anaphylactic shock

See Chapter 11 for the features of anaphylaxis. The major problems are airway obstruction, bronchospasm and shock.

A protocol for management is shown in Fig. 26.28.

Septicaemic shock

Septicaemia is an important cause of shock in children. The main pathogens include:

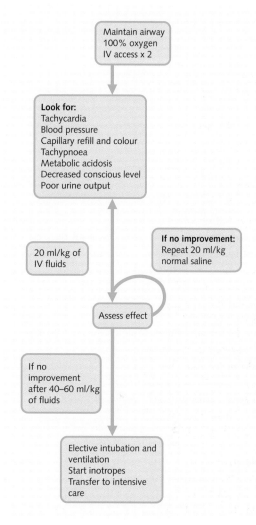

Fig. 26.27 Management of shock (ABC).

- *Neisseria meningitidis.*
- *Haemophilus influenzae* (rare if Hib immunized).
- Staphylococci, pneumococci, streptococci.
- Gram-negative bacteria.

Meningococcal septicaemia is the most fulminant variety. Death can occur within 12 hours of the first symptom; early diagnosis is vital.

Bacterial toxins trigger the release of various mediators and activators, which can:

- Cause vasodilatation or vasoconstriction.
- Depress cardiac function.
- Disturb cellular oxygen consumption.
- Cause 'capillary leak' with hypovolaemia.
- Promote disseminated intravascular coagulation.

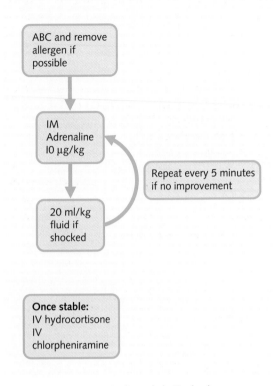

ABC and remove allergen if possible

↓

IM Adrenaline 10 µg/kg

↓

20 ml/kg fluid if shocked

Repeat every 5 minutes if no improvement

Once stable:
IV hydrocortisone
IV chlorpheniramine

Fig. 26.28 Management of anaphylactic shock.

Clinical features The clinical features progress from early (compensated) to late (decompensated) shock:

• 'Early' shock: increased cardiac output, decreased systemic resistance, warm extremities, high fever and mental confusion.

• 'Late' shock: reduced cardiac output, hypotension, cool peripheries and metabolic acidosis.

The cardinal sign of meningococcal septicaemia is a petechial or purpuric rash. This might be subtle in the early stages and a careful search for petechiae is required (in 10% of cases a blanching erythematous rash might occur first). An injection of benzylpenicillin should be given immediately if a diagnosis of meningococcal septicaemia or meningitis is suspected.

Management Key points in initial management include:

• Oxygen: 100% O_2 by face mask.
• Fluids: 20 mL/kg of colloid or crystalloid given as a bolus. This can be repeated but if more than 40 mL/kg is required then assisted ventilation is indicated.
• Antibiotics: IV ceftriaxone.
• Investigations (Fig. 26.29).

Outcome in septic shock is improved with aggressive fluid resuscitation and early referral to intensive care.

In severe illness, intensive care facilities are required to allow continuous monitoring of circulatory parameters (including central venous pressure),

Fig. 26.29 Investigations in septic shock.

Investigations in septic shock	
FBC Electrolytes and liver function Glucose Blood gas Lactate Coagulation screen	These define the severity of disease
Blood culture Urine culture Throat swab Rapid antigen testing and PCR Chest X-ray Abdominal ultrasound if indicated	Looking for the focus of infection

urine output and pulse oximetry. Assisted ventilation, inotropic agents and renal replacement therapy might be required.

Diabetic ketoacidosis

This is an important and life-threatening complication of insulin-dependent diabetes mellitus. It is now relatively uncommon for new cases of diabetes to present in a ketoacidotic state. The majority of episodes are seen in patients known to have type 1 diabetes mellitus.

Diabetic ketoacidosis represents the end stage of insulin deficiency. Deficiency of insulin blocks use of glucose leading to hyperglycaemia. As glucose levels exceed the renal threshold, an osmotic diuresis ensues with severe dehydration and electrolytes losses (sodium and potassium). Without insulin, fat is used as a source of energy leading to the generation of ketones and metabolic acidosis.

Clinical features   The clinical features evolve as the severity of dehydration and acidosis worsens.

- The new diabetic has a history of polyuria, polydipsia and weight loss. This is followed by the rapid development of vomiting, lethargy and abdominal pain.
- The known diabetic might have an intercurrent illness with vomiting, poor control and documented hyperglycaemia and ketonuria.

Characteristic physical signs are listed in Fig. 26.30.

Diagnosis   Essential initial investigations include:

- Blood glucose.
- Urea and electrolytes.
- Arterial blood gas analysis.
- Urine glucose and ketones.

Physical signs in diabetic ketoacidosis	
Dehydration	Dry mucous membranes Loss of skin turgor Tachycardia, hypotension if severe
Acidosis	Ketones on breath Kussmaul breathing: Rapid, deep, sighing respiration
Cerebral oedema	Headache Slowing of pulse rate and hypertension Decreased conscious level Seizures and focal neurological signs

Fig. 26.30 Physical signs in diabetic ketoacidosis.

The typical metabolic abnormalities in diabetic ketoacidosis, which will be revealed by these investigations, include:

- Hyperglycaemia: blood glucose over 15 mmol/L and glycosuria.
- Ketoacidosis: ketonuria, metabolic acidosis on arterial blood gas analysis (ABG) (pH is low, $[HCO_3]$ is reduced, $PaCO_2$ is low, there is respiratory compensation with hypocapnia).
- Dehydration: raised urea.
- Sodium and potassium depletion: serum sodium concentration is often slightly reduced; serum potassium concentration might be low, normal or high, depending on renal function and the degree of acidosis.

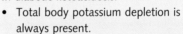

In diabetic ketoacidosis:
- Total body potassium depletion is always present.
- Cerebral oedema is rare but associated with a high mortality. Its prevention is by slow metabolic correction and rehydration.
- Serum potassium concentration falls with treatment as potassium is driven into cells (with insulin action and correction of acidosis) and renal function improves.
- IV fluids need to include potassium to avoid hypokalaemia as treatment proceeds.

Management   The mainstays of management are the slow and careful restoration of fluid and electrolyte status, and insulin (Fig. 26.31).

The acidosis will usually correct with correction of fluid balance and insulin therapy. Administration of bicarbonate is rarely used. A nasogastric tube should be passed if there is vomiting or evidence of gastric dilatation.

Careful monitoring is required of:

- Fluid status: weight, input and output.
- Electrolytes: check urea and electrolytes 2–4-hourly initially.
- Acid–base status: check ABG 2–4-hourly initially.
- Blood glucose: monitor hourly.

Management of diabetic ketoacidosis	
Fluids	Treat shock Maintenance fluids: rehydrate over 48 h 0.9% saline with potassium initially Change to 0.45% saline once glucose has fallen <15mmol/L
Insulin	Start IV at 0.1 units/kg/h Adjust depending on glucose: avoid drops >5mmol/L/h
Additional	Monitor electrolytes regularly Monitor conscious level

Fig. 26.31 Management of diabetic ketoacidosis.

- ECG monitoring allows early identification dysrhythmias secondary to electrolyte imbalances.
- Vital signs and neurological observations.

Complications   Major complications include:

- Cerebral oedema: manifested by reduced conscious level, headache, irritability and fits. Attempt to prevent this by avoiding *rapid* falls in blood glucose or serum sodium concentrations.
- Cardiac dysrhythmias: usually secondary to electrolyte (potassium) disturbances. Acute renal failure is uncommon.

After the initial 24–48 hours, it is usually possible to switch to oral fluids and 4-hourly subcutaneous soluble insulin on a sliding scale determined by the blood glucose concentration.

Further reading

British Medical Association. *Advanced Paediatric Life Support. A practical approach*, 3rd edn. London: BMJ Books, 2001.

Nutrition, fluids and prescribing

Objectives

At the end of this chapter you should be able to

- Know the different types of infant feeds and their advantages and disadvantages.
- Understand various malnutrition and deficiency states.
- Calculate the normal fluid requirements in children.
- Understand the metabolism of drugs in children.

Infants and children are more vulnerable than adults to inadequate nutrition or the derangement of fluid and electrolyte balance. Their high surface area to volume ratio is associated with a high metabolic rate, large calorific requirements and corresponding rapid fluid turnover.

Globally, malnutrition is probably directly or indirectly responsible for half of all deaths of children under 5 years of age. In the developed world, nutrition is a vital consideration in the management of many diseases (such as cystic fibrosis) and special diets are indicated for some disorders (such as coeliac disease, phenylketonuria and food allergy).

Breastfeeding in early infancy saves lives in developing countries. Its benefits are seen in babies who are exclusively breastfed; the addition of formula in early feeding can negate many of its benefits.

Dehydration associated with diarrhoeal diseases is a major killer worldwide and its treatment with oral rehydration solution represented a major advance. However, attention to fluid and electrolyte status is an important aspect of a wide spectrum of disorders, including diabetes mellitus, pyloric stenosis and postoperative care.

Prescribing for infants and children involves many considerations unique to this age group. The route and frequency of administration must be adapted to the age, and dosage must take into account bodyweight, surface area and age-dependent changes in drug metabolism and excretion.

NUTRITION

Normal nutritional requirements

A satisfactory dietary intake should meet the normal requirements for energy and protein, together with providing an adequate supply of vitamins and trace elements. Reference values for energy and protein requirements are shown in Fig. 27.1.

Infants and children are vulnerable to undernutrition because of:

- Low nutritional stores of fat and protein.
- Growth creating high nutritional demands (at 4 months of age, 30% of an infant's energy intake is used for growth; by 3 years of age this has fallen to 2%).
- Brain growth: the brain is proportionally larger in infants and is growing rapidly during the last trimester and first 2 years of life. It is vulnerable to energy deprivation during this period.

Infant feeding

An infant's primary source of nutrition is milk, either human breast milk or so-called 'formula' milk, usually based on modified cow's milk. Weaning, the introduction of solid foods, is usually initiated between the ages of 3 and 6 months.

Breastfeeding

This is the preferred method for most infants. Galactosaemia is the only contraindication but it is advised that HIV-positive mothers should not breastfeed in the Western world. The many advantages, and few disadvantages, of breastfeeding are listed in Fig. 27.2.

Establishing breastfeeding:
- The baby should be put to the breast as soon as possible after birth.
- Thereafter the baby should be fed on demand (indicated by crying).
- Frequent suckling promotes lactation.
- The baby's mouth needs to be well applied round the areola, with the nipple drawn into the back of the baby's mouth.
- Colostrum (high content of protein and immunoglobulin) rather than milk is produced in first few days.
- The interval between feeds gradually lengthens from 2–3 hours to approximately a 4-hourly schedule.

Fig. 27.2 Advantages and disadvantages of breastfeeding.

The composition of breast milk, cow's milk and infant formula differs significantly (Fig. 27.3). Unmodified, whole, pasteurized cow's milk is unsuitable as a main diet for infants under the age of 1 year because it:

- Contains too much protein and sodium.
- Is deficient in iron and vitamins.

Modified cow's milk formulas have a modified casein to whey ratio, reduced mineral content and are fortified with iron and vitamins.

Reference values for energy and protein requirements		
Age	Energy (kcal/kg/day)	Protein (g/kg/day)
0–6 months	115	2.2
6–12 months	95	2.0
1–3 years	95	1.8
4–6 years	90	1.5
7–10 years	75	1.2
11–14 years	60	1.0
15–18 years	50	0.8

Fig. 27.1 Reference values for energy and protein requirements.

Advantages and disadvantages of breastfeeding
Advantages
Quality:
• Breast milk has anti-infective properties including secretory IgA, lysozyme, phagocytic cells, lactoferrin (iron-binding agent), a factor that promotes growth of non-pathogenic flora
• Breast milk has better nutritional qualities, including easily digested protein, low renal solute load, and a favourable calcium to phosphate ratio
Emotional—if successful, promotes maternal–infant bonding
Reduction in risk of maternal breast cancer
Disadvantages
Volume of intake uncertain
Transmission of drugs, e.g. laxatives, anticoagulants, antineoplastics
Nutrient deficiencies:
• Insufficient vitamin K to prevent haemorrhagic disease of the newborn
• Vitamin D deficiency (rickets) may occur if there is prolonged breastfeeding and delayed weaning
Emotional—failure to establish breast-feeding may be a cause of emotional upset

Fig. 27.3 Composition of different milks (per 100 mL).

Composition of different milks (per 100 mL)			
	Breast milk	Cow's milk	Infant formula
Protein (g)	1.3	3.3	1.5
Casein:whey	40:60	60:40	Variable
Carbohydrate (g)	7.0	4.5	7.0–8.0
Fat (g)	4.2	3.6	2.6–3.8
Energy (kcal)	70	65	65
Sodium (mmol)	0.65	2.3	0.65–1.1
Calcium (mmol)	0.87	3.0	1.4
Iron (μmol)	1.36	0.9	10
Vitamin D (μg)	0.6	0.03	1.0

Breastfeeding mothers might be concerned about whether their baby has had an adequate milk intake and this is best measured by the baby's weight gain. Poor weight gain, or weight loss might mean inadequate lactation.

Bottle-feeding:

- Is less restrictive for mothers as others can do the feeding.
- Available as a dry powder requiring reconstitution or as ready made liquid feeds.
- Changing 'brands' in response to feeding difficulties is usually a futile gesture.

Soya formulas

Soya-based milks have been used to prevent atopic conditions in infants and in the treatment of colic, although evidence of this effect is lacking. Infants with cow's milk intolerance often develop intolerance to soya milk.

Weaning

The introduction of solid foods (weaning) is usually undertaken after 4 months of age. At this age the infant can coordinate swallowing and has reasonable head control. After 6 months of age, breast milk alone becomes nutritionally inadequate and continued breastfeeding without introduction of solids will lead to energy, vitamin and iron deficiency. Evidence is conflicting on late feeding and prevention of atopy.

A typical scheme for the introduction of solids is shown in Fig. 27.4.

Special milks

A variety of specialized milks exist that are used in infants who are intolerant of specific constituents. Examples include:

- Low phenylalanine milk: phenylketonuria.
- Low lactose milk: lactose intolerance.
- Soya milk: cow's milk protein intolerance.

Introduction of solids	
Age	Feeding
3–4 months	Cereals, e.g. baby rice
4–5 months	Pureed fruit and vegetables, meat (e.g. chicken)
6–7 months	Able to chew, e.g. rusks Introduce lumpy foods and variety of tastes and textures
8–9 months	Bread and butter, fruit
12 months	'Real' food in small bits

Fig. 27.4 Introduction of solids.

Malnutrition in childhood—causes
Inadequate intake Starvation due to famine Poverty Restrictive diets—parental, iatrogenic, self-inflicted Anorexia nervosa Anorexia due to chronic illness **Malabsorption** Pancreatic disease, e.g. cystic fibrosis Coeliac disease Short gut (postoperative) **Increased energy requirements** Cystic fibrosis Malignant disease Burns Trauma

Fig. 27.5 Malnutrition in childhood—causes.

Consequences of severe malnutrition
Impaired immunity Delayed wound healing Apathy and inactivity Impaired intellectual development

Fig. 27.6 Consequences of severe malnutrition.

Malnutrition

Worldwide, malnutrition due to inadequate intake (starvation) is responsible for millions of childhood deaths. However, malnutrition can also complicate many childhood diseases (Fig. 27.5) and specific nutritional deficiencies such as iron deficiency are not uncommon in the developed world.

Severe malnutrition affects many body systems (Fig. 27.6).

Assessment of nutritional status

Evaluation involves:

- Dietary history.
- Anthropometry and clinical examination.
- Laboratory investigations.

Dietary history

The food intake, as recalled by the parents or recorded in a diary, is determined over a period of several days.

Anthropometry

This involves measurement of:

- Height: height for age is reduced (stunted growth) in chronic malnutrition.
- Weight: reduced weight with normal height (wasting) is an index of acute malnutrition.
- Midarm circumference: an indication of skeletal muscle mass.
- Skinfold thickness: triceps skinfold thickness is a measure of subcutaneous fat stores.

Clinical syndromes of protein-energy malnutrition include:

- Marasmus: wasted (weight less than 60% of mean for age), wizened appearance, withdrawn, and apathetic.
- Kwashiorkor: occurs in children weaned late from the breast and fed on a relatively high-starch diet. It can be precipitated by an acute intercurrent infection. Features include wasting, oedema, sparse hair and depigmented skin, angular stomatitis and hepatomegaly.

Laboratory investigations

Useful laboratory tests include:

- Serum albumin: reduced in severe malnutrition.
- FBC: low haemoglobin and lymphocyte count.
- Blood glucose.
- Calcium, phosphate and vitamin D levels.
- Serum potassium and magnesium levels.

Management

Nutrition can be supplied:

- Enterally, via the gastrointestinal tract: this route is preferred wherever possible.
- Parenterally, directly into the circulation.

In many cases, malnutrition is due to inadequate intake and can be managed by the provision of supplementary enteral feeds given via a nasogastric or gastrostomy tube.

Examples of chronic diseases requiring such supplemental feeding include:

- Cystic fibrosis.
- Congenital heart disease.
- Cerebral palsy.
- Chronic renal failure.
- Malignancy.
- Inflammatory bowel disease.
- Anorexia nervosa.

Vitamin deficiencies

Several important vitamin deficiency diseases still occur in childhood. These include in particular:

- Vitamin D deficiency: rickets.
- Vitamin A deficiency: blindness.
- Vitamin K deficiency: haemorrhagic disease of the newborn.

The most common dietary deficiencies in the UK are of iron and vitamin D.

Scurvy due to vitamin C deficiency is now extremely rare in developed countries.

Vitamin D deficiency: rickets

The effects of vitamin D deficiency on growing bone cause rickets. The bone matrix (osteoid) of the growing bone is inadequately mineralized, giving rise to the clinical features described in Fig. 27.7.

Clinical features of rickets
General
Misery
Hypotonia
Developmental delay
Growth failure
Skeletal
Craniotabes (thin, soft, skull bones)
Enlarged metaphyses (especially wrists and knees)
Rickety rosary (enlarged costochondral junctions)
Bowing of legs (caused by weight bearing)

Fig. 27.7 Clinical features of rickets.

The undermineralized bone is less rigid and bends and twists in an abnormal way.

The normal pathways of vitamin D absorption and metabolism are shown in Fig. 27.8.

The most common cause is nutritional deficiency. The minimum daily requirement of vitamin D is 400 international units (IU) and this might not be attained in infants who are breastfed for a protracted period. An additional important factor is decreased exposure to the sun, because vitamin D is synthesized from precursors in the skin under the effect of ultraviolet light. This can occur especially in:

• Infants with dark skin pigmentation.
• Urban living conditions.
• Winter.

Fig. 27.8 Normal pathways of vitamin D metabolism and action.

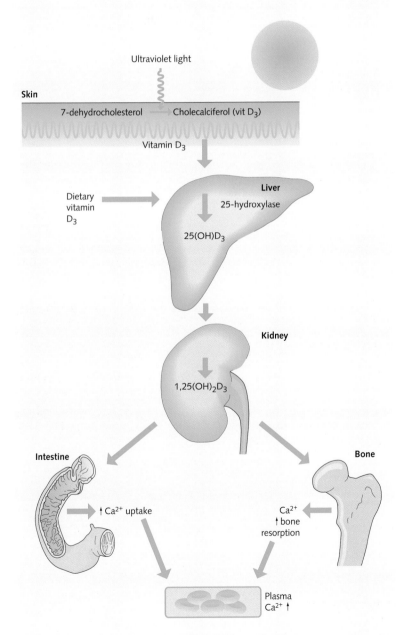

Less common causes of rickets include:

- Inherited abnormalities of vitamin D metabolism or of the vitamin D receptor.
- Mineral deficiency, e.g. X-linked. hypophosphataemia.
- Chronic renal disease.
- Decreased activity of 1α-hydroxylase in the kidneys leads to rickets as one component of renal osteodystrophy.

Rickets of prematurity is a metabolic bone disease in the premature infant that occurs if the milk used contains inadequate calcium and phosphate (1α-dihydroxycholecalciferol levels are elevated because of the hypophosphataemic stimulus, but there is osteopenia and inadequate mineralization of growing bone).

Diagnosis

This is confirmed by X-ray imaging and blood biochemistry. X-ray of the wrist shows cupping and fraying of the metaphysis and a widened metaphyseal plate (Fig. 27.9).

The biochemical changes in classic nutritional rickets include:

- Serum calcium: low or normal (may be normalized by secondary hyperparathyroidism).
- Serum phosphate: low.
- Serum alkaline phosphatase: elevated.
- Serum parathormone (PTH): elevated.
- Serum 1,25-dihydroxycholecalciferol: low.

Treatment

Prevention is obviously preferred and this is achieved by health education, exposure to sunlight and supplementation of the diet with minerals and vitamin D when indicated.

Treatment of nutritional rickets is with vitamin D3 (1,25-dihydroxycholecalciferol) 5000–10 000 IU/day initially for several weeks, followed by provision of 400 IU/day in the diet.

Higher doses might be required in the inherited forms. Biochemistry and radiography monitor the effect of therapy.

Vitamin A (retinol) deficiency

Vitamin A is necessary for membrane stability and it plays a role in vision, keratinization, cornification and placental development. The body's need for vitamin A can be met by milk, butter, eggs, liver and dark green or orange-coloured (e.g. carrots) vegetables.

Worldwide, about 150 million children are at risk of vitamin A deficiency and it has been calculated that up to a third of a million children go blind each year from vitamin A deficiency. In addition, vitamin A deficiency carries increased mortality from infection and poor growth.

The eye disease develops insidiously with impaired dark adaptation followed by drying of the conjunctiva and cornea (xerophthalmia).

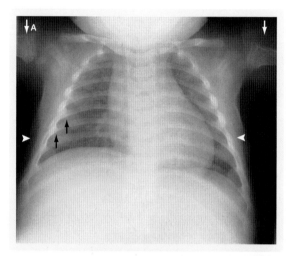

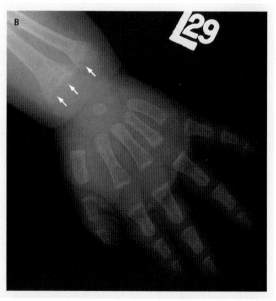

Fig. 27.9 X-ray appearance of rickets. (A) CXR of a young child with partially treated rickets. Note (i) changes at the metaphyses (white arrows), (ii) periosteal reaction on several ribs (white arrowheads), and (iii) bulging of anterior rib ends, the rickety rosary (black arrows). (B) Left wrist X-ray. Note the irregular 'cupped' metaphyses with loss of bone density (white arrows).

Obesity

In 1998 the World Health Organization stated that obesity is a global epidemic. It results from numerous social and environmental factors that are difficult to alter. Obesity in children is increasing in prevalence and treatment is often disappointing. Prevention of obesity remains the optimal solution.

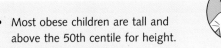

- Most obese children are tall and above the 50th centile for height.
- In Cushing syndrome or hypothyroidism, obesity is associated with low growth velocity and short stature.

The body mass index is a useful measurement of obesity and a BMI >25 is considered obese. Aetiological factors include:

- Genetic factors.
- Excess carbohydrate intake.
- Reduced activity.

Rarely, an endocrine or chromosomal cause is present such as Cushing syndrome, hypothyroidism or Prader–Willi syndrome.

Obesity has several deleterious consequences including:

- Emotional disturbance: many psychological problems are associated with obesity.
- Hypoventilation: obesity is the main cause of obstructive sleep apnoea in the USA.
- Long-term complications: obese children are twice as likely to become obese adults.

Management

A large number of interventions have been tried and involvement of both parents and school is necessary. A reduced-calorie, balanced diet with increased exercise in combination with behavioural modification and psychological support offers the best way to manage obesity.

FLUIDS AND ELECTROLYTES

Important physiological factors render children more vulnerable than adults to disturbances of fluid and electrolyte balance (Fig. 27.10). Such disturbances are common in paediatric practice and occur in a number of important clinical contexts (Fig. 27.11).

Basic physiology

It is useful to know how fluid is distributed between the different compartments of the body and what the normal requirements for fluid and electrolytes are. Important changes occur with age as the ratio of surface area to volume alters.

Fluid compartments

These are shown in Fig. 27.12. Infants are more 'watery' and have a higher proportion of fluid in the

Fluid and electrolyte balance in children
Children have a larger surface area to volume ratio than adults
Total body water is a higher percentage of body weight in children
The rate of turnover of fluids and electrolytes is higher in children

Fig. 27.10 Fluid and electrolyte balance in children.

Clinical conditions associated with fluid and electrolyte disturbance
Gastroenteritis
Major burns
Diabetic ketoacidosis
Renal failure
Sepsis
Trauma

Fig. 27.11 Clinical conditions associated with fluid and electrolyte disturbance.

Fig. 27.12 Body fluid compartments (as a percentage of body weight).

Body fluid compartments (as a percentage of body weight)			
Age	Total body water	Extracellular fluid	Intracellular fluid
Newborn	70	35	35
12 months	65	25	40
Adult	60	20	40

Normal fluid requirements	
Body weight	Fluid requirement per 24 hours
First 10 kg	100 ml/kg
Second 10 kg	50 ml/kg
Further kg	20 ml/kg

Example: 24-hour requirement for child weighing 25 kg

10 kg at 100 ml/kg	= 1000 ml
10 kg at 50 ml/kg	= 500 ml
5 kg at 20 ml/kg	= 100 ml
Total	= 1600 ml

Fig. 27.13 Normal fluid requirements.

Electrolyte content of body fluids			
Fluid	Na+ (mmol/L)	K+ (mmol/L)	Cl− (mmol/L)
Plasma	135–141	3.5–5.5	100–105
Gastric	20–80	5–20	100–150
Intestinal	100–140	5–15	90–130
Diarrhoea	10–90	10–30	10–110

Fig. 27.14 Electrolyte content of body fluids.

Isotonic crystalloid fluids: composition				
Fluid	Sodium (mmol/L)	Potassium (mmol/L)	Chloride (mmol/L)	Energy (kcal/L)
0.9% saline	150	0	150	0
5% dextrose/ 0.45% saline	75	0	75	200

Fig. 27.15 Isotonic crystalloid fluids: composition.

extracellular space than adults. The percentages can be expressed as volumes: e.g. 70% is equivalent to 700 mL/kg bodyweight (see Hints & Tips).

Blood volume is about 100 mL/kg at birth and falls to about 80 mL/kg at 1 year.

- As body density is close to that of water, and 1 litre of water weighs close to 1 kilogram, weights and volumes are freely interchangeable. For example 1000 ml = 1000 g (1 litre = 1 kg).
- Changes in bodyweight are the best guide to short-term changes in fluid balance (e.g. a weight loss of 500 g indicates a fluid deficit of 500 mL).

Normal requirements

Fluid requirement is that needed to make up for normal fluid losses, which include essential urine output and 'insensible' losses through sweat, respiration and the gastrointestinal tract. In pathological states there will be additional abnormal losses, such as those associated with diarrhoea or vomiting.

A simple formula for calculating normal fluid requirements according to bodyweight is shown in Fig. 27.13.

There are obligatory electrolyte losses in the stools, urine and sweat, and these require replacement. The electrolyte composition of various body fluids, which can be lost in excessive amounts, is

shown in Fig. 27.14. The maintenance requirement for sodium is about 3 mmol/kg/day and for potassium is 2 mmol/kg/day.

Intravenous fluids

These can be divided into colloids, which include large molecules such as proteins, and crystalloids, which usually contain dextrose (glucose) and electrolytes. Although concerns about colloids have been raised they are still in widespread use for volume expansion in sepsis.

The compositions of commonly available crystalloid fluids for intravenous use are shown in Fig. 27.15.

Important features of intravenous solutions

- They are isotonic or slightly hypertonic: their osmolality is close to that of plasma—A hypotonic (dilute solution) would lyse red cells and a very hypertonic solution would draw fluid into the circulation. Hypertonic saline has been used in raised intracranial pressure.
- Normal saline: is commonly used for replacing deficits and for rapid volume expansion.
- 5% dextrose and 0.45% sodium with potassium is the usual maintenance fluid. In neonates 10% dextrose solutions are used often with sodium and potassium added depending on serum electrolytes.

- Colloids are less frequently used except in septic shock. The best colloid in trauma is blood.
- 0.18% saline is no longer used in paediatric medicine due to its hypotonicity.

Specific fluid and electrolyte problems

These are mostly considered elsewhere:

- Dehydration (see Chapter 15).
- Diabetic ketoacidosis (see Chapter 26).
- Burns (see Chapter 26).

Important features concerning certain electrolyte disturbances are considered here.

Sodium

Serum sodium levels reflect extracellular water shifts:

- Hyponatraemia is seen in the syndrome of inappropriate secretion of ADH (where excess extracellular water is present) and in gastroenteritis treated with water instead of salt solutions.
- Hypernatraemia is less common but is seen in neonates who become dehydrated as a result of poor breastfeeding and in diabetic ketoacidosis.
- It is important to avoid rapid changes in sodium concentration because cerebral oedema or myelinosis might result.

Potassium

Hypokalaemia is usually a result of gastrointestinal loss (vomiting) or inadequate intake. It is treated by supplementing IV fluids or oral potassium.

Hyperkalaemia is potentially dangerous, but children and neonates are less vulnerable to hyperkalaemia than adults. The most common cause is renal failure, but it also occurs in:

- Severe acidosis.
- Hypoaldosteronism.
- Iatrogenic potassium overload.

Immediate management involves:

- Calcium gluconate to stabilize myocardium: this does not remove potassium
- Promotion of cellular potassium uptake by nebulized or IV salbutamol. An alternative is insulin and dextrose.

- Ion-exchange resins, e.g. oral or PR calcium resonium.
- Dialysis or haemofiltration if the above measures fail.

PAEDIATRIC PHARMACOLOGY AND PRESCRIBING

Great variability exists between children and adults in the pharmacology of drugs; differences also exist between the preterm neonate, neonate and older children. It is therefore important that clinicians recognize that much of the information that applies to adults is not always applicable to children, and must be cautious in extrapolating adult data into paediatric practice. Most paediatric doses are calculated based on the child's weight or body surface area, though the latter is used infrequently (Fig. 27.16).

Water-soluble drugs, e.g. most antibiotics, require a larger initial dose in neonates because they have the greatest amount of total body water. The large volume also means delayed excretion so doses are less frequent

Many drugs currently used in paediatric practice remain unlicensed. Thus, pharmacokinetic and pharmacodynamic data are rarely available. A paediatric formulary published by the Royal College of Paediatrics and Child Health, entitled *Medicines for Children*, is available and currently in its second edition.

Body weight and body surface area by age		
Age	Weight (kg)	BSA (m^2)
Newborn	3.5	0.25
6 months	7.7	0.40
1 year	10	0.50
5 years	18	0.75
12 years	36	1.25
Adult	70	1.80

Fig. 27.16 Body weight and body surface area (BSA) by age.

Absorption and administration

The oral route is most commonly used for administering medication because it is easy, safe and cheap. Its limitations are that many children find certain drugs unpalatable and tablets need to be crushed. High doses are also not always possible and certain drugs, e.g. insulin cannot be absorbed from this route.

The IV route is reliable and effective but requires venepuncture. The PR route is useful in emergencies, and diazepam and paracetamol can be given this way. Intramuscular injections are rarely used except for immunizations.

In neonates and infants, gastric absorption is altered as normal gastric acid secretion is reduced until 3 years of age; gastric motility is also delayed.

Distribution

The concentration of drug at the target organ depends on the solubility and protein binding of the drug and the characteristics of the tissues itself. At birth, there is a greater proportion of water in the extracellular fluid compartments and total body water is greater (85% compared with the adult 60%).

Protein binding of drugs differs as albumin concentrations reach adult levels at 1 year of age and binding capacity is different in children.

Metabolism and excretion

Hepatic metabolism differs from that in adults in that it is slow at birth but increases rapidly with age; the metabolic processes also differ. For example, paracetamol is metabolized by sulphation whereas adults use the glucuronidation pathway. Thus paracetamol toxicity in children is less than in adults.

The renal handling of drugs also differs because the glomerular filtration rate in children does not approach adult levels until 9–12 months age.

HISTORY, EXAMINATION AND COMMON INVESTIGATIONS

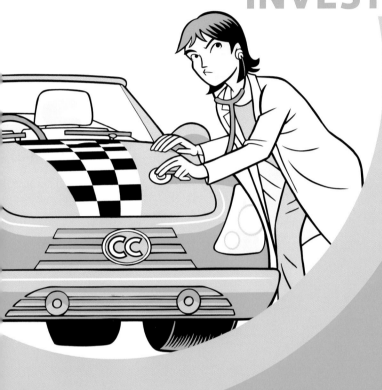

History and examination

Objectives

At the end of this chapter you should be able to

- Take a detailed and appropriate paediatric history.
- Perform a structured clinical examination.
- Perform a routine neonatal examination.
- Document your history, findings and conclusions appropriately.

The art of taking a history from, and examining, a child shares some principles with the corresponding process in adult medicine. The young infant and neonate present special challenges, whereas the older child can often be clerked in a similar manner to an adult. Most clinicians are concerned that children might not cooperate and communicate during the clinical assessment.

In many cases, the history will come predominantly from the parents but it is important not to overlook a communicating child, as he or she might offer a more accurate story than the parents! This is especially important in cases of child protection.

A problem-based approach

It is important to include a summary of clinical problems at the end of your clerking in the notes. This shows that you are able to form a practical plan from your assessment and you have thought about the management of the patient. This is important, even when you are still a student—you may not always be right but it is never too early to train yourself to think like a doctor. Failure to include a problem list and management plan is a common criticism of new house officers!

PAEDIATRIC HISTORY TAKING

The overall format is similar to that in adult medicine but it is important to establish a rapport with parent(s) and child at an early stage. Ignoring the child when taking a history wastes a valuable opportunity to alleviate the anxiety that the child will have in this unfamiliar situation.

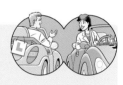

Ask the parents to help if the child is upset or shy.

The beginning

- Introduce yourself to the parents and the child. It is important to find out the name and sex of the child at this point.
- Make sure you know who is accompanying the child; many parents are not married or the child might have been taken to hospital by a relative.

Presenting complaint

Open-ended questions to start will put the parents at ease and at this point they might volunteer both the presenting symptoms and the symptoms that caused them most anxiety. Often the symptoms that they are worried about are not the symptoms that most concern the doctor!

Once the main symptoms are established, details such as the nature of onset, duration and precipitating factors should be obtained by specific questioning. Associated symptoms and previous illnesses should be asked for at this stage.

Past history

Most children are healthy and have only minor illnesses in the past history but an increasing number with significant illnesses such as extreme prematurity, leukaemia and cardiac disease are surviving to older ages. Ask about:

- Immunizations.
- Hospital admissions.

Birth

A birth history includes:

- Gestational age at delivery.
- Mode of delivery.
- Birthweight.
- Problems encountered at birth or during pregnancy.
- Mode of feeding.

Developmental history

- Age at reaching milestones.
- Concerns about vision and hearing.

Family and social history

- Ask about any illnesses that run in the family and about recent infectious contacts.
- Make a family tree and ask about parental consanguinity (this increases the incidence of autosomal recessive conditions, which often present with neurological or metabolic problems).
- Social circumstances: housing, parental occupations and any difficulties at home. The family might be under the care of a social worker.
- Travel history: include foreign travel and contacts.

Systems review

A systems review is not performed routinely because, with experience, the history of the presenting complaint should cover all relevant systems. However, a formal review of systems can be useful if the doctor feels that something might be missing in the history.

The history does not stop at one sitting—repeat questioning might produce information that was not volunteered the first time. There is no shame in reviewing the history and many parents do not give a complete picture at the beginning.

NEONATAL HISTORY

On taking a neonatal history, more emphasis should be on the details of the birth. Many maternal conditions affect the newborn infant and the details of delivery and resuscitation are essential.

Pregnancy

- Maternal medical history, e.g. diabetes, HIV.
- Medication taken during pregnancy including illicit drugs.
- Alcohol and smoking.
- Complications of pregnancy, e.g. pre-eclampsia.
- Results of any amniocentesis, chorionic villus biopsy and ultrasound reports.

Maternal infections

Most mothers in the UK are tested in the antenatal period for HIV, hepatitis B, syphilis and rubella. Ask if a high vaginal swab was taken for group B streptococci and maternal fever.

Birth

Important facts:

- Duration or rupture of membranes.
- Gestational age at delivery.
- Mode of delivery.
- Resuscitation of the baby (if needed).
- Birthweight.

Enquire about any problems after birth, for instance feeding difficulties or admissions to the neonatal unit.

EXAMINATION

Older children are usually cooperative and an approach similar to that used in adults can be employed; young children and infants might be frightened and rather less cooperative. It is important to let the parents help you. They are the people the child is most comfortable with and it should be no surprise if a child is unwilling to let a total stranger approach if the parents are absent.

In children, most of the examination findings are obtained by observing the child interact with their environment. Watching a child play will give you almost all the information you need about his or her neurology!

Examination of the child begins as they enter the room or when they play. Observing their spontaneous movements will provide more information than asking them to perform.

General examination

- Weight and height-plot on a growth chart with head circumference in infants.
- Temperature.
- Colour.
- Posture, movements and conscious level.
- Rashes.

Respiratory system

Count the respiratory rate. Note the different normal values with age. Note any cyanosis or finger clubbing (Fig. 28.1).

Listen for
- Stridor (inspiratory) or wheeze (expiratory) sounds.
- Cough and its nature: barking cough is suggestive of croup.

Look for
- Nasal flaring and use of accessory muscles.
- Intercostal and subcostal recession.
- Chest shape abnormalities and Harrison's sulci.

Percuss
This is more useful in the older child because it can be more sensitive than auscultation alone for detecting pulmonary abnormalities.

Auscultate
This can be done at any time that is suitable because the crying child will make auscultation impossible. Often, upper airway sounds will predominate and mask lung sounds. Listen for:

- Intensity of breath sounds on both sides.
- Presence of bronchial breath sounds.
- Wheeze and crackles.

Cardiovascular system

Similar to adults except that it is done as soon as the child is settled and not crying! (Fig. 28.2). Innocent murmurs are common in children and should be distinguished from pathological murmurs (Fig. 28.3). Palpation of the femoral pulse in neonates is mandatory to detect coarctation of the aorta. Hepatomegaly is one of the signs of cardiac failure.

Do not forget to measure blood pressure!

Abdomen

Observe for jaundice and abdominal distension. It is common for most infants to have a distended abdomen before they are walking. This alone is not pathological.

Respiratory rate at different ages	
Age	Upper limits (breaths per minute)
Neonate	>60
Infant	>40
Young child	>30
Older child	>20

Fig. 28.1 Respiratory rates at different ages.

Normal heart rates in children	
Age	Beats per minute
<1 year	120–160
2–5 years	90–140
5–12 years	80–120
>12 years	60–100

Fig. 28.2 Normal heart rates in children.

Features of innocent heart murmurs
Changes with posture
Localized
Asymptomatic
Normal cardiac examination
Systolic only
No thrill

Fig. 28.3 Features of innocent heart murmurs.

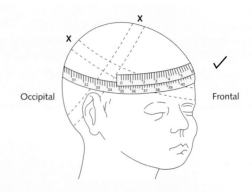

Fig. 28.4 Measuring head circumference.

Palpate

The child must be as relaxed and as comfortable as possible. An unsettled anxious child will unconsciously tense their abdominal muscles.

- Abdominal masses: the liver is usually palpable until puberty.
- Peristalsis: this might represent obstruction or pyloric stenosis.
- Inguinal herniae.
- Umbilical herniae are common and not pathological.
- Watch the child's face for any sign of tenderness.

Nervous system

Most children will give you a lot of information in their play and the examiner must observe how the child interacts with his or her surroundings. The assessment of the cranial nerves, tone, reflexes, power, co-ordination and sensation must be tailored to the individual child.

Observe:

- The gait as the child walks in.
- Postures at rest.
- Level of alertness or conscious level.

Important points:

- In infants, palpation of the fontanelle, sutures and measurement of the head circumference is essential (Fig. 28.4).
- Presence of primitive reflexes in neonates and infants.
- Meningism is usually not detectable until >2 years of age.
- The plantar reflexes are predominantly extensor (down-going) in infants under 6 months and the transition to flexor might be asymmetrical.

Ear, nose and throat

This is often done at the end because it causes the most distress to the child (Fig. 28.5). It is vital that the examiner is helped by a parent who can hold the child still. The neck should be palpated for lymphadenopathy and then the ears should be examined. Looking at the throat should be done at the end because a wooden tongue depressor might be needed to visualize the throat.

Never examine the throat if upper airway obstruction is suspected, e.g. epiglottitis or severe croup.

THE NEONATAL EXAMINATION

Neonatal history includes:

- Present complaint and its history.
- Maternal illness and drugs include smoking and alcohol.
- Pregnancy: details of pregnancy, mode of delivery and labour; include scans and any abnormal tests.
- Birthweight and the need for resuscitation or admission to a neonatal unit.
- Feeding: breast or bottle.

All neonates should undergo a full examination within 24 hours. This allows any abnormalities to be detected early and also reassures parents of the numerous common normal variants that are found (Fig. 28.6).

Vital signs

Look at the baby's:

Fig. 28.5 Throat examination.

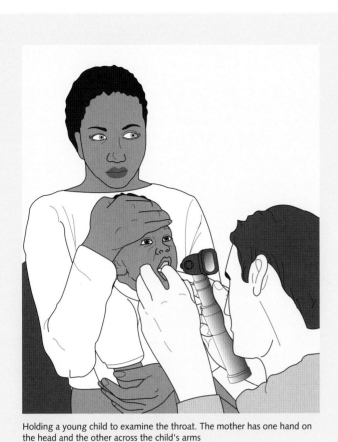

Holding a young child to examine the throat. The mother has one hand on the head and the other across the child's arms

- Colour.
- Heart rate.
- Respiratory rate.
- Weight and head circumference.

Skin

Observe:

- Many neonates show some jaundice but this is pathological if seen in the first day or if severe.
- Erythema toxicum is a benign condition affecting approximately 50% of all infants. It presents as macular lesions with a central yellow papule.
- Cyanosis can be difficult to detect and should be observed on the tongue and lips. Peripheral cyanosis without central cyanosis is not pathological (acrocyanosis).
- Pallor might represent anaemia or illness; plethora might be due to polycythaemia.

- Mongolian blue spots must be documented because they appear identical to bruising.
- Mottling is often seen in healthy infants and alone is not suggestive of pathology.
- Vascular lesions such as strawberry haemangiomas and port wine stains.

Note all Mongolian blue spots for future references.

Head

Note the shape and size of the head and fontanelle. The sutures should be palpable and head trauma from delivery may manifest as:

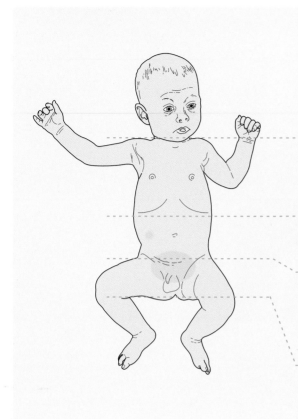

- Birthweight and centile
- Colour
- Skin lesions
- Palpate fontanelle and sutures
- Measure occipito–frontal head circumference
- Check eyes for cataract, red reflex
- Examine facies for dysmorphic features
  —Down syndrome
- Check palate

- Observe breathing rate and chest wall movement
- Palpate precordium
- Auscultate the heart
  —Count heart rate
  —Heart murmurs (see Hints & Tips)

- Palpate abdomen
  Liver 1–2 cms. Spleen tip may be palpable
- Inspect the umbilical cord

- Palpate the femoral pulses
- Inspect genitalia for
  —Inguinal herniae
  —Hypospadias
  —Undescended testes and anus for patency
- Check hips for congenital dislocation (see Hints & Tips)

- Assess muscle tone
  Pick up the baby and hold in ventral suspension
- Inspect back and spine for midline defects
- Moro reflex

Fig. 28.6 Routine neonatal examination.

- Caput succedaneum: diffuse swelling that crosses the suture lines. It resolves in several days.
- Cephalohaematoma: this never crosses the suture lines and is caused by subperiosteal haemorrhage; 5% are associated with fractures.

Neck

Sternocleidomastoid tumours or thyroglossal cysts might be palpable as neck lumps in the midline. The clavicles might be fractured but no treatment is necessary. Palpable lymph nodes are found in 33% of all neonates.

Face

Observe for symmetry when the infant cries or yawns. Facial nerve palsy is common after forceps delivery and is self limiting:

- Eyes: look for the red reflex (if absent think of retinoblastoma) and evidence of conjunctivitis. A blue sclera is normal in <3 months.

- Ears: look at the position and for any skin tags.
- Mouth: loose natal teeth need removal. Palpate *and* look at the palate for cleft palate.

Chest

These often cause concern amongst parents but have no clinical significance:

- Pectus excavatum.
- Breasts and milk production: caused by maternal oestrogens.

Note that the normal respiratory rate in newborns is 40–60 breaths/minute and heart rate is 120–160 beats/minute. Commonly, periodic breathing can be seen, during which there are pauses lasting less than 10 seconds. This is normal and more common in preterm infants.

Auscultation for breath sounds and heart sounds should be done when the infant is quiet.

- Breath sounds: listen for presence and symmetry.

Hospital No. X349282

Baby, A   15/11/03
01/01/04 20:30 6wk old male

PC   Vomiting

1. Presenting complaint should be brief, but it is helpful to mention relevant background information

HPC   Gradual onset over previous five days of intermittent vomiting.
            Usually occurs in period after feed.
            Vomit is milk only – no bile or blood staining
            Forceful vomiting – milk clears mother's lap
            Infant appears hungry and eager to feed. Breast fed
            Stool frequency reduced. No diarrhoea

PMH   Born at St Elsewhere's Hospital
            Full term delivery (FTND)
            Birth weight 3650g
            Mild jaundice 3–5 days
            No significant perinatal problems

2. Past medical history should include details of birth and any neonatal problems

DH   Smiles in response
            Fixing and following
            Responds to sounds

Fam Hx   Siblings   1 brother aged 4 years—mild asthma
                        1 sister aged 2 years—VSD. Under review
            Mother   Age 31 years. Well
            Operated on for 'bowel obstruction' at age 4 weeks
            Father   Age 33 years. Asthmatic

Social Hx   Father electrician.
            Mother a nurse (not working)
            Living in own flat

Drug Hx   Not on medication
            No known allergies

3. Always record the dose and frequency of any drugs – remember you'll be writing the drug chart later! Always document that you have asked about drug allergies

S/E   CVS — No cyanotic episodes
            RS — Episodes of shallow breathing
            GIT — Breast fed. No 'possetting'. Stool frequency
                  previously × 5 per 24 hours
            GU — Good urinary stream

            Medication — Nil

Fig. 28.7 Clerking.

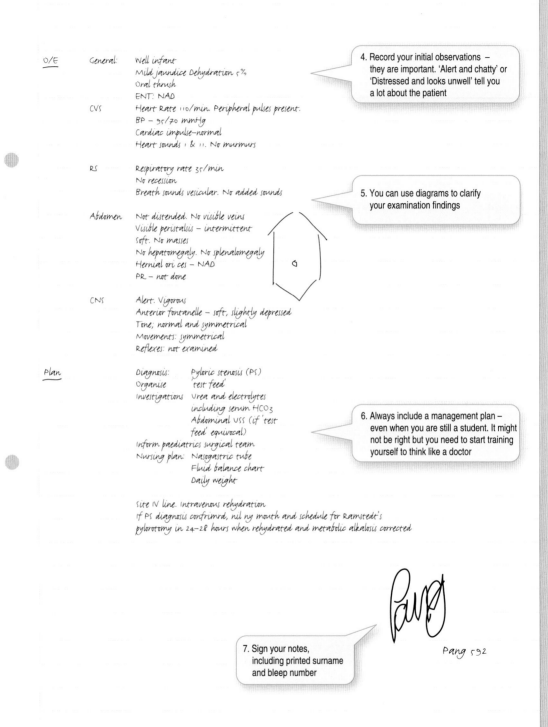

O/E   General: Well infant
                          Mild jaundice Dehydration 5%
                          Oral thrush
                          ENT: NAD

          CVS   Heart Rate 110/min. Peripheral pulses present.
                          BP – 95/70 mmHg
                          Cardiac impulse–normal
                          Heart sounds I & II. No murmurs

          RS   Respiratory rate 35/min
                          No recession
                          Breath sounds vesicular. No added sounds

      Abdomen   Not distended. No visible veins
                          Visible peristalsis – intermittent
                          Soft. No masses
                          No hepatomegaly. No splenomegaly
                          Hernial orifices – NAD
                          PR – not done

          CNS   Alert. Vigorous
                          Anterior fontanelle – soft, slightly depressed
                          Tone; normal and symmetrical
                          Movements: symmetrical
                          Reflexes: not examined

Plan   Diagnosis: Pyloric stenosis (PS)
                     Organise   'test feed'
                     Investigations   Urea and electrolytes
                                  including serum HCO_3
                                  Abdominal USS (if 'test
                                  feed' equivocal)
                     Inform paediatrics surgical team
                     Nursing plan: Nasogastric tube
                                  Fluid balance chart
                                  Daily weight

                     Site IV line. Intravenous rehydration
                     If PS diagnosis confrimrd, nil ny mouth and schedule for Ramstedt's
                     pylorotomy in 24–28 hours when rehydrated and metabolic alkalosis corrected

Pang 592

Fig. 28.7 Cont'd.

- Heart sounds: listen for the quality and intensity of the heart sounds.
- Murmurs might be heard but their presence does not always indicate heart disease.

Murmurs are not always heard in the first 24–48 hours of life and cardiac problems do not usually present at this early stage.

The femoral pulses should be palpated and, if weak or absent, might indicate coarctation of the aorta.

Abdomen

Many infants have a small degree of abdominal distension and this is a normal finding. Observe for:

- Abdominal wall defects.
- Scaphoid abdomen suggests diaphragmatic hernia.
- Examine the umbilicus for three vessels. Single umbilical artery is associated with renal abnormalities. Also look for discharge and inflammation.

Genitalia

The clitoris and labia are normally enlarged and vaginal bleeding might be observed. This is due to maternal oestrogen withdrawal and requires no treatment.

In boys, the testes should be palpable and phimosis is normal. The foreskin should never be retracted. A good urinary stream should be observed.

Anus

Check for patency of anus; meconium should be passed within 48 hours.

Urine should be passed within 24 h and meconium within 48 h.

Extremities

Examine all digits and for palmar creases. Supernumary digits (polydactyly) and abnormal fusion of the digits (syndactyly) are often familial.

Trunk and spine

Hips

Palpate the vertebrae, looking for scoliosis. Any abnormal pigmentation, dimples or hairs over the lumbar region should raise the suspicion of spina bifida. A sacral dimple is common and usually normal if the base is seen.

The Barlow and Ortolani test should be performed. Observe for leg length discrepancy and range of abduction; only gentle force is needed.

Nervous system

The spontaneous movements of the infant should be observed and then examination of:

- Tone: look for both hypo and hypertonia.
- Reflexes: both primitive and deep tendon reflexes.
- Cranial nerves.

A fine tremor and ankle clonus for 5–10 beats is normal.

MEDICAL SAMPLE CLERKING

A sample medical clerking is shown in Fig. 28.7. It illustrates some of the points discussed earlier in this chapter.

Further reading

Gupta A, Gupta P. Neonatal plantar response revisited. *Journal of Paediatric Child Health* 2003; **39**(5):349–351.
Kumhar GD, Dua T, Gupta P. Plantar response in infancy. *European Journal of Paediatric Neurology* 2002; **6**(6):321–325.

Developmental assessment

Growing up involves the acquisition of new abilities and skills, as well as physical growth. The process by which an immobile, incontinent and speechless baby develops into a mobile, communicating, socially interactive and (hopefully!) well-behaved child involves a complex interaction between genes (nature) and environment (nurture).

Much study over many years has established the average rate and pattern of development and identified a very wide range of normal variation. A child might be far from average but still normal. A major challenge is to distinguish such normal variation from a significant problem requiring active intervention.

Developmental screening is offered routinely to all children in the UK. It is one component of child health surveillance, which also encompasses physical health and growth.

The aim is to identify developmental problems at an early stage to allow appropriate intervention. Any delay might be global or specific (see Chapter 8) but it is important to bear in mind the close interrelationships involved, e.g. hearing impairment can cause a delay in speech and language, with consequent disruption of social interaction and behaviour.

Clinical assessment of a child's developmental status is based on a thorough history, physical examination, and observation of the child's performance and play.

HISTORY

Certain aspects of the history clearly assume special importance in assessing development. In particular, it is important to enquire about and document 'risk factors' that contribute to vulnerability and poor outcome (Fig. 29.1). The history should therefore include inquiry into:

- Pregnancy and birth.
- Developmental milestones: depending on age.
- Family and social history.
- Specific parental concerns.
- Parent-held personal child health record.

Milestones reflect the average age that a child acquires a particular ability:
- Motor problems often manifest in the first year.
- Talking and coordination problems often manifest in the second year.
- Behavioural and social problems often manifest in the third year.

EXAMINATION

Four aspects of development are routinely assessed:

- Gross motor.
- Fine motor and vision.
- Hearing and speech.
- Social behaviour.

Routine surveillance is carried out during well-recognized stages of development:

- Newborn.
- Supine infant (6 weeks).

- Sitting infant (8–9 months).
- Mobile toddler (18–24 months).
- Communicating child (3–4 years).
- School-age child (5 years).

The milestones for each area in each of the above age groups are considered below.

Risk factors for developmental delay
Prematurity Birth asphyxia Dysmorphology Psychosocial deprivation

Fig. 29.1 Risk factors for development.

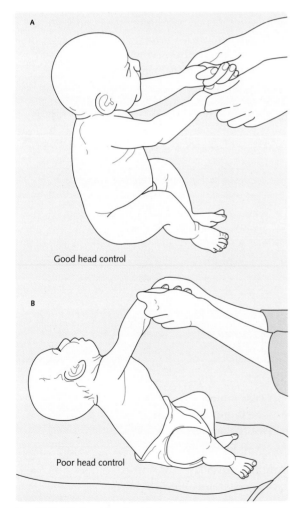

Good head control

Poor head control

Fig. 29.2 (A) Good head control compared with (B) poor head control at 6 weeks.

Newborn

Gross motor

- Symmetrical movements in all four limbs.
- Normal muscle tone.

Fine motor and vision:

- Fixes on mother's face and follows through 90°.

Hearing and speech

- Cries.

Social

- Responds to being picked up.

Six weeks

Gross motor

- Good head control when pulled up to sitting (Fig. 29.2).
- When held in ventral suspension holds head transiently in horizontal plane (Fig. 29.3).
- Presence of the Moro response (Fig. 29.4).

The Moro response consists of extension of the arms, then brisk adduction towards the chest when the infant is startled or the baby's head allowed to drop back slightly (see Fig. 29.4). It should be symmetrical and should have disappeared by 6 months. Persistence of this or any of the primitive reflexes beyond 6 months might indicate a cerebral disorder.

Fine motor and vision

- Stares at and follows mother's face.

Hearing and speech

- Coos.
- Startles to loud noises.

Social

- Smiles in response.

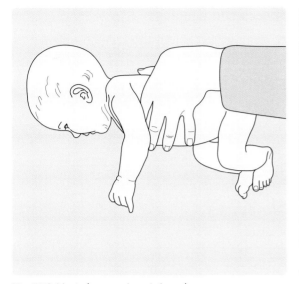

Fig. 29.3 Ventral suspension at 6 weeks.

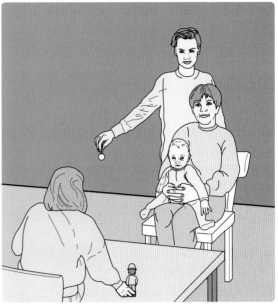

Fig. 29.5 Distraction test.

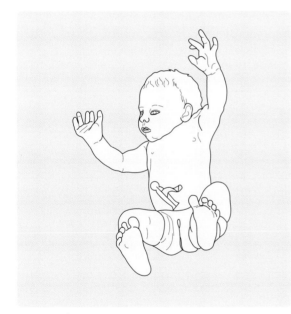

Fig. 29.4 The Moro response.

At 4–6 months the ability to roll, sit and use of both hands is dependent on the disappearance of primitive reflexes and the appearance of head and trunk righting.

Eight months

Gross motor

- Sits unsupported.
- Weight bears on legs.
- Rolls. Starting to crawl.

Fine motor and vision

- Reaches out for toys and has a palmar grasp.
- Transfers objects hand to hand or hand to mouth.
- Follows fallen toys (and points).
- Fixes on small objects.

Hearing and speech

- Babbles, e.g. 'dada'.
- Responds to own name.
- Distraction test (turns to sound) (Fig. 29.5).

Social

- Puts objects into mouth.
- Hand and foot regard.
- Plays peekaboo.
- Stranger awareness.
- Separation anxiety.

Eighteen months

Gross motor

- Walking.
- Climbs stairs two feet to a step.
- Climbs onto and sits on a chair.

Fine motor and vision

- Pincer grip (Fig. 29.6).
- Turns pages.
- Builds a three-brick tower.
- Picks up '100s-and-1000s'.

Hearing and speech

- Uses three or more words.
- Points to parts of body or named objects.
- Understands simple instructions.

Social

- Uses a spoon.
- Domestic mimicry.
- Takes off socks and shoes.
- Developing toilet awareness.

Three years

Gross motor

- Runs, jumps.
- Throws and kicks a ball.
- Pedals a tricycle.
- Climbs stairs (like an adult).

Fine motor and vision

- Threads beads on a string.
- Builds an eight-brick tower.
- Copies a line and a circle.
- Letter matching using charts.

Speech and language

- Short sentences—using and understanding prepositions, e.g. 'on'.

Social

- Toilet trained: dry by day.
- Dresses with supervision.
- Plays with other children.
- Matches two colours.

Five years

Gross motor

- Skips.
- Catches a ball.
- Heel–toe walking.

Fine motor and vision

- Draws a man with all features.
- Copies alphabet letters.
- Snellen's chart test (by name or matching).

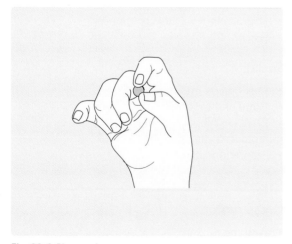

Fig. 29.6 Pincer grip.

Worrying signs	
Age	**Developmental sign**
6–8 weeks	Asymmetrical Moro Excess head lag No visual fixation/following No startle or quietening to sound No responsive smiling
8 months	Persisting primitive reflexes Not weight bearing on legs Not reaching out for toys Not fixing on small objects Not vocalizing
10 months	Unable to sit unsupported
1 year	Showing a hand preference Not responding to own name
18 months	Not walking No pincer grip Persistence of casting
3 years	Inaccurate use of a spoon Not speaking in sentences Unable to understand simple commands Unable to use the toilet alone Not interacting with other children

Fig. 29.7 Worrying signs at various ages.

Hand preference develops at 18–24 months and is fixed at 5 years. Handedness in <1 year indicates a problem with the non-dominant side.

Management options for concern over development:
- Reassure if within normal range.
- Review again.
- Refer for expert assessment.

Hearing and speech

- Comprehensive speech.

Social

- Plays games.
- Learning to read.
- Can tell the time.

Babies who were preterm need their development corrected for their gestational age but this becomes less important after 2 years of age.

SIGNS OF ABNORMAL DEVELOPMENT: 'LIMIT AGES'

Figure 29.7 lists the worrying signs at the ages given.

Investigations

Objectives

At the end of this chapter you should be able to

- Interpret the results of common blood tests.
- Understand the indications, advantages and disadvantages of common imaging studies.
- Understand the indications for certain special investigations and their interpretation.

Special investigations are often used to confirm, or refute, a diagnosis that is clinically uncertain and to monitor the progress of a disease or its treatment. They should be performed only when there are specific indications, not as a 'routine'. In all cases, the potential benefits must be weighed against any associated pain or discomfort.

'Routine' investigation is rarely good practice.

In this chapter, the indications for and interpretation of the following common and important special investigations are considered.

Tests should be done for the benefit of the patient, not the doctor.

Imaging

- Ionizing radiation: chest X-rays (CXR), abdominal X-rays (AXR), skull X-rays (SXR), computed tomography (CT) and radionuclide scanning.
- Ultrasound: antenatal ultrasound, cranial ultrasound (newborn) and abdominal and renal ultrasound.
- Magnetic resonance imaging (MRI).

Blood tests

- Haematological tests: full blood count (FBC), peripheral blood film, sickle test, haemoglobin electrophoresis, coagulation studies.
- Biochemical tests: urea and electrolytes, creatinine, liver function tests, albumin, glucose, calcium and phosphate, magnesium, blood gases and acid–base status.
- Immunology tests: tests for immunodeficiency, autoantibodies, diagnostic serology and acute phase reactants.
- Microbiology tests: blood culture.

Urine tests

- Dipstick for protein, blood, glucose and ketones.
- Microscopy and culture.

Cerebrospinal fluid

- Microscopy and culture.
- Protein and glucose levels.
- Virology.

IMAGING

All the major imaging methods are used in paediatric practice:

- Ionizing radiation: X-rays: simple or computed X-ray tomography and nuclear medicine.
- Ultrasound.
- MRI.

The main circumstances in which each of these tests can be used are described in the following sections.

X-rays

Most commonly requested are:

- CXR.
- Plain AXR.
- SXR.
- CT.

Chest X-ray

When inspecting a CXR, adopt a systematic approach for viewing and presentation:

- Check patient name, date, L/R orientation, posterior–anterior (PA), or anterior–posterior (AP).
- Note any striking abnormalities.
- Heart and mediastinum.
- Lung fields and pulmonary vessels.
- Diaphragm and subdiaphragmatic areas.
- Bony thorax.
- Soft tissues.

The cardiac shadow is not always reliable in diagnosing heart disease. Look at the lung fields and hilar shadows.

Indications for doing a CXR

Acute:

- Pneumonia.
- Severe bronchiolitis.
- Asthma: severe or first presentation.
- Cardiac failure.
- Foreign body inhalation.
- Non-accidental injury (old fractures).

Non-urgent investigation of:

- Cervical lymphadenopathy.
- TB.
- Cystic fibrosis.
- Cardiac disease.
- Malignant disease.

Abdominal X-ray

Supine AP is the standard plain film. An erect AP (or decubitus) often adds little to diagnosis. There is wide variation in the normal appearance of these X-rays.

The checklist for an AXR includes:

- Check patient name, date, erect, or supine.
- Note striking abnormalities.
- Hollow organs: stomach, bowel and bladder.
- Solid organs: liver, spleen and kidneys.
- Diaphragm.
- Bones.

Skull X-ray

The most common indication for skull radiography used to be head injury but CT scanning provides much more useful information (Fig. 30.1). These days, its primary use is in the diagnosis of non-accidental injury and craniosynostosis.

The presence of a skull fracture and/or neurological signs increases the likelihood of intracranial damage.

Computed tomography

CT scanning uses multidirectional X-rays that, instead of falling onto film, are quantified by a detector and fed into a computer. Different readings are produced as the X-ray beam rotates round the body and the information is then presented as a two-dimensional image.

CT is a useful and widely available imaging modality for evaluating brain, chest and abdominal disorders. These include:

Indication for head CT in trauma
GCS less than 15
Any skull fracture
Focal neurological signs or post traumatic seizures
Clinical features of basal skull fracture
Persistent vomiting
Anterograde amnesia

Fig. 30.1 Indication for head CT in trauma.

- Brain: intracranial haemorrhage (e.g. head injury), tumours, intracranial calcification (e.g. tuberous sclerosis).
- Chest: mediastinal masses (e.g. lymphoma), lungs (e.g. bronchiectasis).
- Abdomen: masses (e.g. neuroblastoma or Wilms'), injury (e.g. splenic rupture).

CT accurately assesses the nature of a mass, e.g. fluid, fat, necrosis or calcification. Disadvantages include a disappointing lack of contrast between different organs. Intravenous contrast enhances the resolution between tissue planes.

Stabilization of any ill child must be done prior to a CT.

Ultrasound

Ultrasound scanning (USS) uses ultra-high frequency sound waves to provide cross-sectional images of the body. In addition, Doppler ultrasound can be used for estimating the direction and velocity of blood flow.

The advantages of USS include:

- Non-invasive—no ionizing radiation involved.
- Portable equipment.

Body tissues reflect sound waves to different degrees and are therefore said to be of different echogenicity:

- Hyperechoic tissues appear white (e.g. fat).
- Hypoechoic tissues appear dark (e.g. fluid).

Ultrasound does not penetrate gas or bone and is therefore less useful for assessment of bony lesions. Intracranial contents are only accessible to ultrasound examination in young infants in whom the anterior fontanelle is still open.

The main applications include:

- Antenatal ultrasound.
- Cranial ultrasound in the neonate.
- Abdominal and renal ultrasound.
- Hip ultrasound.

Antenatal ultrasound

Initial ultrasound screening is carried out at 12 weeks (in some units) with a detailed scan at 18–20 weeks' gestation. Antenatal USS allows:

- Estimation of gestational age (less than 20 weeks).
- Identification of multiple pregnancies.
- Monitoring of fetal growth.
- Detection of structural malformations.
- Amniotic fluid volume estimation.

Neonatal cranial ultrasound

This is useful for the detection and evaluation of intracranial pathology (Fig. 30.2), including:

- Intracranial haemorrhage, e.g. intraventricular haemorrhage (IVH).
- Periventricular leucomalacia.
- Hydrocephalus.
- Cerebral malformations.

A cranial ultrasound is routine in all preterm babies under 32 weeks to look for haemorrhages.

Abdominal and renal ultrasound

Abdominal ultrasound is useful in the evaluation of:

- Abdominal pain: acute (e.g. identification of appendix abscess, intussception).
- Vomiting infant: ultrasound is the imaging of choice in pyloric stenosis.
- Liver disease: provides information on size and consistency of both the liver and spleen. The gall bladder and extrahepatic bile ducts can be visualized.

Renal ultrasound is very useful in the investigation of disorders of the genitourinary tract (Fig. 30.3). It provides information on:

- Kidney size.
- Structural abnormalities of the urinary tract, e.g. hydronephrosis, hydroureter, or increased bladder size.

Fig. 30.2 (A) A parasagittal neonatal cranial ultrasound scan showing extensive intraventricular haemorrhage. (B) Coronal ultrasound scan of a neonatal brain with hydrocephalus.

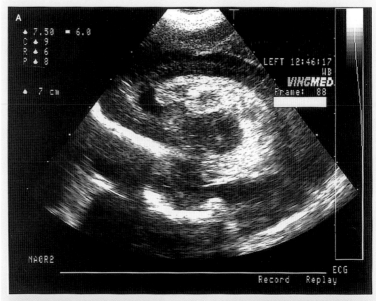

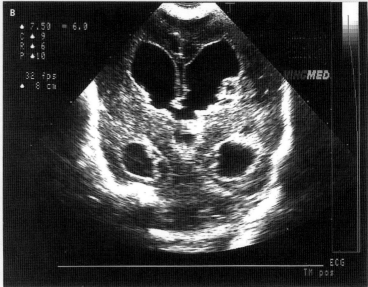

- Gross renal scarring.
- Renal calculi.
- Tumours (e.g. Wilms').

All infants and young children should have a renal USS after a confirmed UTI. Its main role is to reveal structural abnormalities and it does not reliably detect vesicoureteric reflux or minor renal scars.

Hip ultrasound

Ultrasound is a useful modality for the investigation of hip disease. It is the imaging method of choice for assessing neonatal hip instability and is more reliable than plain radiography up to the age of 6 months. It allows evaluation of:

- Acetabular morphology.
- The degree to which the acetabulum covers the femoral head.

Ultrasound is also useful in the investigation of suspected hip pathology in young children. Even small

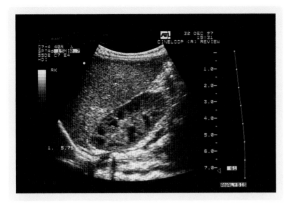

Fig. 30.3 Normal renal ultrasound. Normal prominent pyramids are demonstrated.

effusions can be detected, and needle aspiration can be carried out under ultrasound guidance.

Magnetic resonance imaging

Magnetic resonance imaging (MRI) has several distinctive features that confer a number of useful advantages:

- No ionizing radiation.
- Images can be obtained in any plane.
- Excellent soft tissue contrast.

It is the imaging modality of choice for many disorders of the brain and spine (in which sagittal views are particularly useful). MRI is also helpful in the evaluation of musculoskeletal disorders. It has not replaced other approaches, such as CT or ultrasound, in the imaging of many thoracic and abdominal disorders. Its main disadvantage in children is the need for sedation or general anaesthesia.

BLOOD TESTS

Venous or capillary blood is usually satisfactory and can be obtained by venepuncture or capillary sampling. Arterial blood sampling is only occasionally necessary for blood gas analysis or estimation of acid–base status. (Pulse oximetry has rendered arterial sampling for determination of oxygenation rarely necessary.) With experience, skill and local anaesthetic cream, blood can be obtained quickly and with minimal discomfort from most infants and children.

Blood tests fall into the following general categories. See Fig. 30.4 for clinical chemistry reference values.

Haematology

Full blood count

This provides information on:

- Haemoglobin, Hb (g/dL).
- Total white cell count, WBC ($\times 10^9$/L).
- Platelet count ($\times 10^9$/L).

Haemoglobin concentration and white cell counts must be interpreted in relation to age:
- Hb concentration is high at birth (15–19 g/dL) and falls to a nadir at 3 months (9–13 g/dL).
- The total white cell count is high at birth and rapidly falls to normal adult levels. There is a relative lymphocytosis during the first 4 years of life after the neonatal period.

It can also provide:

- Red cell indices: MCV (fl), MCH (pg), MCHC (%).
- Reticulocytes (%).
- Differential white cell count: neutrophils, lymphocytes, eosinophils, monocytes (% or 10^9/L).

The examination of the film allows evaluation of:

- Red cell morphology (Fig. 30.5).
- Differential white cell count.
- Platelet numbers and morphology.
- Presence or absence of abnormal cells (e.g. blast cells).

See also Fig. 30.6, which shows important abnormalities that can be identified from a FBC.

Sickle test

This is a screening test for the sickle cell trait or disease. Sickle cells are seen when the blood is deoxygenated with Na_2HPO_4.

291

Clinical chemistry		
Test	**Normal range (plasma or serum)**	
Sodium		133–145 mmol/L
Potassium	Infant	3.5–6.0 mmol/L
	Child	3.3–5.0 mmol/L
Urea	Neonate	1.0–5.0 mmol/L
	Infant	2.5–8.0 mmol/L
	Child	2.5–6.5 mmol/L
Creatinine	Infant	20–65 µmol/L
	1–10 years	20–80 µmol/L
Osmolality		275–295 mosm/kg
Calcium (total)	24–48 h	1.8–3.0 mmol/L
	Child	2.15–2.60 mmol/L
Calcium (ionized)	24–48 h	1.00–1.17 mmol/L
	Child	1.18–1.32 mmol/L
Phosphate	Neonate	1.4–2.6 mmol/L
	Infant	1.3–2.1 mmol/L
	Child	1.0–1.8 mmol/L
Alkaline phosphatase	Neonate	150–700 U/L
	1–12 months	250–1000 U/L
	2–9 years	250–850 U/L
	Years	females males
	10–11	250–950 U/L 250–730 U/L
	14–15	170–460 U/L 170–970 U/L
	>18	60–250 U/L 50–200 U/L
Albumin	Neonate	25–35 g/L
	Child	35–55 g/L
Creatine kinase	Infant/child	60–300 U/L
Glucose	I day	2.2–3.3 mmol/L
	>I day	2.6–5.5 mmol/L
	Child	3.0–6.0 mmol/L
Iron	Infant	5–25 µmol/L
	Child	10–30 µmol/L
Ferritin	Child	<150 µg/L
C-reactive protein		<10 mg/L
Blood gas (arterial, not preterm)	pH	7.35–7.45
	pO_2	11–14 kPa (82–105 mmHg)
	pCO_2	4.5–6.0 kPa (32–45 mmHg)
	Bicarbonate	18–25 mmol/L
	Base excess	−4 to +4 mmol/L

Fig. 30.4 Normal ranges for blood tests (normal range for some tests varies between laboratories and must be checked with the local laboratory).

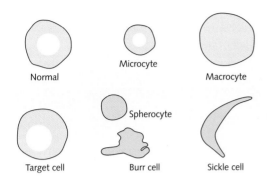

Fig. 30.5 Red cell morphology.

Important problems identifiable on a full blood count
Anaemia, e.g. iron deficiency Thrombocytopenia, e.g. idiopathic thrombocytopenic purpura Neutropenia, e.g. immunosuppression Pancytopenia, e.g. bone marrow failure Neutrophil leucocytosis, e.g. bacterial infection Lymphocytosis, e.g. *Bordetella pertussis*

Fig. 30.6 Important problems identifiable on FBC.

Structure of haemoglobin:
- Fetal haemoglobin (HbF): $\alpha_2 \gamma_2$
- Adult haemoglobin: HbA, $\alpha_2 \beta_2$; HbA2 $\alpha_2 \delta_2$
- Sickle haemoglobin (HbS): $\alpha_2 \beta_2^s$

Haemoglobin electrophoresis

The pattern of haemoglobin electrophoresis at different ages (birth and adult) and in different haemoglobinopathies is shown in Fig. 30.7.

Coagulation studies

Basic screening tests include:

- Prothrombin time (PT): usually expressed as 'international normalized ratio': INR.
- Activated partial thromboplastin time (APTT).
- Thrombin time (TT).

The evaluation of a bleeding disorder also requires an estimation of platelet numbers, morphology and function.

Common patterns of abnormality include:

- PT prolonged: liver disease.
- APTT prolonged: haemophilia (factor VIII), Christmas disease (factor IX).
- PT and APTT prolonged: vitamin K deficiency, liver disease.
- PT, APTT, TT prolonged: disseminated intravascular coagulation (DIC).

von Willebrand's disease (VWD)

This is a heterogeneous group of inherited disorders with a defect in the von Willebrand factor (which is important in platelet adhesion and as a carrier molecule for factor VIII). Bleeding time and APTT are prolonged. VWF levels can be measured directly.

Fig. 30.7 Haemoglobin (Hb) electrophoresis.

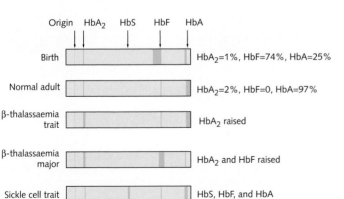

Disseminated intravascular coagulation (DIC)

Uncontrolled activation of coagulation causes:

- Widespread intravascular fibrin deposition.
- Consumption of coagulation factors and platelets.
- Accelerated degradation of fibrin and fibrinogen.

In DIC the constellation of laboratory findings includes:

- Prolonged PT, APTT, TT.
- Low fibrinogen.
- Elevated fibrinogen degradation products (FDPs) or D-dimers.
- Low platelets.
- Red cell fragmentation.

Further detailed investigations might be required, e.g. when clinical evidence indicates a bleeding disorder but screening tests are normal. These tests might include:

- Assays of individual factors (e.g. factor XIII).
- Tests for the presence of endogenous anticoagulants.

Biochemical analysis

Most biochemical analyses are carried out on plasma rather than serum (the sample must be placed in a bottle containing anticoagulant). This is heparin in most cases—glucose estimations are a notable exception and should be in fluoride oxalate. It is important to know that reference values for children are quite different to those in adults.

Urea and electrolytes (U&Es)

U&Es (urea, Na^+, K^+, Cl^-) are the most commonly requested biochemical analysis and can be useful in a host of circumstances including:

- Dehydration-diarrhoea, vomiting.
- Ill patients on IV fluids—monitoring electrolyte status.
- Diabetic ketoacidosis.
- Renal disease.
- Diuretic therapy.

Urea

Urea is a major metabolite of protein catabolism. It is synthesized in the liver and excreted by the kidneys. The plasma concentration is influenced by:

- State of hydration.
- Protein intake.
- Catabolism.
- Glomerular filtration rate (GFR).

The creatinine concentration is a more reliable indicator of renal function. The most commonly encountered cause of a raised plasma urea is dehydration.

Sodium (Na^+)

Changes in the plasma sodium concentration can reflect changes in either the sodium or water balance. Causes are shown in Figs 30.8 and 30.9.

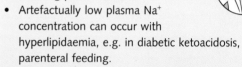

Concerning plasma sodium:
- Artefactually low plasma Na^+ concentration can occur with hyperlipidaemia, e.g. in diabetic ketoacidosis, parenteral feeding.
- A normal plasma Na^+ concentration might be found in salt depletion or overload if associated parallel changes in body water have occurred.
- Rapid falls in plasma Na^+ cause brain swelling.

Potassium (K^+)

This is a predominantly intracellular cation. Plasma concentration is therefore influenced by exchange with the intracellular compartment as well as the whole-body potassium status. The causes of changes in plasma potassium are shown in Figs 30.10 and 30.11.

Causes of hyponatraemia (Na^+ <130 mmol/L)	
Mechanism	**Cause**
Water excess	Iatrogenic: excess hypotonic IV fluids Water retention due to inappropriate ADH secretion, e.g. postoperative, meningitis, head injury
Sodium depletion	Diarrhoea Diuretics Adrenal insufficiency (rare) Cystic fibrosis/sweating (rare)

Fig. 30.8 Causes of hyponatraemia (Na^+ <130 mmol/L).

Causes of hypernatraemia (Na$^+$ >150 mmol/L)	
Mechanism	**Cause**
Water deficit	Diarrhoea
	Diabetes insipidus
	Excessive insensible water loss, e.g. overhead heater
Sodium excess	High solute intake
	Iatrogenic: excess hypertonic IV fluids
	Child abuse: salt poisoning (rare)

Fig. 30.9 Causes of hypernatraemia (Na$^+$ >150 mmol/L).

Causes of hypokalaemia (K$^+$ <3.4 mmol/L)	
Mechanism	**Cause**
Potassium depletion	Diarrhoea
	Diuretics
Inadequate intake	Daily need 2–3 mmol/kg
Redistribution	Metabolic alkalosis
	Glucose and insulin

Fig. 30.10 Causes of hypokalaemia (K$^+$ <3.4 mmol/L).

Causes of hyperkalaemia (K$^+$ >5.5 mmol/L)	
Mechanism	**Cause**
Failure of renal excretion	Renal failure
	Adrenocortical insufficiency
Redistribution	Metabolic acidosis, e.g. diabetic Ketoacidosis
Excess intake	Iatrogenic
Tissue injury	Hypoxia, catabolism
Artefact	Haemolyzed specimen

Fig. 30.11 Causes of hyperkalaemia (K$^+$ >5.5 mmol/L).

Concerning plasma potassium:
- The intracellular K$^+$ concentration is very high: >100 mmol/L.
- Acidosis brings K$^+$ out of cells in exchange for H$^+$.
- Haemolysis releases K$^+$ from red cells and causes artefactual hyperkalaemia.
- ECG changes reflect plasma K$^+$ concentration.

Plasma K$^+$ in diabetic ketoacidosis:
- Whole-body K$^+$ is always depleted.
- Plasma K$^+$ concentration might be normal, high or low, depending on the balance between acidosis and diuresis.
- Plasma K$^+$ falls with treatment as redistribution into cells occurs.

Chloride (Cl$^-$)

Hypochloraemia is seen particularly in vomiting associated with pyloric stenosis and leads to a metabolic alkalosis.

Creatinine

Creatinine is a naturally occurring substance that is formed in muscles. The normal plasma concentration increases with age as muscle mass increases with growth. The plasma concentration of creatinine is a useful indirect measure of the glomerular filtration rate (GFR). In renal failure, the creatinine concentration increases steadily by more than 30 mmol/L/day.

Liver function tests

The basic biochemical tests of liver function include bilirubin, enzymes and albumin and are outlined below.

Bilirubin
- Conjugated and unconjugated.

Enzymes
- Aspartate transaminase (AST).
- Alanine transaminase (ALT).
- Alkaline phosphatase (ALP).
- γ-glutamyltranspeptidase (γGT).

Additional investigations, which are useful for evaluating hepatic function (and are deranged in liver failure), include:

- Coagulation tests: PT, PTT.
- Ammonia.
- Glucose.

Bilirubin

Clinical evaluation of the severity of jaundice is unreliable, so it is important to document plasma levels of unconjugated and conjugated bilirubin.

The normal proportion of conjugated bilirubin should not exceed 15% in infants. The causes of hyperbilirubinaemia are considered elsewhere (see Chapter 9).

Excess conjugated hyperbilirubinaemia is a worrying sign in young infants as it might indicate biliary atresia.

Liver enzymes

Transaminases (aminotransferases) These intracellular enzymes occur in many tissues including the liver, heart and skeletal muscle. Normal plasma activity reflects release of enzymes during cell turnover and increases occur with tissue injury. Elevated serum aminotransferase activity is therefore primarily seen in hepatocyte damage, e.g. hepatitis (infection, drugs).

Raised transaminases indicate hepatocellular damage.

However, elevation is not a specific marker of primary hepatocellular disease as it occurs in other forms of hepatobiliary disease (e.g. biliary atresia, cholecystitis) and also in non-hepatic conditions such as myocarditis and pancreatitis.

AST is the more sensitive indicator of liver injury but ALT is more specific.

Alkaline phosphatase Isoenzymes of alkaline phosphatase are widely distributed in many organs including liver and bone. Normal activity levels change markedly throughout childhood and reference ranges are both age- and method-dependent. Activity is increased in:

- Biliary obstruction: intrahepatic or extrahepatic.
- Hepatocellular damage.
- Increased osteoblastic activity, e.g. rickets normal growth and pubertal growth spurt.

γ-glutamyltranspeptidase Serum activity is commonly raised in liver disease especially when there is cholestasis. It might also be raised in the absence of liver disease in patients taking certain drugs, e.g. phenytoin, phenobarbitone and rifampicin (as a result of enzyme induction).

Albumin

Albumin is synthesized in the liver and is the main contributor to plasma oncotic pressure. It also has an important role as the protein to which many circulating substances are bound such as:

- Bilirubin.
- Calcium.
- Drugs.
- Hormones.

Albumin has a long half-life of about 20 days.

Plasma albumin levels are a useful indicator of hepatic function. Low levels occur in several important clinical contexts (Fig. 30.12).

Prolonged hypoalbuminaemia (e.g. in nephrotic syndrome) is associated with oedema because fluid leaks into the extravascular space and hypovolaemia triggers renal salt and water retention.

Glucose

Blood glucose concentrations are normally maintained within fairly narrow limits, which are lower in the newborn. Blood glucose can be estimated very rapidly at the bedside using test sticks but values should be verified by laboratory investigation.

Causes of hypoalbuminaemia (<30 g/L)	
Type	**Cause**
Decreased synthesis	Chronic liver disease Malnutrition (protein–energy malnutrition) Malabsorption
Increased losses	Nephrotic syndrome Burns Protein-losing enteropathy

Fig. 30.12 Causes of hypoalbuminaemia (albumin <30 g/L).

Always measure the blood glucose urgently in a fitting or unconscious child.

The only common causes of hyperglycaemia in children is insulin-dependent type 1 diabetes mellitus and severe stress states. There are, however, many causes of hypoglycaemia (Fig. 30.13).

Calcium and phosphate

Disorders of calcium and phosphate metabolism in childhood are uncommon and usually reflect abnormalities in the major controlling hormones, vitamin D and parathormone. Laboratory estimations provide a measure of both total and ionized calcium. Changes in plasma albumin concentration affect total calcium levels independently of ionized calcium, leading to misinterpretation if serum albumin is outside the normal range. Therefore, the total calcium concentration needs to be corrected to give the expected value if albumin were in the normal range. Major causes of hypercalcaemia and hypocalcaemia are shown in Fig. 30.14.

Calcium (and magnesium) levels should be measured in infants with seizures.

Blood gases and acid–base metabolism

Metabolism generates acid, which is eliminated via the lungs as carbon dioxide and via the kidneys as hydrogen ions. Acidosis, from whatever cause, is a much more common problem than alkalosis. Ideally, estimations of blood gas and acid–base status are made on an arterial sample from an indwelling catheter, but capillary or venous blood can be useful for pH and PCO_2 measurements.

Where the main concern is oxygenation, non-invasive pulse oximetry is a valuable alternative to arterial blood gas analysis.

The pattern of changes seen in different forms of acidosis and alkalosis are shown in Fig. 30.15.

Common clinical contexts in which these disturbances occur include:

- Respiratory acidosis: hypoventilation (e.g. respiratory distress syndrome, severe asthma, neuromuscular diseases).
- Metabolic acidosis: diabetic ketoacidosis, hypoxia, circulatory failure.
- Respiratory alkalosis: hyperventilation, e.g. hysterical (rare in children), iatrogenic (ventilated patients).
- Metabolic alkalosis: pyloric stenosis.

Immunology

Tests of the immune system carried out on the blood might be required in the following clinical contexts:

Causes of hypercalcaemia and hypocalcaemia	
Hypocalcaemia	**Hypercalcaemia**
Rickets (low phosphate, high alkaline phosphatase) Hypoparathyroidism, e.g. DiGeorge syndrome Hypoalbuminaemia	Hyperparathyroidism Syndromic (Williams syndrome) Vitamin D excess

Fig. 30.14 Causes of hypocalcaemia and hypercalcaemia.

Causes of hyperglycaemia and hypoglycaemia	
Hyperglycaemia	**Hypoglycaemia**
Diabetes mellitus • IDDM (most common) • Secondary—pancreatic disease, Cushing syndrome Stress-related, e.g. postconvulsive iatrogenic • Drugs, e.g. corticosteroids • Total parenteral nutrition	Neonatal • Infant of diabetic mother • Small for gestational age Postneonatal • Ketotic hypoglycaemia • Hyperinsulinaemia—known diabetic, pancreatic tumour (rare) • ↓GH, ACTH, cortisol—hypopituitarism (rare), adrenal failure (rare)

Fig. 30.13 Causes of hyperglycaemia and hypoglycaemia.

Fig. 30.15 Acid-base disturbances.

	pH	PaCO$_2$	HCO$_3^-$
Acid−base disturbances			
Acidosis Respiratory	Low	High	Normal or high (compensation)
Metabolic	Low	Normal or low (compensation)	Low
Alkalosis Respiratory	High	Low	Normal or low (compensation)
Metabolic	High	Normal or high (compensation)	High

- Immunodeficiency.
- Autoimmune disease.
- Infection: diagnostic serology, acute-phase reactants.

Tests for immunodeficiency

Immunodeficiencies can be primary or secondary. The inherited primary deficiencies are rare; secondary causes are far more common (Fig. 30.16).

Immunodeficiency should be suspected in the following clinical circumstances:

- Recurrent severe infections.
- Infections with atypical organisms.
- Common infections with a severe or atypical clinical course.
- Failure to thrive.

Basic screening tests of immune function should include:

- Immunoglobulins.
- FBC including differential WCC and lymphocyte subsets.

Immunoglobulins

Serum immunoglobulin levels vary with age. Maternally transferred IgG is present at high levels at birth but has mostly disappeared by 6 months of age. This decline occurs before endogenous synthesis has fully developed, creating a physiological trough between 3 and 6 months of age. This is shown in Fig. 30.17.

IgG is the major immunoglobulin in normal human serum accounting for about 70% of the total pool. There are four distinct subclasses (IgG-1 to

Causes of immunodeficiency

Primary
  Primary antibody deficiencies:
  - Common variable immune deficiency
  - X-linked antibody deficiency
  - IgG subclass deficiency
  - Specific antibody deficiency
  - Selective IgA deficiency
  Severe combined immunodeficiency
  Chronic granulomatous disease
Secondary
  Malnutrition
  Infections, e.g. HIV, measles
  Immunosuppressive therapy, e.g. steroids, cytotoxic drugs
  Hyposplenism, e.g. sickle cell disease, splenectomy

Fig. 30.16 Causes of immunodeficiency.

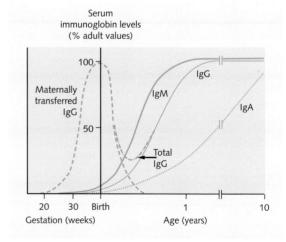

Fig. 30.17 Serum immunoglobulin (Ig) levels in fetus and infant.

IgG-4), which have different functions. Specific IgM changes are very useful in the diagnosis of viral infections, e.g. rubella.

- IgG2 is the most common subclass deficiency and might be associated with IgA deficiency. The total IgG level might be normal. It causes recurrent respiratory infections, e.g. sinusitis, pneumonia.
- Selective IgA deficiency is common (1 : 700 population) and might cause no symptoms.

Differential white cell count

Immunodeficiency caused by marrow-suppressive cytotoxic or immunosuppressive therapy is related to the absolute neutrophil count. Patients with absolute neutrophil counts below 1.0×10^9/L are at increased risk of Gram-negative septicaemia.

Lymphocyte subsets

Lymphocytes are further subdivided into T cells and B cells. T cells are categorized into:

- Cytotoxic T cells (TC), which are mostly CD8$^+$.
- Helper T cells (TH), which are mostly CD4$^+$.

Cytotoxic T cells recognize infected target cells and lyse them. Helper T cells secrete regulatory molecules (lymphokines) that affect other T cells and cells of various lineages.

Monitoring absolute numbers of CD4$^+$ helper cells is useful in monitoring the progression of HIV-related diseases.

Autoantibodies

Autoimmune disease is uncommon in childhood but includes such entities as juvenile chronic arthritis (JIA), systemic lupus erythematosus (SLE) and autoimmune thyroiditis causing juvenile hypothyroidism.

The following tests might be of value.

Antinuclear antibodies (ANA)

A broad group of antibodies present in 5% of normal children and induced by a wide spectrum of inflammatory conditions.

- High titres of ANA occur in 95% of SLE patients.

- The presence of ANA in subgroups of JIA is a risk factor for chronic anterior uveitis.

SLE is associated with antibodies against specific nuclear antigens such as double-stranded DNA.

Rheumatoid factors (RFs)

These are IgM autoantibodies against IgG. They should not be used to screen for JIA because they are neither sensitive nor specific. The majority of children with JIA are rheumatoid factor negative. Rheumatoid factors can be useful as a prognostic indicator in polyarticular JIA (their persistent presence is a poor prognostic factor).

Thyroid antibodies

Thyroid microsomal (peroxisomal) and thyroglobulin titres should be measured in suspected autoimmune thyroiditis.

Diagnostic serology

This is most widely used in the diagnosis of viral infections but is also of value in certain specific non-viral infections such as *Mycoplasma pneumoniae*, group A β-haemolytic streptococci and *Salmonella* spp.

Viral antibody tests

Serological diagnosis depends on the detection of virus antibody. Diagnosis of recent infection requires the demonstration of a rising titre of specific IgM between the acute phase and convalescence. Methods used include:

- Immunofluorescence.
- Enzyme-linked immunoabsorbent assay (ELISA).
- Radioimmune assay (RIA).

Epstein–Barr virus (EBV)

Specific EBV serology is the most reliable diagnostic test. Antibodies to viral capsid antigen (VCA) are detected. IgG anti-VCA merely indicates a past infection. A positive IgM to VCA is diagnostic and is found early in the disease.

Tests for heterophile antibody, which agglutinates sheep red blood cells, are the basis of slide agglutination tests (monospot and Paul–Bunnell). However, this antibody does not appear until the second week or even later, and may not be produced at all in young children.

Mycoplasma pneumoniae

Diagnosis of infection with *Mycoplasma pneumoniae* is most quickly established by acute and convalescent serology: a four-fold rise in complement-fixing antibodies is diagnostic.

Antistreptolysin O titre (ASOT)

Estimation of antibody to streptolysin O is a useful means of retrospectively diagnosing infection by group A β-haemolytic streptococci. The ASOT is a valuable investigation in the evaluation of:

- Suspected acute nephritis.
- Rheumatic fever.
- Scarlet fever.

This test is being replaced by antiDNAseB.

Acute-phase reactants

An inflammatory stimulus provokes the production of proteins in the liver known as the acute-phase reactants. This response is documented by the measurement of:

- C-reactive protein (CRP).
- Erythrocyte sedimentation rate (ESR).

The response is non-specific and does not help in identifying aetiology. However, if acute phase reactants are elevated at the onset of disease, serial measurements are useful for monitoring progress.

The response times vary:

- CRP: elevated within 6 hours.
- ESR: peaks at 3–4 days.

Microbiology

Blood is normally sterile. Transient asymptomatic bacteraemia can occur after dental treatment, or invasive procedures such as catheterization. However, bacteraemia leading to septicaemia and shock can accompany a number of important childhood diseases such as pneumonia, meningitis and typhoid fever.

Blood culture should be taken under the following circumstances:

- Pyrexia of unknown origin.
- Clinical signs of septicaemia.
- Febrile illness: in an immunodeficient child (e.g. sickle-cell disease, nephrotic syndrome, neutropenia) or in patients with a central catheter.

- Investigation of specific infections: meningitis, pneumonia, pyelonephritis, enteric fever.

The most common pathogens recovered from the blood are shown in Figs 30.18 and 30.19. Most significant isolates will be obtained within 48 hours of inoculation, especially in septic neonates.

Upper respiratory culture

- Nasopharyngeal aspirates are best for diagnosing viral respiratory tract infections. They are sent for immunofluorescence and results are usually back on the same day. Rapid antigen tests for influenza are available and can offer a bedside diagnosis.
- Throat swabs are useful to diagnose pharyngeal infections.
- A pernasal swab is used to diagnose pertussis infection.

URINE TESTS

Urine samples are examined in the following ways:

- Dipsticks (sticks are available that test for: protein, glucose, ketones, blood, pH, urobilinogen, leucocytes and nitrites).
- Microscopy and culture (bacteria are easily identified on microscopy of an uncentrifuged

Common causes of septicaemia in children after the newborn period
Streptococcus pneumoniae Neisseria meningitidis Staphylococcus aureus Salmonella spp. Haemophilus influenzae type B

Fig. 30.18 Common causes of septicaemia in children after the newborn period.

Common causes of septicaemia in the newborn
Group B streptococcus Staphylococcus aureus Coagulase-negative staphylococci Coliforms • Enterococcus • E. coli • Klebsiella

Fig. 30.19 Common causes of septicaemia in the newborn.

sample; a centrifuged sample is necessary to examine the urinary sediment).

Dipstick testing

In certain clinical contexts, urine testing by dipstick is mandatory. These include:

- History of polyuria, polydipsia: diabetes mellitus?
- Generalized oedema: nephrotic syndrome?

Microscopy and culture

Microscopy is required to look for casts and red cells in suspected glomerular disease, and is combined with culture in the investigation of suspected urinary tract infection (UTI).

Collection of an uncontaminated urine sample presents a problem in infants and young children. Alternative methods for collection in babies include:

- A clean-catch sample into a sterile pot.
- A pad system or an adhesive plastic bag applied to the perineum after careful washing ('bag' urine). The pad system reduces the false positives that are common with the bag system.
- Suprapubic aspiration (SPA): appropriate in a severely ill infant less than 6 months requiring urgent diagnosis.

The urine should be examined microscopically and cultured immediately, or refrigerated (to prevent overgrowth of contaminants) if there is unavoidable delay.

In UTI, pus cells and bacteria might be seen on microscopy. However, pyuria can occur with fever in the absence of UTI, and cell lysis might obscure pyuria if the sample is not examined immediately. The urine white cell count is not therefore a reliable feature in the diagnosis of UTI.

A mixed growth in the absence of pyuria usually represents contamination. Confident diagnosis of a UTI requires a bacterial culture of more than 10^8/L colony-forming units of a single species in a properly collected specimen.

CEREBROSPINAL FLUID

Cerebrospinal fluid (CSF) is usually obtained by lumbar puncture. This is the critical investigation for the diagnosis of meningitis. The CSF can be evaluated in several ways including (Fig. 30.20):

- Appearance.
- Pressure.
- Microbiology: microscopy (white cell count/ mm^3, organisms—Gram stain or acid-fast?), culture and sensitivity.
- Biochemistry: protein (g/L), glucose (mmol/L).
- Rapid diagnostic techniques: countercurrent immunoelectrophoresis, latex agglutination, polymerase chain reaction.

Concerning meningitis:
- Infants might have non-specific clinical signs; a high index of suspicion is therefore required, and a low threshold for performing a lumbar puncture.
- A missed diagnosis can be catastrophic.

Type	Appearance	WBC (mm³)	Protein (g/L)	Glucose
Normal CSF (not neonatal)	Clear	0–5	0.15–0.4	>50% blood glucose
Bacterial meningitis	Turbid	500–10 000 polymorphs	0.4–3	Low
Viral meningitis	Clear	<1000	<10	Normal
TB meningitis	Clear/viscous	Up to 500 Usually <100	>10	Low

A summary of the content and appearance of CSF in different types of meningitis

Fig. 30.20 A summary of the content and appearance of cerebrospinal fluid in different types of meningitis.

Lumbar puncture is contraindicated in the following circumstances:
- Signs of raised intracranial pressure.
- Focal neurological signs.
- Rapidly deteriorating conscious level.
- Bradycardia.
- A coagulation defect.
- Skin infection at the lumbar puncture site.

Appearance

Normal CSF is clear. If the cell count increases to more than 500 cells/mm^3, it becomes turbid. Typically, this occurs in bacterial meningitis.

Microbiology

Microscopy

Normally, a few (<5 cells/mm^3) white cells can be found in CSF. The presence of polymorphs is always abnormal except in the neonatal period when up to 30 white cells/mm^3 can be physiological. In the early stages of meningitis, white cells might not be detectable but classically very high counts are found.

Spun CSF is routinely Gram stained:

- Gram-negative cocci: *Neisseria meningitidis*.
- Gram-positive cocci: *Streptococcus pneumoniae*.
- Gram-negative coccobacilli: *Haemophilus influenzae*.

Culture and sensitivity

This is always carried out even if the sample is clear and no white cells were detected on microscopy. Viral studies should be sent in encephalitis.

Biochemistry

Protein

Protein content of the CSF rises in bacterial meningitis. Note that in neonates the normal levels are high compared with older children and adults.

Glucose

Normal CSF glucose is approximately two-thirds of the blood glucose level. In bacterial meningitis, it drops to less than 40% of the blood glucose level.

Rapid diagnostic techniques

Bacterial antigens can now be detected by sensitive and rapid tests including:

- Countercurrent immunoelectrophoresis.
- Latex agglutination.

Sufficient antigen remains present even after treatment with antibiotics has been initiated and when direct culture is no longer possible. Unfortunately, neither test is reliable at detecting group B meningococcus, which is the most common type in the UK.

Polymerase chain reaction and DNA hybridization

New techniques that detect bacterial DNA, and viral DNA or RNA are becoming available. These tests are having an increasing role in early and more sensitive detection of infection.

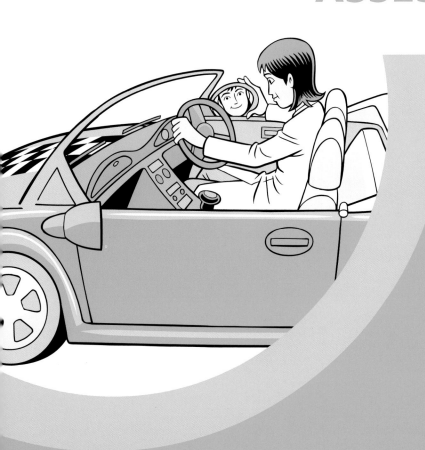

SELF-ASSESSMENT

Multiple-choice questions (MCQs)

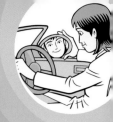

Indicate whether each answer is true or false.

1. **In a febrile child:**
   a. Sepsis is excluded by blood tests.
   b. Lumbar puncture should be done in all <2 months.
   c. A low white cell count is reassuring.
   d. Antibiotics should be withheld until a cause is known.
   e. The condition is commonly due to self-limiting viral infections.

2. **The rash of meningococcal sepsis:**
   a. Is usually non-blanching.
   b. Is pathognomic of meningococcus.
   c. Can be macular.
   d. All cases warrant an immediate lumbar puncture to detect meningitis.
   e. Is usually a late sign.

3. **In a child with stridor:**
   a. Croup is commonly caused by parainfluenza virus.
   b. The cause can be an inhaled foreign body.
   c. The sound is caused by upper airway obstruction.
   d. Epiglottitis is associated with rapid deterioration.
   e. The voice is unaffected in croup.

4. **In the wheezy child:**
   a. Asthma is the most common cause in children under 2 years of age.
   b. It can be caused by a viral respiratory infection.
   c. Sudden onset suggests asthma.
   d. The wheeze is caused by lower airway obstruction.
   e. Poor weight gain and steatorrhoea may suggest cystic fibrosis.

5. **In a comatose child:**
   a. Response only to pain is associated with a GCS of less than 8.
   b. If febrile, lumbar puncture should be done immediately to rule out meningitis.
   c. Seizures are always indicative of meningitis.
   d. Blood sugar measurement is a priority.
   e. Raised intracranial pressure is diagnosed by examination of the pupils alone.

6. **Seizures in a child:**
   a. Should always be treated with anticonvulsants.
   b. Can be caused by minor trauma.
   c. Are associated with migraine.
   d. Can occur in an awake child.
   e. Epilepsy improves with age in most children.

7. **Septic arthritis:**
   a. Is ruled out by normal white cell counts.
   b. Can cause joint damage if not treated urgently.
   c. Is caused by haematogenous spread.
   d. Produces early changes on X-ray.
   e. Can be caused by TB.

8. **Anaemia in childhood:**
   a. Is commonly symptomatic.
   b. Is always treated by transfusion.
   c. A haemoglobin of 9 gdl in a 6 month old is always abnormal
   d. With subcutaneous bleeding like petechiae, purpura suggests bone marrow failure.
   e. Is most commonly due to iron deficiency.

9. **Clotting defects in children:**
   a. Are always due to a genetic defect.
   b. Thrombolic events in childhood warrant further investigation for an underlying disorder.
   c. Haemophilia can be acquired.
   d. Should be checked if non-accidental injury suspected.
   e. Improves with age.

10. **Regarding developmental delay:**
    a. It can be caused by thyroid problems.
    b. It is seen in Down syndrome.
    c. Late walkers have lower IQs in later life.
    d. Walking is not delayed unless >2 years.
    e. Hearing abnormalities can lead to delayed speech development.

11. **Regarding short stature:**
    a. It can be caused by corticosteroids.
    b. Bone age is a useful investigation.
    c. Correction for prematurity should always be done in children over 2 years.
    d. Growth velocity obtained by yearly measurements.
    e. It is the same as failure to thrive.

12. **A 9-month-old child:**
    a. Can sit unsupported.
    b. Has a palmar grip.
    c. Produces babbling noises.
    d. Can fix on small objects.
    e. Cannot transfer objects between their hands.

13. **Worrying developmental signs are:**
    a. Not walking at 18 months.
    b. Handedness fixed at 1 years of age.
    c. Moro reflex at 6 months.
    d. Bottom shuffling.
    e. Head lag at 2 weeks.

14. **In childhood HIV:**
    a. Vertical transmission is decreasing.
    b. Breastfeeding is contraindicated.
    c. Diagnosis is by serology in all cases.
    d. MMR should not be given because it is live vaccine.
    e. Antiviral treatment should not be given to neonates with HIV.

15. **Measles:**
    a. Can mimic Kawasaki disease.
    b. Is associated with neurological sequelae.
    c. Is a leading cause of death in children.
    d. Vaccination requires high uptake for herd immunity.
    e. Lymphadenopathy is common.

16. **In childhood anaphylaxis:**
    a. Intravenous adrenaline (epinephrine) is the treatment of choice.
    b. Insect venom is an uncommon cause.
    c. Epipens should be given to all with previous anaphylaxis.
    d. Cardiovascular symptoms are more common than respiratory.
    e. MMR should not be given if there is a history of anaphylaxis to egg.

17. **Skin-prick testing:**
    a. Antihistamines should be stopped before testing.
    b. A negative test definitely rules out allergy.
    c. Can be done on all ages.
    d. Has similar sensitivity and specificity as RAST testing.
    e. Severity of reaction correlates with clinical symptoms.

18. **Regarding symptoms of allergy:**
    a. They diminish with age.
    b. In infants they are commonly caused by inhalation antigens.
    c. Latex allergy is associated with banana allergy.
    d. They are always caused by IgE.
    e. They can manifest as failure to thrive.

19. **In a child with itchy skin:**
    a. Scabies can be seen on the feet in infants.
    b. Seborrhoeic eczema is the commonest cause.
    c. Antihistamines are useful.
    d. Head lice might be seen on the scalp.
    e. Molluscum contagiosum might be a cause.

20. **Atopic eczema:**
    a. Persists into adulthood in 60%.
    b. Requires treatment with systemic steroids.
    c. Might require antibiotics.
    d. Is associated with asthma.
    e. Emollients can be used continuously.

21. **Patent ductus arteriosus:**
    a. Is common in preterm infants.
    b. Can be associated with endocarditis.
    c. Can spontaneously resolve in preterm infants.
    d. Closes at 24–48 h in term infants.
    e. Has a continuous murmur.

22. **A ventricular septal defect:**
    a. Is not usually haemodynamically significant.
    b. The murmur corresponds to clinical severity.
    c. Is common in trisomy 21.
    d. Has an ejection systolic murmur.
    e. Causes a left to right shunt.

23. **In cyanotic heart disease:**
    a. The presence of a PDA might be essential.
    b. There is always decreased pulmonary blood flow.
    c. Infants might be normal on examination at birth.
    d. Tetralogy of Fallot is complicated by congestive cardiac failure.
    e. Prostaglandin infusion might be lifesaving.

24. **Regarding gastro-oesophageal reflux:**
    a. Most resolve after 1 year of age.
    b. A 24-h pH study is diagnostic in all children.
    c. It might cause apnoea.
    d. It might cause failure to thrive.
    e. Should be treated with cisapride.

25. **Pyloric stenosis:**
    a. Presents with projectile vomiting.
    b. Usually requires surgery.
    c. Is associated with alkalosis.
    d. Occurs more commonly in girls.
    e. Causes bilious vomiting.

26. **In a child with haematuria:**
    a. There might be a preceding sore throat.
    b. Blood pressure might be raised.
    c. Abdominal X-ray is not indicated.
    d. Henoch–Schönlein purpura may be a cause.
    e. Abdominal ultrasound is not usually useful.

27. **All children with proven urinary infection:**
    a. Require micturating cystography.
    b. Need a blood pressure measurement.
    c. Need prophylactic antibiotics.
    d. Require treatment even if asymptomatic.
    e. Have dysuria.

28. Regarding haemolytic-uraemic syndrome (HUS):

a. It is the most common cause of acute renal failure.
b. It is caused by a specific *Escherichia coli*.
c. Jaundice might be present.
d. Platelet levels are high.
e. It requires prompt antibiotics.

29. In childhood Guillain–Barré syndrome:

a. Prognosis is better than for adults.
b. Treatment is always with steroids.
c. Neurological sequelae are common.
d. Dysrhythmias might occur.
e. *Campylobacter* infection might precede illness.

30. Regarding a child who presents with seizures:

a. Anticonvulsants should always be started.
b. The EEG might be normal.
c. 50% will have no cause.
d. The condition improves with age.
e. Checking blood glucose should be routine.

31. Regarding muscular dystrophies:

a. Becker is associated with a better prognosis than Duchenne.
b. They might be asymptomatic at birth.
c. Creatinine kinase levels are always raised in all muscular dystrophies.
d. Respiratory failure is untreatable.
e. Duchenne is autosomal recessive.

32. Sudden infant death syndrome:

a. Is associated with sleeping supine.
b. Is associated with bed-sharing.
c. Occurs up to 5 years of age.
d. Is prevented by apnoea alarms.
e. Is caused by viruses.

33. In suspected child abuse:

a. Failure to thrive might be present.
b. Clotting studies should be carried out if bruising is present.
c. All cases will require hospital admission.
d. Physical findings are present in all sexual abuse cases.
e. Younger children are at higher risk.

34. In Down syndrome:

a. Echocardiography is indicated in all cases after diagnosis.
b. The genetic abnormality is always trisomy 21.
c. IQ is usually normal.
d. There is an association with adrenal abnormalities.
e. Hypotonia in the neonatal period is a frequent physical feature.

35. Regarding autosomal dominant disorders:

a. They include achondroplasia.
b. They can skip generations.
c. Male-to-male transmission does not occur.
d. Males outnumber females.
e. They are associated with parental consanguinity.

36. When feeding the neonate:

a. Breastfeeding is contraindicated in galactosaemia.
b. Soya milks are useful if allergies are a concern.
c. Weight gain is the best measure of adequate calorie intake.
d. Preterm infants might need supplemental feeds.
e. Breast milk is protective against infection.

37. Prescribing in young children:

a. The intramuscular route is commonly used.
b. Oral medications in neonates are reliable.
c. Paracetamol toxicity is more common than in adults.
d. Many drugs in daily use are unlicensed.
e. The per rectum route is useful in status epilepticus.

38. In head injuries:

a. Skull X-rays are indicated.
b. CT should be carried out in all with a GCS <13.
c. CSF otorrhoea, Panda eyes and haemotympanum suggest basal skull fracture.
d. Cranial sutures can mimic fractures.
e. Occipital fractures are associated with abuse.

39. Regarding the collection of microbiological cultures:

a. This should be prior to antibiotic treatment.
b. Lumbar puncture is always indicated immediately in comatose children
c. Urine should be collected by suprapubic aspirate in <3 months.
d. PCR of the CSF is useful in meningitis.
e. Blood cultures are often positive in septic neonates.

40. Regarding childhood diabetes:

a. Type 1 is more common.
b. Intensive control does not lead to hypoglycaemia.
c. Insulin requirements decrease during puberty.
d. Oral glucose tolerance test is needed for diagnosis.
e. Hypoglycaemic awareness is decreased in children.

41. In congenital adrenal hyperplasia:

a. Neonatal screening is routine part of the Guthrie test.
b. Mineralcorticoid function is unaffected.
c. Inheritance is autosomal recessive.
d. Treatment is life long.
e. Most common defect is 11-hydroxylase deficiency.

307

42. In neonates:

 a. Galactosaemia is associated with jaundice.
 b. Coarse facies are seen in mucopolysaccharidosis.
 c. Phenylketonuria is symptomatic.
 d. Ketonuria is common.
 e. Hypoglycaemia is commonly asymptomatic.

43. Regarding haemophilia:

 a. Haemophilia A is due to factor IX deficiency.
 b. Diagnosis is confirmed by specific factor assay.
 c. APTT is usually normal.
 d. Inheritance is autosomal dominant.
 e. Bleeding due to haemophilia B is treated with prothrombin complex concentrate.

44. Regarding nocturnal enuresis:

 a. A 4 year old who regularly wets the bed needs treatment.
 b. Constipation can be a causative factor.
 c. Examination of the spine is important.
 d. Urinalysis should be done in all children for proteinuria and glycosuria.
 e. Star charts can be useful in treatment.

45. Developmental dysplasia of the hip:

 a. Was previously called congenital dislocation of the hip.
 b. Always requires treatment with a hip spica.
 c. Is increased in breech deliveries.
 d. Clinical assessment will detect all cases.
 e. Can be associated with asymmetrical skin creases.

46. Regarding hip pain in children:

 a. The cause can be detected on plain radiographs.
 b. Perthes' disease usually affects girls in adolescence.
 c. It might present with knee pain.
 d. Transient synovitis is self-limiting.
 e. Septic arthritis should always be ruled out.

47. In childhood arthritis:

 a. There is an association with autoimmune diseases.
 b. The use of non-steroidal anti-inflammatory drugs is contraindicated.
 c. Methotrexate is a second-line drug.
 d. Ocular symptoms might be present.
 e. The child might be Rheumatoid Factor negative.

48. Regarding iron deficiency anaemia:

 a. Iron stores are adequate until 1 year of age.
 b. A macrocytic anaemia is present.
 c. The cause could be a bleeding Meckel's diverticulum.
 d. Formula milk has more iron than breast milk.
 e. 50% of all dietary iron is absorbed.

49. Regarding haemophilia:

 a. Factor VII deficiency is seen in haemophilia A.
 b. It can be treated with desmopressin.
 c. There is always a family history.
 d. Diagnosis is by measuring APTT.
 e. Haemophilia B is caused by factor IX deficiency.

50. Low platelet levels in children:

 a. Always require treatment.
 b. Might be associated with infection.
 c. Can be caused by autoantibodies.
 d. Can manifest as petechiae.
 e. Are seen in von Willebrand's disease.

51. Childhood leukaemia:

 a. Carries a worse prognosis than adult leukaemia.
 b. Requires bone marrow transplantation in the majority.
 c. Requires CNS therapy in the early stages.
 d. Requires bone marrow analysis for diagnosis.
 e. Has a worse prognosis in <1-year-old infants.

52. Regarding solid tumours in childhood:

 a. Most are CNS tumours.
 b. Wilms' tumour causes hypotension.
 c. Bone tumours are seen mostly in long bones.
 d. They have a worse prognosis than leukaemias.
 e. Brain tumours are found mainly in the posterior fossa.

53. Attention Deficit Hyperactivity Disorder:

 a. Affects 1 in 200 children.
 b. Is treated by stimulant drugs.
 c. Is not commonly associated with other psychiatric disorders.
 d. Can be caused by obstructive sleep apnoea.
 e. Symptoms continue into adulthood in 50%.

54. Regarding HIV in pregnancy:

 a. Caesarean section reduces vertical transmission.
 b. AZT should be given to all babies born to an HIV-positive mother.
 c. The incidence of vertical transmission is 10%.
 d. Breastfeeding should be discouraged.
 e. Diagnosis can be reliable by serology in children less than 1 year of age.

55. During neonatal resuscitation:

 a. Active babies with meconium staining should be suctioned.
 b. CPR should be started if the heart rate <60 beats/minute.
 c. The Apgar score is done at the time of birth.
 d. Maternal drugs can cause depressed respiration at birth.
 e. All preterm babies need to be admitted to a neonatal unit.

56. Regarding necrotizing enterocolitis:

a. It affects only preterm babies.
b. Breast milk is protective.
c. It is always caused by infections.
d. It can be associated with bowel perforation.
e. Total parenteral nutrition and nil by mouth is part of the treatment.

57. In shock:

a. Children decompensate earlier than adults.
b. Fluids are one of the first lines of treatment.
c. Hypotension is a late sign.
d. AVPU assessment is useful?
e. Viruses can be a cause.

58. Regarding paediatric cardiac arrest:

a. Asystole is the most common rhythm.
b. It can be caused by hypovolaemia.
c. It is treated by early high-dose adrenaline (epinephrine).
d. It can be caused by insect stings.
e. Outcome is poor if longer than 20 minutes.

59. In the normal neonate:

a. Breathing is regular and without pauses.
b. Sacral dimples are always abnormal.
c. The foreskin should never be pulled back.
d. A single umbilical artery is not associated with other anomalies
e. Respiratory rate of 60/min is normal.

60. Regarding a child with a murmur:

a. A diastolic murmur is always pathological.
b. A palpable thrill is not always pathological.
c. Innocent murmurs commonly vary with posture.
d. Innocent murmurs are most commonly ejection systolic.
e. A venous hum is most prominent when lying flat.

61. In a child with stridor:

a. A toxic, unwell appearance suggests croup.
b. Intravenous antibiotics is the priority if epiglottitis is suspected.
c. Vascular rings are common causes of acute stridor.
d. Drooling is a feature of acute epiglottitis.
e. Antibiotics should be given if croup is suspected.

62. In a child with vomiting:

a. Bilious vomiting is always significant.
b. Pyloric stenosis is a common cause of bilious vomiting.
c. Gastrooesophageal reflux is a common cause of vomiting in infants.
d. Pyloric stenosis usually presents in babies between 3 weeks and 3 months of age.
e. Increased intracranial pressure can be a cause of vomiting.

63. In a child with haematuria:

a. It is very important to check the blood pressure.
b. Associated loin pain suggests pyelonephritis.
c. A history of sore throat is always present in poststreptococcal glomerulonephritis.
d. Presence of purpuric rash along the extensor aspects suggests Henoch–Schönlein purpura.
e. UTI can be a cause.

64. Vasovagal syncope:

a. Commonly affects teenagers.
b. Attacks usually last for more than 30 minutes.
c. An ECG should be an important part of the investigation in a child with a fainting attack.
d. Can be associated with nausea and dizziness.
e. Can be precipitated by prolonged standing in a hot environment.

65. Breath holding attacks:

a. Is common in babies under 6 months.
b. Can be associated with few jerky movements.
c. An EEG is diagnostic.
d. Can lead to developmental delay if untreated.
e. Sodium valproate is the drug of choice for treatment.

66. In an unconscious child:

a. Checking blood sugar is part of the initial assessment.
b. Unequal pupils suggest raised intracranial pressure.
c. Lumbar puncture should be performed immediately to rule out meningitis.
d. Consider intubation if GCS is less than 8.
e. A normal CT scan safely rules out raised intracranial pressure.

67. In a child with bruising:

a. Bruising on the shins is usually accidental.
b. Coagulation screen should be done before diagnosing non-accidental injury.
c. Henoch–Schönlein purpura can present with bruising and purpura along the back of the thighs and buttocks.
d. Haemophilia is a common cause for bruising.
e. Steroid therapy can be a cause of easy bruising.

68. Regarding short stature:

a. It is defined as height less than the 0.4th centile.
b. Growth velocity is a more important parameter in its evaluation than a single height measurement.
c. Bone age assessment is important in the evaluation of short stature.
d. An endocrine evaluation is always indicated.
e. Turner syndrome is a cause of short stature in girls.

69. Regarding delayed speech:

a. Hearing should be assessed in all children with delayed speech.
b. Autism can be a cause of delayed speech.
c. Poor environmental stimulation can lead to poor language development.
d. Tongue tie is a common cause.
e. First true words appear around 1 year of age.

70. Regarding MMR vaccination:

a. It is a live attenuated vaccine.
b. It is associated with increased risk of autism.
c. Current UK immunization schedule recommends only one dose, at 9 months.
d. It is contraindicated in individuals with egg allergy.
e. Usually provides lifelong protection.

71. Congenital rubella:

a. Usually follows maternal rubella infection in the third trimester.
b. Deafness is a common feature.
c. Infection during pregnancy is an indication for offering termination.
d. Non-immune pregnant women should be given MMR during pregnancy.
e. All pregnant women are routinely tested for antirubella IgG.

72. Chicken pox in children:

a. Is characterized by Koplik spots.
b. Has an incubation period of about 14–21 days.
c. Children can be infective even before the appearance of the rash.
d. Varicella immunoglobulin should be given to newborns if mum develops chickenpox within 7 days of delivery.
e. Infection during early pregnancy can cause congenital malformations.

73. Scarlet fever:

a. Is caused by group A streptococci.
b. Tonsillitis and cervical lymphadenopathy are uncommon.
c. The rash produces characteristic streaks along skin folds.
d. Peeling of skin occurs once rash begins to fade.
e. Penicillin is the drug of choice.

74. Regarding Kawasaki disease:

a. Is the commonest cause of acquired heart disease in the UK.
b. Commonly affects teenagers.
c. Coronary aneurysms occur in about 30% of untreated cases.
d. IVIG significantly reduces the risk of aneurysms if given early.
e. Routine steroid administration improves the outcome.

75. Regarding anaphylaxis:

a. Foods are the commonest cause of anaphylaxis in the UK.
b. Stridor is a common clinical feature.
c. IM adrenaline (epinephrine) is the treatment of choice.
d. Hydrocortisone has no role in its management.
e. Epipen should not be prescribed to children.

76. Regarding eczema:

a. A family history of asthma increases the risk of getting eczema.
b. Biological detergents can worsen eczema.
c. Eosinophilia is a feature of atopic eczema.
d. Wet wraps are used for the treatment of mild eczema.
e. Tacrolimus and pimecrolimus are topical immunomodulators used in the treatment of eczema.

77. In a child with cyanosis:

a. If the oxygen saturation and colour normalizes in oxygen, the cause is most likely to be cardiac.
b. Tetralogy of Fallot is an example of increased pulmonary blood flow.
c. Tetralogy of Fallot usually presents after few weeks of life.
d. Prostaglandin infusion should be started to close the ductus arteriosus.
e. Total anomalous pulmonary venous drainage (TAPVD) is an example of cyanotic heart disease.

78. Regarding arrhythmias:

a. A heart rate of 180 in a newborn is usually due to supraventricular tachycardia.
b. The commonest cause of SVT is the presence of an accessory pathway.
c. A delta wave in the ECG is characteristic of Wolf–Parkinson–White syndrome.
d. Adenosine given as a rapid IV bolus will usually terminate an attack of SVT.
e. Radio ablation is needed in almost all children with SVT.

79. Regarding otitis media:

a. Recurrent glue ear is a cause of delayed speech.
b. Can lead to sensorineural hearing loss.
c. Antibiotics are not routinely indicated in acute otitis media.
d. Meningitis is a potential complication of acute otitis media.
e. *Streptococcus pneumoniae* is the commonest bacteria causing otitis media.

80. In a child with pneumonia:

a. Chest X-ray will help to differentiate a bacterial pneumonia from a viral one.
b. *Mycoplasma* pneumonia is commoner in older children.
c. Pleural effusion is more common in viral pneumonia.
d. Recurrent pneumonia can be a presenting feature of cystic fibrosis.
e. A repeat chest X-ray is needed at the end of treatment to confirm the eradication of infection.

81. In children with asthma on inhaled corticosteroids:

a. A spacer device is routinely recommended for use with steroid inhaler.
b. Long term use can affect growth.
c. In older children, dry powder inhalers are an effective alternative.
d. Double the dose of inhaled steroids is recommended during an acute exacerbation.
e. Adrenal insufficiency is never a complication of inhaled steroids.

82. Regarding cystic fibrosis:

a. It is part of the neonatal screening programme in UK.
b. Chest physiotherapy is an important part of management.
c. In most centres, flucloxacillin is given prophylactically in all infants diagnosed with cystic fibrosis.
d. The inheritance is autosomal dominant.
e. Intestinal fibrosis is a complication of long term use of high dose pancreatic enzyme supplements.

83. Bronchiolitis:

a. Is more severe in infants born preterm.
b. Severity and incidence can be reduced by giving prophylactic RSV antibody to all at risk infants during winter months.
c. Infants with congenital heart disease have a higher risk of severe bronchiolitis.
d. Apnoea can be a clinical feature of bronchiolitis.
e. Chest X-ray often reveals hyperinflated lung fields.

84. Regarding gastroenteritis:

a. Rotavirus is the commonest pathogen causing diarrhoea in the UK.
b. Antibiotics are indicated for all bacterial gastroenteritis.
c. Antidiarrhoeals can reduce the duration of the illness.
d. Transient lactose intolerance can occur following gastroenteritis.
e. In the presence of circulatory failure immediate administration of 5 ml/kg of 0.45% saline is indicated.

85. Renal tract anomalies can present with the following clinical features:

a. Recurrent urinary tract infections.
b. Palpable abdominal mass.
c. Failure to thrive.
d. Haematuria.
e. Recurrent abdominal pain.

86. Antenatally detected renal pelvic dilatation:

a. May be due to an obstructive lesion of the urinary tract.
b. Most will resolve spontaneously in subsequent scans or after birth.
c. Observation of a good urinary stream is important before discharge.
d. Trimethoprim prophylaxis is indicated until further investigations are normal.
e. Vesicoureteric reflux is a cause.

87. Regarding urinary tract infections:

a. *E. coli* is the commonest pathogen in children.
b. Can present with neonatal jaundice.
c. Renal ultrasound is indicated in all infants after the first UTI.
d. MCUG is indicated in all children after the initial UTI.
e. Prophylactic trimethoprim is indicated in all children under 1 year until investigations are complete.

88. The following is a feature of poststreptococcal glomerulonephritis:

a. Haematuria.
b. Hypertension.
c. Facial puffiness.
d. Elevated complement C3.
e. Proteinuria.

89. Increased intracranial pressure may present with:

a. Unequal pupils.
b. Altered sensorium.
c. Headache.
d. Seizures.
e. Hypertension, bradycardia, abnormal respiration (Cushing's triad).

90. In meningitis:

a. Type B meningococcal meningitis is the commonest in UK.
b. Neck stiffness is a common feature in infants.
c. Characteristic purpuric rash is always present in meningococcal meningitis.
d. Lumbar puncture should be performed immediately if a diagnosis of meningitis is made.
e. All children should have a hearing test following recovery from meningitis.

91. **Regarding cerebral palsy:**
    a. The commonest cause is birth asphyxia.
    b. A motor dysfunction is always present.
    c. In spastic quadriplegia, arms are worse affected than legs.
    d. In kernicterus, the damage occurs in the basal ganglia.
    e. Botulinum toxin injection is one of the options for treating spasticity.

92. **The following are risk factors for developmental dysplasia of the hip:**
    a. Breech presentation.
    b. Male sex.
    c. Congenital talipes equinovarus deformity.
    d. Family history.
    e. Neuromuscular disorders.

93. **Regarding osteomyelitis:**
    a. The commonest pathogen is *S. aureus*.
    b. *Salmonella* osteomyelitis is common in children with sickle cell disease.
    c. X-rays are always diagnostic.
    d. The usual site of infection is in the diaphysis.
    e. Surgical drainage is necessary in most instances.

94. **Iron deficiency anaemia:**
    a. Is common in children born prematurely.
    b. Excessive intake of unmodified cow's milk can be a cause.
    c. Iron supplementation can be stopped immediately after the anaemia is corrected.
    d. Irritability and delayed milestones can be a presenting feature.
    e. A blood film usually shows macrocytic anaemia.

95. **Regarding haemolytic anaemias:**
    a. Lifelong iron supplementation is necessary.
    b. High reticulocyte count is common.
    c. Unconjugated jaundice can be a presenting feature.
    d. Splenomegaly is not a feature of longstanding sickle cell disease.
    e. Aseptic necrosis of long bones is a complication of sickle cell disease.

96. **Regarding childhood malignancy:**
    a. Brain tumours are the commonest neoplasms in childhood.
    b. ALL accounts for over 80% of childhood leukaemias.
    c. Wilms' tumour usually presents in early teens.
    d. Neuroblastomas can sometimes regress spontaneously.
    e. Hodgkin's lymphoma is the commonest type of lymphoma in young children.

97. **Childhood leukaemia can present with:**
    a. Anaemia.
    b. Purpura, bleeding diathesis.
    c. Bone pain.
    d. Hepatosplenomegaly.
    e. Severe infection.

98. **Regarding diabetes mellitus:**
    a. A glucose tolerance test is always needed for diagnosis.
    b. Multiple daily injection regimes result in more physiological insulin levels.
    c. Diabetic ketoacidosis is always treated with a soluble insulin.
    d. Mixtard is a biphasic insulin.
    e. Hypostop is an oral glucose polymer used to treat hypoglycaemia.

99. **Congenital hypothyroidism:**
    a. Can be picked up by Guthrie test.
    b. Early treatment results in near normal development.
    c. One of the clinical presentations is with prolonged neonatal jaundice.
    d. Investigations include a thyroid scan.
    e. Treatment is monitored by assessment of T4 and TSH.

100. **Regarding immunization:**
    a. Pneumococcal vaccination is part of the routine immunization schedule in the UK.
    b. Acute febrile illness is a contraindication to immunization.
    c. BCG is given to all schoolchildren following a negative Heaf test.
    d. It is common for children to develop a mild febrile illness following vaccination.
    e. Cerebral palsy is a contraindication for DTP vaccine.

Short-answer questions (SAQs)

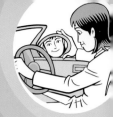

1. How do you manage diabetic ketoacidosis?

2. Describe the common problems encountered by a preterm infant of 26 weeks' gestational age and 800 g birthweight. How are they treated?

3. How would you assess a limping 3-year-old child?

4. Write brief notes on the management of leukaemia in childhood.

5. How is Kawasaki disease diagnosed?

6. What are false contraindications to vaccination?

7. List the features of non-accidental injury?

8. What are the differences between children and adults respiratory systems?

9. Describe the management of the mother with HIV and how HIV infection is diagnosed in young children.

10. How might an infant with inborn error of metabolism present?

11. What are the advantages and disadvantages of breastfeeding?

12. Write short notes on acute viral bronchiolitis.

13. Describe the aetiology and management of jaundice in the newborn.

14. Discuss the diagnosis and management of short stature.

15. Describe the clinical features and diagnosis of Down syndrome.

16. Write brief notes on cerebral palsy.

17. Give an account of the causes of iron deficiency anaemia in infancy and childhood.

18. Write brief notes on attention-deficit hyperactivity disorder.

19. Discuss the management of nocturnal enuresis ('bedwetting') in childhood.

20. How would you manage moderately severe atopic eczema in a 9-month-old infant?

Extended-matching questions (EMQs)

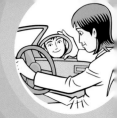

1.

(a) Innocent murmur
(b) Tetralogy of Fallot
(c) Coarctation of the aorta
(d) Atrial septal defect
(e) Ventricular septal defect
(f) Mitral stenosis
(g) Primary pulmonary hypertension
(h) Transposition of the great arteries
(i) Aortic stenosis
(j) Patent ductus arteriosus

Instruction: For each scenario described below, choose the SINGLE most likely diagnosis from the above list of options. Each option may be used once, more than once or not at all.

1. A 2-day-old baby develops cyanosis on the postnatal ward and despite oxygen therapy the cyanosis does not resolve. A pansystolic murmur is heard. Femoral pulses normal. CXR shows increased prominence of pulmonary vessels. ECG is normal. ☐

2. A 1-year-old child is noted to be cyanotic and has spells where he becomes increasingly blue which are relieved by squatting. ☐

3. A 3-week-old boy presents with an ejection systolic murmur and hypertension. Femoral pulsations are difficult to feel. ☐

2.

(a) Kawasaki disease
(b) Scarlet fever
(c) SLE
(d) Measles
(e) Leukaemia
(f) Stills disease
(g) Chickenpox
(h) Herpes simplex type 1
(i) HIV
(j) Rubella

Instruction: For each scenario described below, choose the SINGLE most likely diagnosis from the above list of options. Each option may be used once, more than once or not at all.

1. A 3-year-old child has a persistent fever, irritability and a macular rash. There is also bilateral non-purulent conjunctivitis, unilateral lymphadenopathy and a red tongue. ☐

2. A 4-year-old boy develops high spiking fevers, a salmon-like rash with knee, wrist and ankle pain and swelling. There is also hepatosplenomegaly. ☐

3. A 6-year-old girl has a high fever, generalized itchy vesicular rash which crusts on day 5 of her illness. ☐

3.

(a) Respiratory distress syndrome
(b) Apnoea of prematurity
(c) Transient tachypnoea of the newborn
(d) Pneumothorax
(e) Sepsis
(f) Congenital diaphragmatic hernia
(g) Congenital pneumonia
(h) Laryngomalacia
(i) Gastro-oesophageal reflux
(j) Inhaled foreign body

Instruction: For each scenario described below, choose the SINGLE most likely diagnosis from the above list of options. Each option may be used once, more than once or not at all.

1. A male term infant is seen at 8 hours on the postnatal ward with respiratory distress. He is grunting and has a respiratory rate of 90/min. Subcostal recessions are present and he is tachycardic but afebrile. A CXR shows fluid in the horizontal fissure. Subsequent blood cultures are negative. ☐

2. A 1-week-old preterm infant of 28 weeks' gestational age has recently been weaned off ventilatory support but develops attacks of apnoea and bradycardia. He is well in between these attacks. ☐

3. A 2-hour-old baby of 30 weeks' gestational age develops respiratory distress and requires oxygen therapy on the neonatal unit. The CXR shows a ground glass appearance and he requires mechanical ventilation. ☐

4.

(a) Anti-gliadin antibodies
(b) Sweat test
(c) Barium swallow
(d) Pulmonary function testing
(e) Broncho-alveolar lavage
(f) CT chest
(g) Cervical X-ray
(h) Skin prick testing
(i) Bronchoscopy
(j) Echocardiography

Instruction: For each scenario described below, choose the SINGLE most likely diagnosis from the above list of options. Each option may be used once, more than once or not at all.

1. A 2-year-old boy presents with poor weight gain, abdominal distension and loose smelly stools. He has frequent courses of antibiotics for chest infections. ☐

2. A 5-year-old boy with HIV develops increasing respiratory distress, fever and is placed on high flow oxygen. He has had a course of antibiotics recently for a chest infection. ☐

3. A 4-year-old girl develops a sudden onset of wheeze and breathlessness while playing in the garden with her toys. She is afebrile and a CXR shows collapse of her middle lobe. ☐

5.

(a) Macular rash
(b) Olive-shaped mass in abdomen
(c) Bulging fontanelle
(d) Papilloedema
(e) Bilious vomiting
(f) Low birth weight
(g) TB contact in family
(h) Smell of acetone in breath
(i) Eczema
(j) Wheeze and crackles on auscultation

Instruction: For each scenario described below, choose the SINGLE most likely diagnosis from the above list of options. Each option may be used once, more than once or not at all.

1. A 3-month-old child with fever, irritability and seizures. ☐

2. A 1-month-old child with poor weight gain despite a good appetite, vomiting and always being hungry. ☐

3. A 5-month-old child with wheeze, respiratory distress after a cold-like illness. ☐

6.

(a) Sepsis
(b) Acute leukaemia
(c) Malaria
(d) Autoimmune hepatitis
(e) HIV
(f) Spherocytosis
(g) Infective hepatitis
(h) Thalassaemia
(i) Sickle cell disease
(j) Pyruvate kinase deficiency

Instruction: For each scenario described below, choose the SINGLE most likely diagnosis from the above list of options. Each option may be used once, more than once or not at all.

1. A 7-year-old boy with hepatosplenomegaly and a non-blanching rash. He has a Hb of 7 g/dl and a platelet count of 30×10^9/L. ☐

2. A 5-year-old caucasian boy with jaundice. He is anaemic with a Hb of 9 g/dl and he was noted to be jaundiced as a baby. ☐

3. A 10-year-old African girl with breathlessness and severe chest pain. Her Hb is 6 g/dl and her spleen is not palpable. ☐

7.

(a) Duodenal ulcer
(b) Crohn's disease
(c) Ulcerative colitis
(d) Psychogenic
(e) Irritable bowel syndrome
(f) Hypercalcaemia
(g) Cystic fibrosis
(h) Coeliac disease
(i) Pancreatitis
(j) Food intolerance

Instruction: For each scenario described below, choose the SINGLE most likely diagnosis from the above list of options. Each option may be used once, more than once or not at all.

1. A 13-year-old boy has recurrent abdominal pain, loose stools, mouth ulcers and a right side lower abdominal mass. ☐

2. An 18-month-old toddler with eczema and frequent wheezy episodes presents with loose stools despite changing from cow's milk to soya. ☐

3. A 14-year-old male with epigastric pain radiating to the back, which is worst at night and relieved with eating. ☐

8.

(a) Hypsarrythmia
(b) 3-Hz spike wave on EEG
(c) Associated with minor head injury
(d) Meningitis
(e) Visual field disturbances
(f) Decorticate posturing
(g) Temporal lobe involvement on EEG
(h) Hypoglycaemia
(i) Burst suppression on EEG
(j) Shock-like jerks

Instruction: For each scenario described below, choose the SINGLE most likely diagnosis from the above list of options. Each option may be used once, more than once or not at all.

1. A 6-month-old child with infantile spasms. ☐

2. A 6-year-old child with absence seizures. ☐

3. A 9-year-old child with herpes simplex encephalitis. ☐

317

9.

(a) Slipped upper femoral capital epiphysis
(b) Perthes disease
(c) Toddlers fracture
(d) Irritable hip
(e) Osgood–Schlatters disease
(f) Osteosarcoma
(g) Leukaemia
(h) Osteochondritis dissecans
(i) Growing pains
(j) Developmental dysplasia of the hip

Instruction: For each scenario described below, choose the SINGLE most likely diagnosis from the above list of options. Each option may be used once, more than once or not at all.

1. A 2-year-old child with a limp but weight bearing. She is afebrile but has recently had a cold.

2. A 13-year-old male with knee pain. He is obese and examination shows decreased hip movement. He is afebrile.

3. A 7-year-old child with a limp and pain in the hip and knee. He has an antalgic gait and a X-ray shows collapse of the femoral head.

10.

(a) 0–3 months
(b) 3–6 months
(c) 6–9 months
(d) 9–12 months
(e) 12–15 months
(f) 15–18 months
(g) 18–21 months
(h) 21–24 months
(i) 2–4 years
(j) >4 years

Instruction: For each scenario described below, choose the SINGLE most likely diagnosis from the above list of options. Each option may be used once, more than once or not at all.

1. Can pedal a tricycle, builds an 8 brick tall tower, is dry by day and can dress with supervision.

2. Can sit unsupported and weight bear on legs, transfer objects from hand to hand, will respond to own name and plays peek-a-boo.

3. This child can walk, has a pincer grip, uses two to three words and can use a spoon.

11.

(a) Paramyxovirus
(b) Enterovirus
(c) *Staphylococcus aureus*
(d) Ebstein–Barr virus
(e) Herpes simplex type 1
(f) *Streptococcus pyogenes*
(g) *Haemophilus influenzae*
(h) Hepadnavirus
(i) Rotavirus
(j) Human Herpes Virus 6

Instruction: For each scenario described below, choose the SINGLE most specific answer from the above list of options. Each option may be used once, more than once or not at all.

1. Mumps.

2. Infectious mononucleosis.

3. Scarlet fever.

12.

(a) Ceftriaxone
(b) No treatment required
(c) Oral erythromycin
(d) Nystatin cream
(e) Hydrocortisone ointment
(f) Topical emollient
(g) 5% permethrin cream
(h) Aciclovir
(i) Penicillin V
(j) Methotrexate

Instruction: For each scenario described below, choose the SINGLE most specific answer from the above list of options. Each option may be used once, more than once or not at all.

1. A 10-day-old baby on the neonatal unit has developed weeping erythematous rash in the nappy area. There are few satellite lesions around this region.

2. A 5-year-old boy presented to the A&E with fever, myalgia and a rash. On examination, he looked unwell and had a petechial rash, with few purpuric spots.

3. A 7-year-old boy presents with few pearly white papules with central dimples on the chest.

13.

(a) Pneumonia
(b) Bronchiolitis
(c) Laryngotracheobronchitis
(d) Acute asthma
(e) Tracheal foreign body
(f) Acute epiglottitis
(g) Vascular ring
(h) Pertussis
(i) Laryngomalacia
(j) Cystic fibrosis

Instruction: For each scenario described below, choose the SINGLE most specific answer from the above list of options. Each option may be used once, more than once or not at all.

1. A 3-month old infant presents in the winter months with a history of being snuffly for 2 days. She has fed poorly over the last few hours being breathless. On examination she is tachypnoeic, has subcostal recession and on auscultation inspiratory crepitations and widespread wheeze. ☐

2. A 13-month-old unimmunized boy presents to the A&E with history of noisy breathing and high temperature. On examination, he looks unwell, drooling saliva and has quiet stridor. ☐

3. A 2-year-old toddler with eczema presents with a history of shortness of breath for one day. On examination, he has chest recessions and bilateral reduced air entry and wheeze. There is a family history of hay fever and eczema. ☐

14.

(a) Cystic fibrosis
(b) Chronic asthma
(c) Vesicoureteric reflux
(d) Splenectomy
(e) HIV
(f) ALL
(g) Long-term steroid therapy
(h) Hodgkin's lymphoma
(i) ITP
(j) Haemolytic uraemic syndrome

Instruction: For each scenario described below, choose the SINGLE most specific answer from the above list of options. Each option may be used once, more than once or not at all.

1. Trimethoprim prophylaxis. ☐

2. Penicillin prophylaxis. ☐

3. Flucloxacillin prophylaxis. ☐

15.

(a) Gastrooesophageal reflux
(b) Duodenal atresia
(c) Sigmoid volvulus
(d) Acute gastroenteritis
(e) Pyloric stenosis
(f) Meckel's diverticulum
(g) Intussusception
(h) Cow's milk allergy
(i) Crohn's disease
(j) Necrotizing enterocolitis

Instruction: For each scenario described below, choose the SINGLE most specific answer from the above list of options. Each option may be used once, more than once or not at all.

1. A 4-week-old male infant presents with history of non-bilious projectile vomiting. On a test feed there is visible peristalsis and on palpation an olive-sized mass is felt in the right upper quadrant. ☐

2. A 8-month-old boy presents with history of abdominal pain and vomiting. A sausage-shaped mass is palpable in the abdomen and he has passed blood-stained stools. ☐

3. A 15-day-old infant, born at 30 weeks' gestation, now fully formula fed develops abdominal distension and bilious aspirates from nasogastric tube. His abdominal X-ray showed dilated bowel loops with gas in the bowel wall. ☐

16.

  (a) Chronic lung disease
  (b) Respiratory distress syndrome
  (c) Bronchiolitis
  (d) Transient tachypnoea of the newborn
  (e) Physiological jaundice
  (f) Rh incompatibility
  (g) Biliary atresia
  (h) ABO incompatibility
  (i) Hereditary spherocytosis
  (j) G6PD deficiency

Instruction: For each scenario described below, choose the SINGLE most specific answer from the above list of options. Each option may be used once, more than once or not at all.

1. A 3-month-old infant, born at 25 weeks' gestation on special care, still requiring oxygen. ☐

2. A 1-day-old neonate admitted for jaundice. Her blood group is A positive and her mother's group is O positive. A Coomb's test is positive. ☐

3. A 3-week-old infant is investigated for prolonged jaundice. He passes clay coloured stools and has a conjugated hyperbilirubinaemia. ☐

17.

  (a) Guillain–Barré syndrome
  (b) Myotonic dystrophy
  (c) Duchenne muscular dystrophy
  (d) Dyskinetic cerebral palsy
  (e) Spastic cerebral palsy
  (f) Transverse myelitis
  (g) Cord compression
  (h) Spinal muscular atrophy
  (i) Hereditary neuropathy
  (j) Congenital muscular dystrophy

Instruction: For each scenario described below, choose the SINGLE most specific answer from the above list of options. Each option may be used once, more than once or not at all.

1. A 4-year-old boy with a history of abnormal gait. On examination, he has hypertrophy of calf muscles and a positive Gower sign. ☐

2. A 16-month-old with a history of delayed motor milestones. On examination he has increased tone in all limbs and brisk reflexes, but no abnormal movements. An MRI of his brain is normal. ☐

3. A 10-year-old boy with a history of weakness starting in both legs, now involving upper limbs as well. His tone is reduced in all limbs and tendon reflexes could not be elicited. ☐

18.

  (a) Down syndrome
  (b) Angelman syndrome
  (c) Prader–Willi syndrome
  (d) Achondroplasia
  (e) Turner syndrome
  (f) Edward syndrome
  (g) Patau syndrome
  (h) Russell–Silver syndrome
  (i) Simple obesity
  (j) Fragile X syndrome

Instruction: For each scenario described below, choose the SINGLE most specific answer from the above list of options. Each option may be used once, more than once or not at all.

1. A 15-year-old girl with short stature, delayed puberty. ☐

2. A 13-year-old boy with obesity, short stature, learning difficulties. ☐

3. A 2-day-old infant with hypotonia, single palmar crease, epicanthal folds, Bruschfield spots and heart murmur. ☐

19.

(a) Oral dexamethasone
(b) IV hydrocortisone
(c) IV adenosine
(d) IV ceftriaxone
(e) Oral amoxicillin
(f) Insulin infusion
(g) Nebulized salbutamol
(h) IV digoxin
(i) Oral prednisolone
(j) Oral azithromycin

Instruction: For each scenario described below, choose the SINGLE most specific answer from the above list of options. Each option may be used once, more than once or not at all.

1. A 13-month-old with barking cough, and stridor.

2. A 8-month-old with tachypnoea, tachycardia, ECG—heart rate >300/min.

3. A 5-year-old with vomiting, abdominal pain, dehydration, blood gas—pH 7.1; base deficit—24; blood sugar—28.

20.

(a) Streptococcal impetigo
(b) Head injury
(c) MMR vaccination
(d) Kawasaki disease
(e) Haemophilia
(f) Congenital rubella
(g) Otitis media
(h) Diabetes mellitus
(i) Rheumatic fever
(j) Staphylococcal scalded skin syndrome

Instruction: For each scenario described below, choose the SINGLE most specific answer from the above list of options. Each option may be used once, more than once or not at all.

1. Sensorineural hearing loss.

2. Coronary aneurysm.

3. Acute glomerulonephritis.

21.

(a) Echocardiography
(b) Full blood count
(c) Urea & electrolytes
(d) Amylase
(e) Sputum culture and spirometry
(f) HbA1C
(g) Autoantibody screen
(h) Urine culture
(i) Blood culture
(j) ECG

Instruction: For each scenario described below, choose the SINGLE most specific answer from the above list of options. Each option may be used once, more than once or not at all.

1. Cystic fibrosis.

2. Diabetes mellitus.

3. Kawasaki disease.

22.

(a) Congenital hypothyroidism
(b) Hereditary spherocytosis
(c) Congenital adrenal hyperplasia
(d) Suspected non-accidental injury
(e) Sudden infant death syndrome
(f) Septic arthritis
(g) Osteomyelitis
(h) Spina bifida
(i) Congenital torticollis
(j) Thalassaemia

Instruction: For each scenario described below, choose the SINGLE most specific answer from the above list of options. Each option may be used once, more than once or not at all.

1. Neonatal screening.

2. Skeletal survey.

3. Prone sleeping position.

23.

    (a) Diabetes mellitus
    (b) Diabetes insipidus
    (c) Water intoxication
    (d) Congenital adrenal hyperplasia
    (e) Addison disease
    (f) Cushing syndrome
    (g) Hypothyroidism
    (h) Hyperthyroidism
    (i) SIADH
    (j) Craniopharyngioma

Instruction: For each scenario described below, choose the SINGLE most specific answer from the above list of options. Each option may be used once, more than once or not at all.

1. Short stature, truncal obesity, striae, moon facies, hypertension.

2. Ambiguous genitalia, hypoglycaemia, hypotension, hyponatraemia, hyperkalaemia.

3. Polyuria, polydipsia, polyphagia, weight loss.

24.

    (a) Sickle cell disease
    (b) Folate deficiency
    (c) Iron deficiency anaemia
    (d) Acute leukaemia
    (e) Idiopathic thrombocytopenic purpura
    (f) Hereditary spherocytosis
    (g) Polyarteritis nodosa
    (h) Vitamin B_{12} deficiency
    (i) Meningococcal septicaemia
    (j) Trauma

Instruction: For each scenario described below, choose the SINGLE most specific answer from the above list of options. Each option may be used once, more than once or not at all.

1. Hypochromic microcytic anaemia.

2. A well child presents with petechiae, thrombocytopenia, normal haemoglobin, white cell count and blood film.

3. Vaso-occlusive crisis.

25.

    (a) Food intolerance
    (b) Peptic ulcer disease
    (c) Crohn's disease
    (d) Ulcerative colitis
    (e) Coeliac disease
    (f) Pyloric stenosis
    (g) Gastrooesophageal reflux
    (h) Autoimmune hepatitis
    (i) Pernicious anaemia
    (j) *H. pylori* infection

Instruction: For each scenario described below, choose the SINGLE most specific answer from the above list of options. Each option may be used once, more than once or not at all.

1. 24 hour pH monitoring.

2. IgA antigliadin antibodies.

3. RAST testing.

26.

(a) Pneumonia
(b) Congenital diaphragmatic hernia
(c) Cystic fibrosis
(d) Chronic asthma
(e) Pertussis
(f) Diphtheria
(g) Bronchiolitis
(h) Croup
(i) Non-specific cough
(j) Chronic lung disease

Instruction: For each scenario described below, choose the SINGLE most specific answer from the above list of options. Each option may be used once, more than once or not at all.

1. A 2-month-old infant is admitted with history of coryza over the last week. He has developed a cough since then, which comes in bouts and can last for a few seconds, sometimes associated with vomiting in the end. He is breathless and takes a deep breath at the end of the bout, often with a whoop.

2. A 1-year-old boy is seen in the outpatients with a history of recurrent chest infections. He has had over four episodes of chest infections in the last 6 months, all needing antibiotics. On examination, his weight is below the 0.4th centile and has chest recessions. On auscultation, he has scattered wheeze and coarse crepitations all over the chest.

3. A 1-month-old infant is seen in A&E with history of shortness of breath. He had been well until 2 days ago when he became snuffly. On examination, he looks alert and active, but has mild chest recessions. On auscultation, he has reduced air entry on the left side. A chest X-ray showed multiple loopy shadows on the left side of the chest with heart shadow shifted to the right.

27.

(a) Chronic renal failure
(b) Acute renal failure
(c) Haemolytic uraemic syndrome
(d) Henoch–Schönlein purpura
(e) Meningococcal septicaemia
(f) Poststreptococcal glomerulonephritis
(g) Nephrotic syndrome
(h) Congestive cardiac failure
(i) Urinary tract infection
(j) Idiopathic thrombocytopenic purpura

Instruction: For each scenario described below, choose the SINGLE most specific answer from the above list of options. Each option may be used once, more than once or not at all.

1. A 4-year-old boy is seen on the ward with a history of 'smoky' urine for the last 4 days. On examination, he has mild facial puffiness and his blood pressure is 139/90 mmHg. There is a history of sore throat about 3 weeks ago and his urine was positive for blood.

2. A 5-year-old girl was brought with a history of gradual onset of facial puffiness over the last 1 week. On examination, she has generalized oedema with ascites and normal blood pressure. Her urine had 4+ of protein and no blood. Her serum albumin was 20 g/L (low).

3. A 2-year-old boy is brought with history of a rash on his lower limbs for the last 2 days and abdominal pain. On examination, he has a purpuric rash over the back of his thighs, legs and buttocks. His blood pressure is normal and urinalysis showed traces of blood.

28.

(a) Acute severe asthma
(b) Pneumonia
(c) Shock
(d) Raised intracranial pressure
(e) Salicylate poisoning
(f) Seizure disorder
(g) Dehydration
(h) Diabetic ketoacidosis
(i) Pneumothorax
(j) Acute epiglottitis

Instruction: For each scenario described below, choose the SINGLE most specific answer from the above list of options. Each option may be used once, more than once or not at all.

1. Headache, vomiting, unequal and poorly reacting pupils. ☐

2. Drowsy, pale, cold clammy skin, tachycardia, capillary refill about 4 seconds (normal <2 s). ☐

3. Conscious, severe chest recession, not able to speak, prolonged expiration, silent chest bilaterally on auscultation, no h/o choking, chest X-ray—hyperinflated lung fields. ☐

29.

(a) Breathholding spell
(b) Long QT syndrome
(c) Vasovagal syncope
(d) Absence seizure
(e) Generalized tonic clonic convulsion
(f) Myoclonic epilepsy
(g) Meningitis
(h) Cyanotic spell
(i) Choking episode
(j) Infantile spasms

Instruction: For each scenario described below, choose the SINGLE most specific answer from the above list of options. Each option may be used once, more than once or not at all.

1. A 12-year-old, who had been standing under the sun for a while suddenly becomes dizzy and collapses. She regains consciousness after a few seconds and is brought to A&E. She looks normal on examination and an ECG is normal. ☐

2. A 1-year-old infant continues to cry and then stops breathing, turns blue. After a few seconds, he starts breathing and is back to normal colour. ☐

3. A 6-year-old boy brought to outpatients with history of a period of lack of awareness lasting a few seconds. This happens several times a day and is not associated with any abnormal movements. On hyperventilating in the clinic, he becomes still and does not respond when called. He becomes normal in a few seconds. ☐

30.

(a) Quinine
(b) Piperazine
(c) Nystatin
(d) Ceftriaxone
(e) Permethrin
(f) Chloroquine
(g) Co-trimoxazole
(h) Rifampicin
(i) Isoniazid
(j) Pyrazinamide

Instruction: For each scenario described below, choose the SINGLE most specific answer from the above list of options. Each option may be used once, more than once or not at all.

1. Scabies. ☐

2. *Enterobius vermicularis.* ☐

3. *Plasmodium falciparum vivax.* ☐

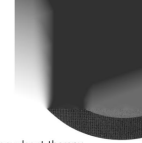

1. a. F   Blood tests done early in the course of the illness may be normal
    b. T   In younger infants infections can be generalized and meningitis needs to be ruled out
    c. F   A low white cell count may suggest a serious infection or immune dysfunction
    d. F
    e. T

2. a. T
    b. F   A purpuric rash can also occur in other conditions, but in an unwell child it suggests a serious infection like meningococcal sepsis
    c. T
    d. F
    e. T

3. a. T
    b. T
    c. T   Lower airway obstruction commonly results in a wheeze
    d. T
    e. F

4. a. F   Viral-induced wheeze is more common in this age group; a diagnosis of asthma is made only if the wheezy episodes are recurrent
    b. T
    c. F   This is seen commonly with foreign body inhalation
    d. T
    e. T

5. a. T
    b. F   Lumbar puncture should never be done in an unstable child. A raised intracranial pressure should be ruled out before this is undertaken
    c. F
    d. T
    e. F

6. a. F   The need for anticonvulsant therapy depends on the seizure type or syndrome, frequency of attacks and the risk–benefit of treatment itself
    b. T
    c. F
    d. T
    e. T

7. a. F
    b. T
    c. T   Rarely it may result from trauma or from osteomyelitis of an adjacent bone
    d. F
    e. T

8. a. F
    b. F   Transfusion is reserved for children with severe anaemia with symptoms, certain haemolytic anaemias or in the presence of acute blood loss
    c. F   A low Hb in this age group is usually physiological
    d. T
    e. T

9. a. F
    b. T
    c. F
    d. T
    e. F

10. a. T
    b. T
    c. F   Late walking may be just a deviation from normal; delay in one sphere of development can occur independently of others
    d. F   Usually walking is attained by 18 months of age
    e. T

11. a. T
    b. T
    c. F   Correction is made for children under 2 years
    d. T
    e. F

12. a. T
b. F
c. T
d. T
e. F

13. a. T
b. T This may suggest an underlying weakness of the non-dominant side
c. T
d. F This is a normal developmental deviation
e. F

14. a. T
b. T
c. F Diagnosis is by viral detection, usually by PCR or culture
d. T
e. F Intrapartum therapy is a way of reducing vertical transmission. This is continued into the neonatal period

15. a. T
b. T
c. T
d. T
e. F This is more common in German measles (Rubella)

16. a. F In anaphylaxis, adrenaline (epinephrine) is given by the intramuscular route
b. T
c. T
d. F
e. F Egg allergy is not a contraindication for any of the vaccines in the routine immunization schedule

17. a. T Antihistamines can diminish the response to the test antigens
b. F Neither RAST nor skin prick testing can definitely rule out allergy
c. T
d. T
e. F

18. a. T
b. F Allergy to one or more food is more common
c. T
d. F Allergic reactions can be IgE mediated or non IgE mediated
e. T

19. a. T
b. F
c. T
d. T
e. F Neither molluscum contagiosum nor seborrhoeic dermatitis cause pruritis

20. a. T
b. F
c. T
d. T
e. T

21. a. T
b. T
c. T
d. T
e. T

22. a. T
b. F Sometimes a tiny defect can cause a loud murmur (Maladie Roger)
c. T
d. F The murmur is usually pansystolic
e. T

23. a. T
b. F The cyanosis may also occur due to a mixing defect in the absence of pulmonary stenosis, in which case the pulmonary blood flow is increased (e.g. transposition of great arteries without pulmonic stenosis)
c. T
d. F
e. T

24. a. T
b. F Not all reflux episodes are acidic and these non-acid reflux are not picked up on pH studies
c. T
d. T
e. F Cisapride can cause prolonged QT syndrome and is no longer recommended for the treatment of reflux

25. a. T
b. T
c. T
d. F
e. F

26.
a. T
b. T
c. F
d. T
e. F

27.
a. F
b. T
c. F — The new NICE guidelines does not recommend prophylactic antibiotics routinely for all children
d. T
e. F

28.
a. T
b. T — It is caused by *E. coli* O157:H7
c. T
d. F
e. F

29.
a. T
b. F
c. F
d. T
e. T

30.
a. F — Anticonvulsants are not usually started following a single episode of seizure
b. T — Interictal EEG can be normal in nearly half the children with seizures. A sleep EEG may give better results but is time consuming
c. T
d. T
e. T

31.
a. T
b. T
c. F — CK is elevated in Duchennne and Becker dystrophies but not so in most other muscular dystrophies
d. F — Respiratory weakness may be irreversible, but it can be managed by invasive and non-invasive respiratory support
e. F

32.
a. F
b. T
c. F
d. F
e. F — There is no evidence for the role of viruses in its aetiology or the use of apnoea alarms to prevent it

33.
a. T
b. T
c. F
d. F
e. T

34.
a. T
b. F
c. F
d. F
e. T

35.
a. T
b. F — This is a feature of autosomal recessive disorders
c. F
d. F
e. F

36.
a. T
b. F — Children with cow's milk intolerance also cross react with soya milk very often
c. T
d. T
e. T

37.
a. F — This is not usually used in children due to the large volume of administration and poor muscle bulk
b. F
c. F
d. T
e. T

38.
a. F
b. T
c. T
d. T
e. T — Multiple fractures, fractures crossing suture line, occipital fractures, etc. imply a significant force and are more suggestive of non-accidental injury

39.
a. T
b. F
c. T
d. T
e. T

40.
a. T
b. F
c. F
d. F
e. T

327

41. a. F
   b. F
   c. T
   d. T
   e. F   The commonest defect is 21-hydroxylase deficiency

42. a. T
   b. F   Coarse facial features are not apparent in the neonatal period
   c. F
   d. F
   e. T

43. a. F
   b. T
   c. F
   d. F
   e. T

44. a. F
   b. T
   c. T
   d. T
   e. T

45. a. T
   b. F   In most children, Pavlik's harness would suffice; hip spica or surgical correction is reserved for the more severe forms
   c. T
   d. F
   e. T

46. a. F
   b. F
   c. T   Hip pain may be referred to the knee and any child presenting with knee pain should also have the hips examined
   d. T
   e. T

47. a. T
   b. F
   c. T
   d. T
   e. T   Most childhood arthritis are rheumatoid factor negative

48. a. F
   b. F
   c. T
   d. T   But the iron contained in breast milk is more readily absorbed
   e. F

49. a. F
   b. T
   c. F
   d. F   Prolonged APTT can suggest the diagnosis, but it is confirmed by specific factor assay
   e. T

50. a. F
   b. T
   c. T
   d. T
   e. F   Here the platelet numbers are usually normal, but their function is affected

51. a. F
   b. F
   c. T
   d. T
   e. T

52. a. T   CNS tumours are the commonest solid tumours in children
   b. F
   c. T
   d. T
   e. T

53. a. T
   b. T
   c. F
   d. F
   e. T

54. a. T
   b. T   Intrapartum prophylaxis is started during labour and continues through the neonatal period
   c. F   With the current interventions to reduce vertical transmission, this has come down from nearly 20% to lower than 2% in the UK
   d. T
   e. F

55. a. F
   b. T
   c. F
   d. T
   e. F   Generally well premature infants born later than 35 weeks' gestation are not admitted to the special care unit, unless they are small for gestation or have problems with feeding or temperature regulation

56. a. F Term babies can rarely be affected
b. T
c. F Infection is contributory, but in most instances, no pathogen is isolated
d. T
e. T

57. a. F
b. T Once the airway and breathing are established, fluid resuscitation remains the next most important step in the management of shock
c. T
d. T
e. T

58. a. T
b. T
c. F High dose adrenaline (epinephrine) has doubtful value and is only indicated in the later stages of resuscitation if the normal doses have been ineffective
d. T
e. T

59. a. F
b. F
c. T
d. F Single umbilical arteries can be associated with other anomalies, especially of the renal tract
e. T

60. a. T
b. F
c. T
d. T
e. F

61. a. F This goes more with a diagnosis of acute epiglottitis
b. F Stabilizing the airway remains the priority in acute epiglottitis
c. F
d. T
e. F

62. a. T
b. F
c. T
d. T
e. T

63. a. T This can indicate a variety of causes including glomerulonephritis, tumours and renal arterial thrombosis
b. T
c. F Poststreptococcal glomerulonephritis more commonly occurs following streptococcal skin infections
d. T
e. T

64. a. T
b. F
c. T
d. T
e. T

65. a. F
b. T
c. F
d. F
e. F They do not need any treatment other than reassurance and advice on not to reinforce the behaviour

66. a. T
b. T
c. F
d. T
e. F

67. a. T
b. T
c. T
d. F Haemophilia is much rarer cause for bruising
e. T

68. a. T
b. T
c. T
d. F
e. T

69. a. T
b. T
c. T
d. F Tongue tie usually does not cause any problems and will not need treatment in most instances
e. T

70.
a. T
b. F
c. F — There are two doses, one at 13 months and a booster between 3.5 and 5 years of age
d. F
e. T

71.
a. F — It usually follows maternal infection in the first trimester
b. T
c. T
d. F — MMR (for that matter, most vaccines) are contraindicated during pregnancy
e. T

72.
a. F — This is a feature of measles
b. T
c. T
d. T
e. T

73.
a. T
b. F
c. T
d. T
e. T

74.
a. T
b. F — It commonly affects under fives
c. T
d. T
e. F

75.
a. T
b. T
c. T
d. F
e. F

76.
a. T
b. T
c. T
d. F
e. T

77.
a. F
b. F
c. T
d. F — Prostagalandin infusion is started to keep the ductus arteriosus open
e. T

78.
a. F
b. T
c. T
d. T
e. F

79.
a. T
b. F
c. T
d. T
e. T

80.
a. F
b. T
c. F — Pleural effusions are usually seen in bacterial pneumonia, especially in staphylococcal pneumonia
d. T
e. F

81.
a. T
b. T — But this impairment in growth is usually transient
c. T
d. F
e. F

82.
a. T
b. T
c. T
d. F
e. T

83.
a. T
b. T
c. T
d. T
e. T

84.
a. T
b. F — Most bacterial gastroenteritis does not require antibiotics, which can, in fact worsen the diarrhoeal illness
c. F
d. T
e. F — The treatment of shock is usually with 20 ml/kg of 0.9% saline, i.e. normal saline

85.
a. T
b. T
c. T
d. T
e. T

86. a. T
b. T
c. T
d. T
e. T

87. a. T
b. T
c. T
d. F
e. T   This remains the practice at the time of publication, although the new NICE guidelines may change that

88. a. T
b. T
c. T
d. F   Complement C3 is usually low in poststreptococcal glomerulonephritis
e. T

89. a. T
b. T
c. T
d. T
e. T

90. a. T
b. F
c. F
d. F
e. T

91. a. F   In most cases the cause is idiopathic
b. T
c. T
d. T
e. T

92. a. T
b. F
c. T
d. T
e. T

93. a. T
b. T
c. F   A bone scan is usually more sensitive
d. F
e. F

94. a. T
b. T
c. F   Usually iron therapy is continued for a few months after the anaemia is corrected to replenish the body's iron stores
d. T
e. F

95. a. F   Iron supplementation is contraindicated in haemolytic anaemias
b. T
c. T
d. T
e. T

96. a. F
b. T
c. F
d. T
e. F

97. a. T
b. T
c. T
d. T
e. T

98. a. F
b. T
c. T   DKA is treated with intravenous insulin infusion and only soluble insulin is compatible with intravenous use
d. T
e. T

99. a. T
b. T
c. T
d. T
e. T

100. a. T
b. T
c. F   This practice has changed recently; the current recommendation is to give BCG to selected groups of children only
d. T
e. F   DTP vaccine is contraindicated in the presence of a progressive neurological illness and not in cerebral palsy

1. The most important aspect of managing all critical illness is ensuring that the ABCs are assessed and treated. In diabetic ketoacidosis (DKA) the airway (A) is usually not at risk unless a decreased level of consciousness is present. Breathing (B) is also unlikely to be a problem but deep rapid breathing is present, which indicates the body's compensatory mechanisms against metabolic acidosis. The main problems are with the circulation (C) as these children are often severely dehydrated with associated metabolic derangements such as hypokalaemia. Rehydration should be slowly done over 48 hours after treatment of shock as rapid fluid shifts are believed to precipitate cerebral oedema. Insulin should be commenced to slowly reduce the blood sugar and antagonise ongoing catabolism.

2. The immaturity of the organ systems lead to numerous problems:
   - Respiratory: deficiency of surfactant leads to respiratory distress syndrome. This is characterized by atelectasis and treatment is by exogenous surfactant and respiratory support.
   - Infection: the immature immune system, lack of maternal antibody and invasive procedures lead to both congenital and acquired infections. Antibiotics, good skin care and neonatal unit infection control are essential to treat and minimize infections.
   - Temperature and skin: the thin and immature epithelial barrier with a high surface area to volume ratio and a decreased ability to generate heat increases the risk of hypothermia and dehydration.
   - Gastrointestinal: immaturity of the gut means that early nutrition is via the parenteral route and feeds have to be introduced slowly. Necrotizing enterocolitis is a major complication. Sucking and feeding reflexes means that nasogastric tube feeds are needed until after 35 weeks gestational age.
   - Central nervous system: preterm infants below 32 weeks gestational age are at risk of intracranial haemorrhage, retinopathy of prematurity and neurodevelopmental problems.
   - Cardiovascular: persistent fetal circulation and patent ductus arteriosus.

3. The most important diagnosis to exclude is septic arthritis and this can be clinically difficult. Warning signs are high fever, inability to weight bear or move the joint and bony tenderness. The presence of these signs should lead to urgent orthopaedic referral and hip imaging. The most common cause of a limp is transient synovitis and this is a reactive arthritis that occurs about 10–14 days after a viral upper respiratory tract infection. The child is usually able to weight bear and might have a mild fever. There is a good range of movement. Blood tests for inflammation are indicated as if they are negative then the diagnosis may be made and treatment is rest and analgesia. If the inflammatory markers are raised then further investigation and imaging might be required.

4. Once the diagnosis of leukaemia is made then chemotherapy is instituted. Six phases are required:
   1. Induction.
   2. CNS directed therapy.
   3. Consolidation.
   4. CNS prophylaxis.
   5. Intensification.
   6. Maintenance.
   It is important to offer psychological support and to be aware of the late consequences of leukaemia, such as poor growth, secondary tumours, endocrine disorders, educational and cognitive problems and reduced fertility.

5. Five out of six criteria are required:
   1. Fever for 5 or more days.
   2. Bilateral non-purulent conjunctivitis.
   3. Polymorphous rash.
   4. Cervical lymphadenopathy.
   5. Lip or oral mucosa changes.
   6. Extremity erythema, oedema or peeling (late).
   Fewer of the above criteria are needed in the presence of coronary artery aneurysms. Other diseases that can mimic Kawasaki disease and need to be excluded are sepsis, scarlet fever, toxic shock syndrome, scalded skin syndrome and certain forms of vasculitis.

6. Many reasons are given for children not to have vaccinations and many of these are based on incorrect reasoning, with the result that harm can occur. The following are *not* reasons to withhold vaccination:
   - Family history of adverse events.
   - Non-progressive neurological disorders.
   - Minor afebrile illness in the child.
   - History of allergy (although egg anaphylaxis is a contraindication to influenza vaccination).
   - Family history of convulsions.
   - Child's mother being pregnant.
   - Prematurity or underweight.
   - Previous history of pertussis, mumps, rubella or measles infection.
   Note that children with HIV should receive MMR.

7. Non-accidental injury is one of the types of child abuse. It has a wide spectrum from clear-cut injury to minor injuries that require a high index of suspicion. The types of injury include bruises, burns, fractures, and head and mouth injury. It is important to distinguish common accidental injuries that occur in mobile young children from deliberate trauma. Features of non-accidental injury include:
   - Delay in reporting injury.
   - Parental indifference.
   - Inconsistent history.
   - Injury that is incompatible with the child's development.
   - Varied and inconsistent account of injury.
   - Previous unexplained injury.
   There might be associated failure to thrive, developmental delay and poor hygiene. The child might appear withdrawn or frightened.

8. A child's airway differs from that of an adult in many ways. This means that obstruction is easier and it has implications in emergencies:
   - Larger tongue.
   - Larynx more anterior and higher.
   - Larynx funnel shaped and narrowest at cricoid (in adults it is narrowest at the vocal cords).
   - Short trachea.
   - Horseshoe-shaped epiglottis.
   - Children are obligate nasal breathers until 5 months age.
   Other respiratory differences:
   - Inefficient respiratory muscles.
   - Compliant chest wall.
   - Increased oxygen consumption and metabolic rate.

9. As antenatal screening has been introduced, with improved methods of preventing vertical transmission, it is now uncommon for HIV to be passed on from the mother to her child. Prevention is by administration of zidovudine (AZT) to the mother during labour and to the baby for 6 weeks. Delivery is by Caesarean section and breastfeeding is not recommended (unless in a developing country) because the virus is detected in breastmilk.

   HIV antibody is diagnostic only if the child is older than 18 months because the presence of maternal antibody will confound the results until then. In younger children HIV can be detected by polymerase chain reactions.

10. Inborn errors of metabolism have non-specific features and might mimic clinical sepsis or encephalopathy with seizures. Features in the history include:
    - Previous sudden death.
    - Parental consanguinity.
    - Previous encephalopathy.
    - Frequent miscarriage.
      Patterns of clinical presentations include:
    - Encephalopathy and seizures.

- Metabolic acidosis.
- Hypoglycaemia.
- Cardiac failure.
- Liver dysfunction.
- Progressive learning difficulties.
Most infants are well and asymptomatic at birth because the placenta provides an effective system for toxin removal. The defective enzymes have sufficient substrates only after feeding has been established.

11. In general, there is no doubt that 'breast is best' but there are, in fact, a number of disadvantages in breastfeeding.

    The quality of breast milk is superior in several respects to that of modified cow's milk formulae. It confers some protection against infection by virtue of containing secretory IgA, lysozyme, phagocytic cells and lactoferrin, an iron-binding agent that promotes growth of non-pathogenic flora. The nutritional content is more suited to newborn infants. The protein is easily digested, there is a low renal solute load and a more favourable ratio of calcium to phosphate.

    Potential disadvantages include uncertainty about the volume of intake and the transmission of maternal drugs, such as anticoagulants and antineoplastic agents, and pathogens such as HIV. Breastfed infants are at risk of two important vitamin deficiencies. Vitamin K deficiency causing haemorrhagic disease of the newborn can occur in breastfed infants unless vitamin K is given prophylactically at birth. Rickets due to vitamin D deficiency might also occur, especially in dark-skinned infants, if breastfeeding is prolonged and weaning delayed.

    Successful breastfeeding is an emotionally positive experience and promotes mother–infant bonding. However, failure of attempts to establish breastfeeding can cause emotional upset. Lastly, breastfeeding mothers have a lower risk of breast cancer in later life.

12. Bronchiolitis is most commonly caused by respiratory syncytial virus (RSV). It occurs in annual winter epidemics, predominantly affecting infants aged 3–9 months. Coryzal symptoms are followed by a cough and increasing difficulty in breathing. Clinical signs include tachypnoea, intercostal recession, chest hyperinflation, bilateral fine crackles and high-pitched rhonchi. CXR shows hyperinflation and/or patchy collapse and oxygen saturation monitoring might reveal hypoxia. A nasopharyngeal aspirate is examined by a fluorescent antibody test to detect RSV. Management is supportive and depends on severity. Most infants require supplemental oxygen and more severely affected infants may require IV fluids. A minority become severely ill (young infants, those who were preterm with chronic lung disease, and babies with congenital heart disease are at high risk) and require

assisted ventilation for respiratory failure or recurrent apnoea. Bronchodilators are frequently administered but are often ineffective.

A new monoclonal antibody called palivizumab is available for high-risk infants. This is administered prophylactically to prevent infection and hospitalization.

13. The aetiology of jaundice in the newborn is best considered according to the age of onset. Persistently high levels may lead to neurological damage (bilirubin encephalopathy).

Jaundice in the first 24 hours: this is always pathological. Haemolysis is the most common cause and may be due to haemolytic disease of the newborn (Rhesus or ABO incompatibility) or intrinsic red cell defects such as congenital spherocytosis or G6PD deficiency.

Jaundice between 2 days and 2 weeks: the most common cause is physiological jaundice due to the combination of liver enzyme immaturity and increased bilirubin load from red cell breakdown.

Jaundice beyond 2 weeks of age: persistent (prolonged, protracted) jaundice is usually an unconjugated hyperbilirubinaemia most commonly caused by 'breast milk' jaundice. An important cause of prolonged conjugated hyperbilirubinaemia is biliary atresia, which requires early surgical treatment. This is suggested by the presence of conjugated bilirubin.

In management, the main concerns are to identify the cause and to prevent kernicterus. Treatment options include phototherapy using blue light (wavelength 450 nm, not UV light), which converts bilirubin into water-soluble metabolites which are excreted. Exchange transfusion might be necessary if bilirubin rises to dangerous levels despite phototherapy but this is uncommon now.

14. A practical definition of short stature is a height below the 0.4th centile for age, a predicted height less than the mid-parental target height, or an abnormal growth velocity as indicated by the height falling by more than the width of the centile band over 1–2 years.

The majority of children whose short stature has triggered concern are normal. They have either familial short stature or constitutional delay of the pubertal growth spurt.

The history should include enquiry about size at birth, parental height and a family history of conditions such as the skeletal dysplasias. The mid-parental height allows calculation of a target centile range. On examination attention is paid to the height and weight, pubertal status and the presence or absence of any dysmorphic features. Growth velocity should be calculated from at least two height measurements 6 months apart.

Potentially useful investigations include the bone age, the karyotype and endocrine investigations such as thyroid function tests and growth hormone secretion (requires a provocation test).

Important organic causes of short stature include endocrine causes (GH deficiency, hypothyroidism), genetic disorders (Turner syndrome, Prader–Willi syndrome) and skeletal dysplasias (achondroplasia).

Management depends on the cause. Effective treatment usually involves hormone replacement, e.g. growth hormone or thyroxine if deficiency is present.

15. Down syndrome due to trisomy 21 is the most common autosomal trisomy compatible with life with an incidence of 1 in 700 live births. The extra chromosomal material might result from non-disjunction, translocation or mosaicism. It is often suspected at birth because of the characteristic facial appearance: round face, flat occiput, flat nasal bridge, epicanthic folds, protruding tongue, small ears and Brushfield spots on the iris. Additional features can include single palmar creases, incurved little fingers, a sandal toe gap and generalized hypotonia. Cardiac defects are present in 50% and duodenal atresia is increased in incidence. Developmental delay occurs and there is usually severe learning impairment. Late medical complications include an increased risk of leukaemia, hypothyroidism and atlantoaxial instability.

Down syndrome can be diagnosed antenatally by screening procedures designed to detect it in pregnancies at increased risk. Risk increases with maternal age from 1 in 900 at 30 years to 1 in 110 at 40 years. Postnatal diagnosis is confirmed by chromosomal analysis, which takes several days because white cells must be examined during mitosis. Ninety-five per cent of children with Down syndrome have trisomy 21 due to non-disjunction.

16. Cerebral palsy is defined as a disorder of motor function due to a non-progressive lesion of the developing brain. In many patients the cause is unknown but risk factors are well recognized and can be classified as:
- Antenatal, e.g. congenital infections.
- Intrapartum, e.g. birth asphyxia.
- Postnatal, e.g. hyperbilirubinaemia.

Cerebral palsy can be classified as spastic (70%), dyskinetic (10%), ataxic (10%) or mixed (10%). Spastic CP is further subdivided into hemiplegic, diplegic (lower limbs predominantly affected) and quadriplegic. It might present with delayed motor milestones, abnormal tone or posturing, feeding difficulties, or speech and language delay.

Associated problems include sensory deficits (vision and hearing), learning impairment and epilepsy. Management requires a multidisciplinary approach.

17. Iron deficiency anaemia in infancy or childhood usually results from inadequate dietary intake rather than loss of iron through haemorrhage. Groups at risk of nutritional deficiency include preterm infants who have limited iron stores and outstrip their

reserves by 8 weeks of age unless supplements are provided. Term infants will develop iron deficiency after 4 months of age if introduction of mixed feeding is delayed or unmodified cow's milk is used in excess (both breast milk and unmodified cow's are low in iron). Children with a poor diet on account of low socioeconomic status or vegetarian diets are at risk. Malabsorption syndrome might be complicated by iron deficiency.

Iron deficiency due to blood loss might occur with hookworm infestation (most common cause worldwide), menstruation, repeated venesection in babies, recurrent epistaxis or gastrointestinal bleeding, e.g. from a Meckel's diverticulum.

18. The hallmarks of attention-deficit hyperactivity disorder (ADHD) are inattention, hyperactivity and impulsiveness. Hyperkinetic syndrome is a more severe subtype in which all three features are present, persist in more than one situation and impair function. Hyperkinetic syndrome is four times more common in boys than girls.

Inattention is manifest as frequent changes of activity, hyperactivity is an excess of movement with persisting fidgeting and restlessness, and impulsiveness leads to erratic and impetuous behaviour.

Physical examination should include a search for developmental delay, clumsiness, sensory deficits and dysmorphic features but most children do not have an identifiable brain disorder and do not need special investigations.

About 50% of children respond to behavioural therapy, including a structured environment, positive reinforcement and measures to enhance relaxation and self-control. If this approach fails, drug therapy can be tried. Paradoxically, CNS stimulants such as dexamphetamine or methylphenidate are most effective. Up to one-third will have another psychiatric disorder.

19. Nocturnal enuresis is the involuntary voiding of urine during sleep beyond the age at which dryness at night has been achieved in a majority of children. In primary nocturnal enuresis dryness has never been achieved.

The physical examination should aim to exclude the rare organic causes: review growth and blood pressure, palpate the abdomen to exclude an enlarged bladder, inspect the spine and examine for neurological signs in the lower limbs. Urine should be cultured and tested for proteinuria and glycosuria.

A good rapport must be established with child and parents. Parental intolerance and 'functional payoffs' should be discouraged. A diary of wetting should be kept. Further management is age-dependent. Under 5 years, reassurance, waterproof sheets and a lifting regimen might suffice. Over 5 years, star charts are useful, and over 7 years, buzzer type alarms are worth a trial.

Desmopressin, a synthetic analogue of ADH, provides effective short-term relief, and a percentage of patients who attain dryness remain dry when it is stopped.

20. Management of moderate atopic eczema in a 9-month-old infant would include:
    1. Avoidance of aggravating factors such as:
       • Synthetic or woollen fabrics (cotton clothing is best).
       • Allergens such as dander from furry pets.
       • Excessive heat.
    2. Emollients (e.g. aqueous cream) to moisturize and soften the skin.
    3. Mild topical steroids, e.g. 1% hydrocortisone to affected areas twice daily.
    4. Oral antihistamines at night to reduce itching and help sleep.
    5. Treatment of complications such as secondary bacterial infection with oral antibiotics.

EMQ 1

1. (h) These features indicate a cyanotic congenital heart disease with increased pulmonary blood flow. The age of this child makes transposition very likely

2. (b)

3. (c)

EMQ 2

1. (a)

2. (f)

3. (g)

EMQ 3

1. (c) This is likely to be transient tachyponea of the newborn in view of term gestation and negative blood cultures. Chest X-ray findings also suggest this diagnosis, although it is difficult to rule out infection at the time of presentation and all such babies need antibiotics until culture results are obtained

2. (b)

3. (a)

EMQ 4

1. (b) This is likely to be cystic fibrosis

2. (e) *Pneumocystis carinii* has to be ruled out in this child

3. (i) This is very suggestive of foreign body aspiration

EMQ 5

1. (c) Any child under 6 months with fever and seizures should be investigated for meningitis. A bulging fontanelle indicates raised intracranial pressure

2. (b) This is probably pyloric stenosis. Vomiting is usually projectile

3. (j) This child has bronchiolitis

EMQ 6

1. (b)

2. (f)

3. (i) This child has acute chest syndrome from sickle cell disease

EMQ 7

1. (b)

2. (j) Most infants with cow's milk intolerance are also allergic to soya

3. (a)

EMQ 8

1. (a)

2. (b)

3. (g)

EMQ 9

1. (d)

2. (a)

3. (b)

EMQ 10

1. (i)

2. (d)

3. (f)

EMQ 11

1. (a)

2. (d)

3. (f)

This lists the causative viruses for each of these infections

EMQ 12

1. (d) This is very suggestive of candidal dermatitis and is usually treated with topical nystatin cream

2. (a)

3. (b) These lesions are caused by molluscum contagiosum and does not need treatment in most instances

EMQ 13

1. (b) The presence of wheeze and crepitations with (a) typical onset in the susceptible age group is very suggestive of bronchiolitis

2. (f)

3. (d) A family history of atopy—asthma, hay fever or eczema—predisposes to asthma

EMQ 14

1. (c)

2. (d) Penicillin prophylaxis is given to splenectemized patients to prevent infections by capsulated bacteria

3. (a)

EMQ 15

1. (e)

2. (g)

3. (j)

EMQ 16

1. (a)

2. (h) These are the most common blood groups implicated in ABO incompatibility

3. (g)

EMQ 17

1. (c)

2. (e) Most children with cerebral palsy do not have any identifiable cause and have normal scans

3. (a)

EMQ 18

1. (e)

2. (c) Obesity with short stature is more likely to be due to an endocrinal or genetic cause and needs investigation. In this child, the choice that fits the features is Prader–Willi syndrome

3. (a)

EMQ 19

1. (a)

2. (c) IV adenosine given as a rapid bolus is the treatment of choice in a haemodynamically stable child with SVT

3. (f) This child is in diabetic ketoacidosis and needs insulin infusion

EMQ 20

1. (f) Sensorineural hearing loss is a feature of congenital rubella; others are postinfectious complications of the respective conditions

2. (d)

3. (a)

EMQ 21

1. (e)

2. (f)

3. (a)

They represent the most appropriate follow-up investigations for these children with these conditions

EMQ 22

1. (a)

2. (d)

3. (e)

EMQ 23

1. (f)

2. (d)

3. (a)

EMQ 24

1. (c)

2. (e)

3. (a)

EMQ 25

1. (g) At present, this remains the gold standard for the diagnosis of gastrooesophageal reflux although it fails to identify non-acid reflux

2. (e)

3. (a) RAST and skin prick testing have similar sensitivity and specificity in identifying food allergies

EMQ 26

1. (e)

2. (c) This child needs investigations to identify an underlying condition like cystic fibrosis, immunodeficiency, congenital malformations of the lung or a ciliary dyskinesia

3. (b) Congenital diaphragmatic hernia can sometimes present beyond the neonatal period

EMQ 27

1. (f)

2. (g) Here proteinuria and hypoalbuminaemia are the major features unlike the previous question. This strongly suggests nephrotic syndrome and needs treatment with steroids

3. (d)

EMQ 28

1. (d)

2. (c)

3. (a) This represents a very severe exacerbation of asthma

EMQ 29

1. (c)

2. (a)

3. (d)

EMQ 30

1. (e)

2. (b)

3. (a) Chloroquine is not recommended for falciparum malaria

Index

NB: page numbers in italics refer to information in self-assessment section; in the form *308/328* these are corresponding questions and answers